Progress in Oncology 2004

Edited by

Vincent T. DeVita, Jr.
Yale Cancer Center
New Haven, Connecticut

Samuel Hellman
Department of Radiation Oncology
University of Chicago
Chicago, Illinois

Steven A. Rosenberg
National Cancer Institute
National Institutes of Health
Bethesda, Maryland

JONES AND BARTLETT PUBLISHERS
Sudbury, Massachusetts
BOSTON TORONTO LONDON SINGAPORE

World Headquarters
Jones and Bartlett Publishers
40 Tall Pine Drive
Sudbury, MA 01776
info@jbpub.com
www.jbpub.com

Jones and Bartlett Publishers
Canada
2406 Nikanna Road
Mississauga, ON L5C 2W6
CANADA

Jones and Bartlett
Publishers International
Barb House, Barb Mews
London W6 7PA
UK

ISSN: 1535-9980

ISBN: 0-7637-4578-2

Production Credits:
Chief Executive Officer: Clayton Jones
Chief Operating Officer: Don W. Jones, Jr.
President, Higher Education and Professional Publishing: Robert W. Holland, Jr.
V.P., Sales and Marketing: William J. Kane
V.P., Design and Production: Anne Spencer
V.P., Manufacturing and Inventory Control: Therese Bräuer
Executive Publisher: Christopher Davis
Special Projects Editor: Elizabeth Platt
Editorial Assistant: Kathy Richardson
Composition: Modern Graphics
Printing and Binding: Malloy Lithographing
Cover Printer: Malloy Lithographing

Printed in the United States of America
08 07 06 05 04 10 9 8 7 6 5 4 3 2 1

Contents

List of Contributors

Robert J. Amato, DO
Scott Department of Urology, Baylor College of Medicine, Houston, Texas

Carlos R Becerra, MD
The University of Texas Southwestern Medical Center at Dallas, Dallas, Texas

Noa Ben-Baruch, MD
Department of Oncology, Kaplan Medical Center, Rehovot, Israel

Vicki Brooks, PA
Division of Colorectal Surgery, Department of Surgery, Beth Israel Medical Center, New York, New York

Prof. Bertrand Coiffier
Hospices Civils de Lyon & Université Claude Bernard, Lyon, France

Dennis Cooper, MD
Stem Cell Transplant Program, Section of Medical Oncology, Yale University School of Medicine, New Haven, Connecticut

William L. Dahut, MD
Genitourinary Clinical Research Section, Medical Oncology Clinical Research Unit, Center for Cancer Research, National Cancer Institute, Bethesda, Maryland

Mark E. Dudley, PhD
Surgery Branch, National Cancer Institute, Bethesda, Maryland

Kieron Dunleavy, MD
Experimental Transplantation and Immunology Branch, Division of Clinical Sciences, National Cancer Institute, Bethesda, Maryland

Warren E. Enker, MD
Division of Colorectal Surgery, Department of Surgery, Beth Israel Medical Center and the Continuum Cancer Centers of New York, New York, New York

Guillermo Garcia-Manero, MD
Department of Leukemia, University of Texas M.D. Anderson Cancer Center, Houston, Texas

Steven G. Gray, PhD
Receptor Biology Laboratory, Novo Nordisk, Hagedorn Research Institute, Gentofte, Denmark

Braden Greer, MA
Advanced Technology Center, National Cancer Institute, National Institutes of Health, Gaithersburg, Maryland

James L. Gulley, MD, PhD
Laboratory of Tumor Immunology and Biology and Genitourinary Clinical Research Section, Medical Oncology Clinical Research Unit, Center for Cancer Research, National Cancer Institute, Bethesda, Maryland

Roy S. Herbst, MD, PhD
The University of Texas M. D. Anderson Cancer Center, Houston, Texas

Clifford Hudis, MD
Memorial Sloan-Kettering Cancer Center, 1275 York Avenue, New York, New York

Kullervo Hynynen, PhD
Department of Radiology, Brigham and Women's Hospital, and Harvard Medical School, Boston, Massachusetts

Jean-Pierre J. Issa, MD
Department of Leukemia, University of Texas M.D. Anderson Cancer Center, Houston, Texas

Javed Khan, MD
Advanced Technology Center, National Cancer Institute, National Institutes of Health, Gaithersburg, Maryland

Joseph Martz, MD
Division of Colorectal Surgery, Department of Surgery, Beth Israel Medical Center, New York, New York

Nathan McDannold, PhD
Department of Radiology, Brigham and Women's Hospital, and Harvard Medical School, Boston, Massachusetts

John Mendelsohn, MD
The University of Texas M. D. Anderson Cancer Center, Houston, Texas

Larry Norton, MD
Memorial Sloan-Kettering Cancer Center, 1275 York Avenue, New York, New York

Amir Onn, MD
The University of Texas M. D. Anderson Cancer Center, Houston, Texas

Steven A. Rosenberg, MD, PhD
Surgery Branch, National Cancer Institute, Bethesda, Maryland

Stuart Seropian, MD
Stem Cell Transplant Program, Section of Medical Oncology, Yale University School of Medicine, New Haven, Connecticut

Louis Staudt, MD, PhD
Metabolism Branch, National Cancer Institute, Bethesda, Maryland

Udit N. Verma, MD
The University of Texas Southwestern Medical Center at Dallas, Dallas, Texas 75390

Wyndham H. Wilson, MD, PhD
Experimental Transplantation and Immunology Branch, Division of Clinical Sciences, National Cancer Institute, Bethesda, Maryland

Yosef Yarden, PhD
Department of Biological Regulation, the Weizmann Institute of Science, Rehovot, Israel

Chapter 1

The Varied Applications of Small Interference RNA

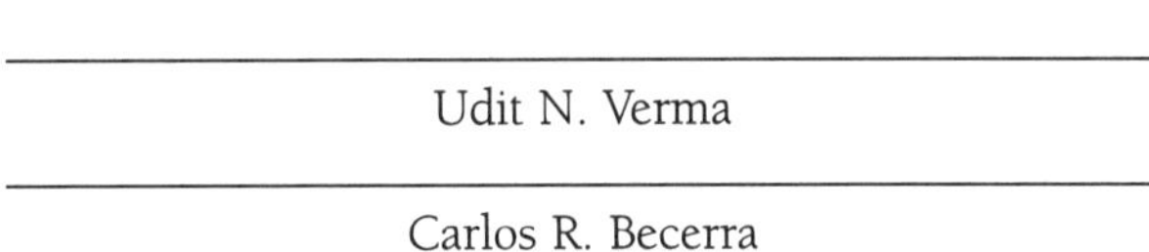

Udit N. Verma

Carlos R. Becerra

RNA interference (RNAi) refers to a process where double stranded RNA (dsRNA) induces degradation of its cognate mRNA. The term RNAi was coined five years ago by Fire et al[1] and its applicability to mammalian cells described in 2001.[2] This naturally-occurring gene silencing technique has generated considerable interest in the scientific community, called the "breakthrough of the year" for 2002 by the journal *Science* and is viewed by many as the most exciting discovery in biology in the past several decades. The interest and excitement about RNAi is due to its ability to efficiently silence genes from diverse species with unique specificity. Gene silencing with RNAi has rapidly been adopted by the scientific community as a tool to study gene function in place of the tedious knock-out techniques and has permitted the dissection of the intricate cell signaling pathways. RNAi also holds promise as an antisense strategy to knock-down genes aberrantly expressed in certain disease states. Cancer is one obvious field where the RNAi technique holds immense promise in understanding the biology of oncogenesis, in discovering new drug targets, and in its use directly as a therapeutic tool. At present, the academic community and the pharmaceutical industry are aggressively pursuing all these potential prospects for RNAi.

Tumors are characterized by an array of genetic changes that confer the neoplastic cell a growth advantage and a malignant phenotype. With the advent of modern molecular techniques, investigators have been able to decipher many of the changes that occur at the molecular level in malignant cells. These changes include loss of function of tumor suppressor genes and/or gain of function of protooncogenes. Usually more than one such change is required for development of neoplasia and this leads to alteration in several cell-signaling pathways. Deciphering the consequences of these genetic or epigenetic changes and developing ways to reverse them have been a major focus of cancer research. Knockout and transgenic techniques have been widely used to study these changes both in vitro and in vivo. Additional tools such as antisense nucleotides directed against specific mRNA targets are being employed both for research and therapeutic purposes. Advancement in anti-sense technology has allowed for a greater stability of the molecule and presently there are numerous trials ongoing using the technology to silence specific genes as part of a combined modality approach. As will be discussed in this review, gene silencing by RNAi provides a more potent and flexible tool to explore these possibilities and has become a major research focus during the past two years in several medical fields such as oncology and infectious disease. In this review, we present the discovery and development of siRNA from prokaryotes to mammalian cells and its potential applications in molecular biology and clinical medicine.

DISCOVERY OF siRNA

In 1990, plant biologists at DNA Plant Technology Corporation[3] wanted to improve the color of petunias by inserting a second copy of the gene chalcone synthetase, which is involved in the coloring of petunias. Instead of obtaining brighter petunias, investigators obtained either multicolored or white plants, indicating that there was silencing of the endogenous gene as well as the transgene. This observed paradoxical effect, named "cosupression,"[3] could be passed on to the next generation of plants.[4,5] In 1995, scientists at Cornell made the surprising observation that "sense" RNA used as a control to "antisense" RNA and expected to have no biologic effect, led to silencing of the corresponding gene in *Caenorhabditis elegans*.[6] However, no satisfactory explanation existed for the observed findings until 1998, when Fire et al[1] elicited a potent gene silencing effect when they injected mixed strands of sense and antisense RNA into *C. elegans*. They coined the term RNA interference after demonstrating that double stranded RNA (dsRNA) was responsible for the silencing effect. This discovery provided an explanation for similar phenomenon observed in plants and fungi called PTGS (posttranscriptional gene silencing) and quelling, respectively.

Early on RNAi was effectively applied to plants, worms, and other invertebrates, including *Drosophila*. However, efforts to elicit RNAi with double stranded RNA that varied in size between 38 and 1662 base pairs in mammalian cells other than mouse oocytes and embryos were unsuccessful[7–10] due to non-specific double-stranded (ds) RNA-activated protein kinase (PKR)-mediated interferon response and global shutdown in protein synthesis and cell death. A turning point in the study of RNAi in mammals was provided by Tuschl and coworkers,[2] who were able to suppress specific genes in cultured mammalian cells by introducing short double-stranded RNAs (siRNA), 21–23 nucleotides in length without initiating PKR-induced global shutdown and cell death. Subsequent studies by the same group revealed that nucleotides shorter than 21 nucleotides or longer than 25 nucleotides were inefficient in the ability to silence genes. Since publication of work by Tuschl and coworkers, RNAi has been adopted widely in different laboratories across the globe, allowing scientist to systematically knockdown genes of interest in an effort to understand different problems in cell biology.

MECHANISMS OF ACTION OF siRNA

Understanding how siRNA works is currently an area of active research. The process of gene silencing by the double stranded RNA is only partially understood and is modeled after the phenomenon of PTGS triggered by the acquisition of double stranded RNA by the cell. This double stranded RNA leads to the degradation of endogenous RNA that has sequence identity with the dsRNA. Early work on *C. elegans* demonstrated that injection of sense or antisense RNA strands into worms was not as effective in inhibiting specific genes as injecting both sense and antisense strands. This finding was followed by subsequent experiments in *C. elegans* in which feeding dsRNA to the worms resulted in long-lasting and specific down-regulation of gene expression that was carried on to the offspring. In cell lines, this effect has been carried for up to nine cell divisions.

The enzymes that have been identified so far in opening up the double strand to allow reading of the sequence have included helicases, RNase III-related nucleases, members of the argonaute family (proteins first identified in mutants of the plant *Arabidopsis* that produce altered leaf morphology) and RNA-dependent RNA polymerase.[11] This enzymes form a ribonucleotide protein complex with siRNA called RNA-induced silencing complex (RISC) and requires consumption of adenosine 5′-triphosphate (ATP). A common characteristic of these enzymes is the ability to cleave long double-stranded RNA by an evolutionary conserved type III RNase with dual catalytic domain, helicase activity and PAZ motifs, named Dicer.[12,13] As a result, there is a fragmentation of the double strand RNA to sizes of 21 to 25 nucleotides in length with two nucleotide overhangs at the 3′ end of the RNA. Dicer also is involved in the fragmentation of 70–nucleotide hairpin RNA precursors to single strand RNAs called micro RNAs (miRNAs), which pair with target mRNAs that contain partially complementary sequences to miRNA repressing mRNA translation without altering mRNA stability.[14–17] These miRNAs also can enter the RNAi pathway and act as siRNA.[18] Two genes involved in the RNAi pathway—*RDE 4* and *RDE 1*—are believed to function together to detect and retain foreign dsRNA and to present the dsRNA to Dicer for processing.[19] Although Dicer is believed to be an important component of the siRNA pathway, it is not indispensable for the activity of siRNA, since *C. elegans* knockouts for Dicer still showed siRNA effect, implying that there is an alternative pathway in siRNA processing.[20] The RNAi pathway is ATP dependent in at least three of its steps: processing of double stranded RNA into small interfering RNA, unwinding of siRNA duplex to generate an active complex, and recognition and cleavage of the RNA target.[21]

A second postulated mechanism in the amplification of the siRNA signal in the cell involves RNA-dependent RNA polymerases (RdRP) primed by existing siRNAs.[22,23] RdRP are believed to convert the single strand mRNA to double strand RNA using the antisense template of the siRNA as a primer.[24] Dicer then cleaves the double stranded RNA to small fragments. These newly formed siRNAs will then attach to their complementary double stranded mRNA and be cleaved further by Dicer. In this particular model RISC does not play a role. An alternative model postulates that siRNAs acts as a guide to cleave the target mRNA. Active siRNAs bind to RNA-binding proteins and form the RISC complex, are activated by the helicase activity of the complex, and then guide the complex to the specific complementary mRNA. The process is amplified and includes other mRNAs with identical sequence. The effect of siRNA appears to be localized to the cytoplasm but not the nucleus in the experimental systems studied thus far.[11,25]

There are additional genes involved in the RNAi pathway. For example, studies in *Drosophila* embryos have shown that mutation in the gene *Argonaute 2* suppresses the effect of RNAi.[26] The effect is due to the reduced ability to degrade mRNA in response to dsRNA in vitro and appears to occur downstream of siRNA production.[27] In *C. elegans*, investigators injected pools of siRNA resulting in the discovery of four genes involved in the siRNA pathway.[28,29] Additional genes involved in the siRNA pathway have been identified in several different models, but to date their functions have not been elucidated.

One of the roles of siRNA in the cell appears to be in the formation and maintenance of heterochromatin since deletion of the genes involved in the siRNA pathway *argonaute, Dicer,* and *RdRP* results in aberrant accumulation of centromeric heterochromic repeats.[30] As a result, there is impairment of centromere function. In addition, it is possible that siRNA affects gene expression by methylating homologous sequences that share sequence identity with the DNA promoter.[31,32] siRNA also might have activity at the translational level, since in *C. elegans* inducers of the siRNA machinery had activity at the level of the protein synthesis. Finally, there might be a link between siRNA and nonsense mediated decay of improperly processed mRNA or in the regulation of mRNA stability, at least in some organisms such as *C. elegans*.[33]

The effect of siRNA appears to be systemic and transmitted by a transmembrane protein called sid-1 (systemic RNA interference deficient loci). This protein has a signal peptide sequence, 11 putative transmembrane domains, and is believed to act as a channel for dsRNA and siRNA. Mutants for the protein in *C. elegans* did not show evidence of gene silencing when exposed to siRNA.[34] PTGS in plants have systemic effects but the mechanism is unclear.[35]

The specificity of siRNA has been tested in human cell lines with gene expression profiling by several investigators. Initial experiments with siRNA-induced gene silencing reported a high specificity with no secondary effects detectable by gene expression profiling.[36] The specificity of the siRNA effect was brought into question by further experiments with lentivirus transfected 21 nucleotide long siRNAs originating from shRNAs after processing by Dicer and transfected into human fibroblast cell lines.[37] Gene expression analysis after transfection revealed that there was a twofold up-regulation of the expression in the genes involved with the interferon pathway.[38] This effect was mediated through PKR, appeared to be dose dependent and more modest than the non-specific interferon activation effect seen with long double-stranded RNAs. A possible explanation for these divergent results relates to the malignant cells used for the first experiments, since many of these cell lines have a defective interferon response. In addition, siRNA might directly target genes containing as few as 11 nucleotides of identity to the siRNA, thus demonstrating cross reactivity with nontargeted genes of limited identical sequences.[39] Thus, investigators should exercise caution when reporting their results with siRNA and consider the potential effect of the interferon pathway activation in the results.

IMPROVEMENTS IN siRNA SILENCING EFFICIENCY AND STABILITY

Investigators have been able to introduce specific siRNA into cultured cells by lipid and viral-based transfection methods, resulting in knock down of the target gene product by at least 90%. In order to further improve on the silencing of the gene in question, investigators have constructed siRNAs directed against several sequences of the gene. The most critical aspects of gene silencing efficiency with this technique involve transfection of the dsRNA into the cell and optimal secondary structure of the target region within the mRNA. By modeling the secondary structure of the target region, it is possible to predict the regions that need to be targeted for gene silencing. The potential pitfall is that this modeling can lead to structures of the lowest energy state that often differ from the natural form of the molecule and thus introduce potential bias into the experiments.

In an effort to improve on the potency, thermal stability and pharmacokinetic properties on siRNA, investigators modified the molecule by introducing phosphodiester, varied the numbers of phosphorothioate linkages, and locked nucleic acid nucleotides and 2′-deoxy-2′fluorouridine.[40] In *Drosophila* cell lysates, 2′-O-methyl modifications to either the sense or antisense strands inactivated the siRNA silencing effect.[13] Removing the 3′-hydroxyl group did not affect the activity of siRNA, but the 5′-hydroxyl groups were essential for its activity.[41,42] Replacing the 3′ two uridine overhangs with two deoxy-thymidine overhangs resulted in decreased gene silencing and replacement of either the sense or antisense strand of the molecule by DNA resulted in reduction or complete loss of RNAi activity. From these studies, it can be inferred that the preferred structure for interaction between the antisense and mRNA appears to be a U-turn motif that enhances the RNA pairing rates.[43]

More recently, investigators have used plasmids expressing siRNAs as dsRNA hairpin inverted repeats (shRNA) with similar potency to trigger RNAi in mammalian cell lines. One of the advantages of this approach is that the gene expression is suppressed for prolonged periods of time and opens the possibility of studying gene function in this model instead of using the more time consuming and costly mouse knockouts.

SIMILARITIES AND DIFFERENCES BETWEEN ANTISENSE DNA AND siRNA

RNase H is a ubiquitously expressed endonuclease that recognizes DNA-RNA structures and hydrolyzes the RNA strand. The RNase H recognizes antisense strands that contain at least five consecutive deoxynucleotides. In contrast, siRNA uses double stranded RNase as the terminating mechanism. Investigators compared phosphorothioate deoxyribonucleotide with 2′-O-methoxyethyl modifications and siRNA in human cell culture assays. Results showed a similar potency, efficacy, specificity, and duration of action between the two methods. Both molecules appeared to work at different stages of the mRNA processing and metabolism.[44]

Comparisons between different anti-sense technologies including siRNA, locked nucleic acids, phosphorotioates and 2′-O-methyl modified oligonucleotides revealed that the most potent inhibitor of the gene in the study, vanilloid receptor 1 tagged to green fluorescent protein expression, was siRNA (IC_{50} 0.06 nmol/L), followed by locked nucleic acids (IC_{50} 0.4 nmol/L), phosphorotioates (IC_{50} 70 nmol/L), and 2′-O-methyl modified oligonucleotides (IC_{50} 220 nmol/L).[45] The luciferase reporter activity of 12 antisense DNA and siRNAs was assessed. The reporter activity was similar but the sites targeted by the antisense DNA and siRNA did not overlap, indicating that the molecules had a different site of activity in the mRNA molecule.[46] In summary, these sets of experiments attest to the potency of siRNA as compared to other current methods of knocking down genes.

PHYSIOLOGICAL FUNCTIONS OF RNAi

RNA-based gene silencing is an evolutionary conserved mechanism that protects the host and its genome from viruses and endogenous threats such as transposons. Recent work in plants and animals from several different groups suggests that RNA-based regulatory mechanisms are more widespread than previously thought. Thus far, the strongest evidence for the physiologic role of RNAi has been in plants, but several observations, as discussed below, imply that RNAi based mechanisms are operative across different species including mammals.

Plant viruses have a diverse genomic organization and gene expression strategies. Over 90% of the plant viruses have a single-strand RNA genome that replicates by using RdRP via a double-stranded replicative intermediate. Plant cells utilize this dsRNA to trigger virus-induced gene silencing (VIGS) by a mechanism analogous to RNAi in animal cells. This phenomenon of pathogen-derived resistance (PDR) had been known for some time; however, its mechanisms were unclear until 1993 when Lindbo et al[47] studied the effect of viral infection with tobacco etch virus in tobacco plants. The infected plants recovered in three to five weeks and became resistant to further infection by the same virus. Although the transcription rate was similar between the uninoculated and recovered plants, the steady-state transgene mRNA level was 12- to 20-fold lower in inoculated plants. This provided the clue that the resistant state in plants was mediated by target specific inactivation of mRNA in the cell cytoplasm. Today we know that plants use this viral-induced siRNA-mediated gene silencing as a mechanism of defense against all major RNA and DNA viruses.

Several different endogenous miRNA species have been identified from plants to human. This points towards much wider role of RNAi or related mechanisms in maintaining genomic integrity, regulation of gene expression during development and possibly other physiological processes. Rapid progress being made in this area should soon define a new chapter in cell biology of RNA dependent gene regulation.

RNAi AS A RESEARCH TOOL

Tuschl's group raised possibility of potential therapeutic applications of siRNA in their first article describing the successful use of the technique in mammalian cells.[2] However, the greatest impact of their discovery has been in its rapid adaptation by the research community. RNAi not only accelerated *C. elegans* and *Drosophila* research, but an increasing number of laboratories are using siRNA to study various aspects of mammalian genetics and cell biology, incorporating RNAi into the already existent laboratory tools to answer novel questions as discussed below.

Functional Genomics

With the unraveling of the human genome, the task ahead lies in understanding how the genes function and their down stream effects. siRNA has been employed successfully in the laboratory to determine the effects of different genes in the cell. Most of the published work thus far has been in *C. elegans*, but work in different models such as *Drosophila melanogaster*, *Arabidopsis thaliana,* and mammalian cells is in progress.

C. elegans was the first animal to have its genome, totaling 19,427 genes, sequenced. Soon afterwards, scientist presented results on the function of the different genes at a much wider scale by using siRNA. For example, Gonczy et al[48] targeted 2174 genes on chromosome III by injecting siRNA into the syncytia of adult worms in order to obtain knockout progeny. The authors found that siRNA directed to 133 genes induced a change in phenotype and included defects in meiotic cell division, nuclear appearance, pace of development and general embryonic appearance. Previous studies using classic genetics found only seven of the 133 chromosome III genes to have a role in early cell division. Importantly, there was no difference observed in the phenotypic changes in *C. elegans* between siRNA and genetic mutant analysis by knocking down these seven genes, thus validating RNAi as a tool for studies in functional genomics. In a second example, Fraser et al[49] fed *C. elegans* with siRNA to 2416 predicted genes on chromosome I and observed for anatomical and motility abnormalities, altered sex ratio and sterility. The group observed an RNAi-induced phenotype change in 13.9% (378) of the genes tested, whereas only 70 genes on chromosome I had been previously known to affect the phenotype of *C. elegans* by standard forward genetic methods.

Functional genomics has been extended to genome wide targeting as reported by Kamath et al[50] using RNAi to inhibit the function of 86% of 19, 757 *C. elegans* genes. The authors created a library of *Escheriscia coli* with plasmids encoding dsRNA, fed the *C. elegans* with these, and observed the knock down-induced phenotypic changes of targeted gene(s). They were able to assign an RNAi-induced phenotype to 1528 genes, two-thirds of which had no known biologic function. Ashrafi et al,[51] using a similar method, performed genome wide RNAi to evaluate for genes involved in body fat regulation in *C. elegans* and identified genes that reduced (305 genes) or increased (112 genes) body fat. Of interest is the fact that most of these genes are conserved in humans and will provide new targets for obesity research with potential therapeutic implications. The work by these groups and the generation of *E. coli* libraries has laid the framework for further research in functional genomics.

The success of functional genomics with siRNA in *C. elegans* and *Drosophila* has not yet been translated to the study of mammalian cells. Systemic large scale analysis of gene function in human or other mammalian cells is likely to be equally informative and more relevant and efforts are underway to create human siRNA based libraries targeting genes on a genome wide scale.[52,53] Several groups are active in developing new methods for high-throughput genome wide screening of gene function and validation. Mousses et al[54] used siRNA arrayed on a glass slide in a transfection matrix overlaid with a monolayer of adherent cells to allow for reverse transfection. Their technique worked well in HeLa cells with the cells expressing green fluorescent protein in a stable fashion. A somewhat similar siRNA microarray technique by Kumar et al[55] validated these results. Aza-Blanc et al[56] applied this screening method to study TNF-related apoptosis inducing ligand (TRAIL) induced apoptosis in HeLa cells by using an array of 510 genes and were able to identify a variety of uncharacterized as well as previously known genes that modulate TRAIL activity.

Genome wide or chromosome wide screening for gene function in human cells has become a feasible task by combining expression profiling, proteomics and RNAi to unravel gene function much more efficiently as compared to classical methods. Widespread use of expression profiling by microarray particularly in different neoplastic disorders has led to the identification of over- or under-expressed expressed sequence tags (ESTs). RNAi against these ESTs in combination with protein-based methods should lead to the identification of novel genes critical in neoplasia. These strategies, technologies to generate data, information analysis, and management systems are evolving at a rapid pace. Researchers in the United Kingdom and The Netherlands already have formed a consortium to systematically uncover function of each gene in the human genome using RNAi by 2004[52] and in the near future we should see the results of these efforts.

Cell Biology

The scientific community working with *C. elegans* and *D. melanogaster* rapidly adopted the RNAi technology placing a special emphasis on functional genomics. However, scientists working on mammalian cells have focused on RNAi as a tool to dissect complexities of cell signaling networks, bridging the gaps in our understanding, identifying potential target molecules for therapy, and using siRNA as a therapeutic agent.

A comprehensive review of siRNA uses in cell biology is beyond the scope of this chapter, however, we will review some important work in this area. Mutations in presenilin genes account for early onset familial Alzheimer disease. Presenilins in association with co-factors nicastrin, APH-1 and PEN-2 form a multi-protein complex to cleave (γ-secretase activity) β-amyloid precursor protein. Takasugi et al used RNAi to define the role of these co-factors in γ-secretase complex.[57] Barnes et al used RNAi to investigate the mammalian circadian rhythms and demonstrated that mammalian timeless (mTim) is required for rhythmicity.[58] Several other neurobiologists have used RNAi to address neuronal growth,[59] survival[60] and modulation of potassium channels.[61,62]

Another area of extensive RNAi use is in filling the gaps in cell signaling pathways. Several breakthrough contributions already have been made during the short span since the technique has been available, and many more discoveries are likely to come during the next several years. Wnt/Wingless pathway is critical for development and its aberrant signaling plays a major role in development of colo-rectal and possibly other cancers. Takemaru et al[63] used siRNA to identify Chibby as a nuclear antagonist of Wnt/Wingless pathway that acts by competitive inhibition of LEF-1 binding to β-catenin. Another group of investigators reported that the PDZ protein tax-interacting protein-1(TIP-1) binds to β-catenin and down-regulates its *trans*activation activity.[64] Axin is a negative regulator of the Wnt/Wingless pathway. A study by Yamazaki and Yanagawa[65] using siRNA in *Drosophila* found that Axin and the Axin/Arrow binding protein DCAP mediates the glucose-glycogen metabolism, raising the possibility of cross-talk between Wnt/Wingless and insulin signaling. Du et al[66]demonstrated that TRB3, a mammalian homologue of *Drosophila* tribbles, disrupts insulin signaling by binding to Akt. Glycogen synthase kinase-3 (GSK-3) is a critical kinase involved in the negative regulation of several cell signaling pathways including Wnt/Wingless. In the past, cell biologists have used lithium chloride to inhibit GSK-3 in spite of its non-specificity. Yu et al[67] demonstrated that it was technically feasible to simultaneously inhibit GSK-3α and GSK-3β with RNAi and Zhang et al[68] used a synthetic inhibitory peptide and RNAi to provide evidence that GSK-3 activity is autoregulated by the N-terminal phosphorylation of the molecule. Phosphatidylinositol 3-phosphate (PI-3) kinase/Akt signaling is critical for cell growth and survival. Small molecule inhibitors are in development to target this pathway as a therapeutic strategy to treat neoplastic disorders. Czauderna et al[69] used siRNA to the p110α catalytic subunit of PI-3 kinase and demonstrated an inhibition of the neoplastic phenotype both in vitro and vivo. Unlike PI-3 and PI-3 kinase, the role of phosphatidylinositol-4 phosphate (PI4P) in mammalian cells was uncertain until recently when Wang et al[70] demonstrated that siRNA to PI4 kinase IIα blocked recruitment of the clathrin adaptor activator protein-1 (AP-1) to Golgi and inhibited AP-1 dependent functions. The importance of arachidonic acid metabolites is well established and pathways leading to synthesis of various prostanoids and eicosanoids are well known. However, events upstream to the activation of phospholipase A2 are not well established. Pettus et al[71] showed that ceramide-1 kinase is activated in response to interleukin (IL)-1β and Ca^{++} ionophore and the levels of ceramide-1 phosphate increased, while siRNA to ceramide-1 kinase blocked these effects. Their results suggest that ceramide-1 phosphate is an upstream modulator of phospholipase A2 activity, thus providing new targets to block the synthesis of prostaglandins.

In addition to the examples cited above, multiple other studies addressed various signal transduction pathways and other aspects of cell biology. Industry is actively involved in developing the siRNA technology, and multiple commercial siRNA oligonucleotides are available to target signal transduction proteins, cell cycle machinery and transcription factors. Currently, scientists are taking advantage of siRNA to answer complex and hitherto unknown aspects of normal cellular physiology and pathogenesis of various disease states at the molecular level.

siRNA AS A THERAPEUTIC TOOL

In the past decade the focus of therapeutic interventions has shifted to target specific treatment modalities, based on the molecular pathology of the disease. Multiple new agents such as small molecules and antibodies are being incorporated into the therapeutic armamentarium, particularly for neoplastic and autoimmune disorders. Discovery of antisense technology has provided a novel method to silence disease-associated genes at the posttranscriptional level. However, enthusiasm over antisense therapy is dampened by its limitations and impractical use for broader therapeutic application. As discussed above, RNAi methods overcome many of the pitfalls associated with DNA based antisense techniques. Most of the work performed in the laboratory thus far provides evidence that siRNA holds promise as a "drug" or a tool for new drug development, with the majority of the work directed towards either neoplastic disorders or viral diseases. In the following section we will briefly discuss the potential applications of siRNA as a therapeutic tool for the treatment of cancer and other conditions.

Use of siRNA to Target Oncogenes/Oncogenic Pathways

The process of carcinogenesis involves activation of proto-oncogenes, loss of tumor suppressor genes, and aberrant cell signaling resulting in abnormal growth, increased proliferation, inhibition of apoptosis, and metastasis. Thus, it was natural for investigators to knock-down different oncogenes and other key targets inducing cell proliferation, inhibiting apoptosis, or promoting metastasis. Most of the work has been performed either in cell culture using cell lines derived from different tumors or in xenograft mice models and is summarized in Table 1.1.

siRNA as a Therapeutic Tool for Viral Induced Neoplasms

Twenty percent of all cancers are related to viral infections. The oncogenic role of human papillomavirus (HPV) in cervical and anal cancers, hepatitis C and B in hepatocellular carcinoma, human lymphotropic virus-1 (HTLV-1) in adult T cell leukemia/lymphoma (ATLL), Epstein-Barr virus (EBV) in Burkitt's, primary central nervous system (CNS) lymphoma (PCNSL) and naso-pharyngeal carcinoma, human herpes virus-8 (HHV-8) in Kaposi, primary effusive lymphoma (PEL), and multi-focal Castleman's disease are a few of the examples of the association between virus and neoplasia. Viruses transform cells by different oncogenic proteins encoded by the viral genome (v-oncogenes), activating host proto-oncogenes or suppressing tumor suppressor genes. Some of these transforming proteins expressed in the neoplastic cells are attractive targets for inhibition at the mRNA level by RNAi and several groups are utilizing siRNA as a therapeutic tool

TABLE 1.1 In Vitro And In Vivo Studies Using siRNA To Silence Oncogenes

Pathway	Gene	Cell Line	Results	Reference
Ras/Raf/MEK/ERK	*K-Ras^{v12}*	CAPAN-1	Inhibition of soft agar colony growth	72
			Inability to form tumor in nude mice	
	H-Ras	MM66	Decrease protein expression	
			Decreased in vitro growth	73
	B-Raf	WM793	Growth arrest, Increased apoptosis	
			Inhibition of soft agar colony growth	74
	C-Raf	Myeloid	Combined with siRNA to bcl-2 led increased apoptosis, Increased sensitivity to VP-16	75
Wnt/Wingless	*β-catenin*	HCT116 SW480	Inhibition of in vitro and in vivo growth in nude mice	76
PI-3K/Akt	*P110β*	HeLa	Inhibition of growth on matrigel	
			Some inhibition of growth in SCID mice	69
	Akt1	HeLa	No significant effect on growth	69
	Akt2	HeLa	No significant effect on growth	69
Receptor PTK	*erbB1*	A431	Decreased proliferation	
			Increased apoptosis	77
	Axl	293	Cell cycle arrest in G0/G1	78
	IGF-IR	MDA-MB231	Decreased clonogenic potential	
			Decreased post-irradiation survival	79
Cytosolic PTK	*Brk*	T-47D	Proliferation inhibition	80
			Decreased BrdU incorporation	
	Btk	Different hematopoietic	Down-regulation of downstream signaling	81
			Decreased histamine release	
	Bcr/abl	K562/others	Induction of apoptosis	82, 83
	Bcr/abl	32Dp210 and mutants	Decreased cell growth, Sensitization to gleevac in bcr/abl His396Pro mutant cell line	84
	NPM/ALK	HeLa	Down-regulation of expression	85
	FAK	MIAPaCa2	Induction of gemcitabine induced chemosensitivity	86
	PLK1	MCf-7, others	Decreased proliferation and increased apoptosis	87

Chemikine Receptors	*CXCR4*	MDA-MB-231	Inhibition of in vitro cell migration	88
Transcription Factors	*c-myc*	HCT116	Decreased proliferation Inhibition of growth in nude mice	89
	AML1/MTG8	Kasumi-1 SKNO-1	Induction of differentiation with TGF(/vitamin D3, decreased clonogenicity	90
	P65	HCT116	Inhibition of in vitro and in vivo growth	165
	Fra-1	Rat pleural/ Mesothelial	Down regulation of CD-44 and c-met	91
	MEF(ELF-4)	NB4–306	Decreased IL-8 production	92
Anti-apoptotic	*Bcl-2*	HeLa	Increase in doxorubicin induced apoptosis	93
	Bcl-2	LNCaP	Induction of apoptosis	94
	Bcl-2/c-raf	Myeloid	Combined with siRNA to c-raf led increased apoptosis, increased sensitivity to VP-16	75
	Bcl-2	HCT116	Induction of p53 dependent apoptosis	95
	Bcl-xL	HCT116	Induction of p53 independent apoptosis	95
	FKBP-38	HeLa	Increased apoptosis in response to etoposide	96
	Survivin	HCT116	Cell cycle block, Decreased in vitro and in vivo growth	89
	Livin	HeLa	Increased sensitivity to pro-apoptotic stimuli	97
	Bax Inhibitor-1	Different Prostate CA lines	Increased spontaneous apoptosis	98
Angiogenesis	*VEGF*	ID8	Reduced levels of VEGF	99
	MIF	Colon 26	Down-regulation of VEGF, decreased tumor growth and angiogenesis	100
Others	*iASPP*	MCF-7	Induction of p53 dependent apoptosis	101
	S100A10	CCL-222	Loss of plasminogen dependent cellular invasiveness	102
	(β-arrestin 2	HeLa, 293	Inhibition of stromal cell derived factor 1α induced migration	
	RPTPzeta	G122,D566	Reduced migration of glioblastoma cells	103
	FASE	LNCaP	Inhibition of growth, induction of apoptosis	104
	Galectin-3	HP75	Decreased proliferation, increased apoptosis	105
	ARA55	LNACaP	Reduction in agonist activity of anti-androgens	106
	Cyclin E	HCC lines	Induction of apoptosis and block in proliferation	107

to validate potential targets in virally induced cancers. Progress in this direction is summarized in Table 1.2.

A promising approach is to target the proteins encoded by the oncogenic strains of HPV that are responsible for cellular transformation and drive a continued neoplastic phenotype.[108,109] Early dysplastic lesions due to HPV infection are routinely identified by PAP smears during screening of women and high risk HIV-positive men. In the future, it might be possible to use a topical approach to treat these lesions using siRNA. Hepatitis C is another attractive target and it might be possible to use siRNA to inhibit viral protein expression in the near future.

siRNA As A Means To Reverse Resistance To Chemotherapy And Enhance Sensitivity of Cells to Chemotherapy and Radiation Therapy

The gene product of *MDR-1*, P-glycoprotein, is a transmembrane phosphoglycoprotein capable of transporting a variety of chemotherapy agents such as paclitaxel, vinblastin and doxorubicin outside the cell and has been implicated as an important mechanism of tumor resistance to chemotherapy agents. In cell line studies, silencing of *MDR* with siRNA resulted in an increase of the chemotherapy agent inside the cell and restoration of the cell line sensitivity.[116,117] Other investigators targeted molecules involved in the DNA repair pathway with siRNA and demonstrated increased sensitivity of prostate cancer cell lines to radiation therapy.[118] Peng and collaborators used siRNA directed against the protein in charge of DNA non-homologous end joining after radiation induced damage in fibroblast cell lines called Prkdc. siRNA directed against Prkdc resulted in down regulation of the protein and a significant increase in cell killing compared to controls.[119] In our lab we have down-regulated with siRNA, the p65 component of nuclear factor-κB (NF-κB) to determine whether it would increase sensitivity to irinotecan. In in vitro and in vivo models with the HCT 116 colon cancer cell line, the sensitivity of irinotecan was enhanced by transfecting siRNA to p65.[165]

siRNA as Anti-Viral Therapy

It is not surprising that there has been a flurry of activity to use siRNA as an antiviral agent, since RNAi was discovered in plants as a host defense mechanism against viruses. Moreover, conventional drugs have a limited efficacy against a few viruses for which drugs exist. For most of the viral diseases, there is no effective drug treatment. Discovery of RNAi provided a greatly needed opportunity to investigate and exploit the use of siRNA to treat viral diseases. There has been considerable progress using siRNA in plants and animals, and several excellent reviews are available on the subject.[120–124] We will limit our discussion to viral diseases affecting humans.

TABLE 1.2 siRNA to Target Virus Induced Neoplasms

Virus	Target Gene	Cell Line	Result	Ref
HPV-16	*E6*	SiHa	Degradation of E6 mRNA	108
	E7	SiHa	Induction of apoptosis	108
HPV-18	*E6, E7*	HeLa	Inhibition of DNA synthesis and induction of cellular senescence	109
HHV-8	*LANA*	BCBL-1	Block in expression of IL-6	110
	vFLIP	BCBL-1	Block in JNK/AP1 pathway	111
Hep C	*NS5A*	HepG2	Inhibition of HCV protein expression	112
	Various	Huh-7	Inhibition of virus specific protein expression Protection of naïve cells from HCV replicon RNA	113
	5' core region	Huh-7.5	Clearance of replicating HCV from infected cells	114
Hep B	Core	Huh-7, HepG2	Reduction in level of replicative intermediates	115

Several published articles address the therapeutic use of RNAi in HIV.[125–133] Though most of the focus has been on HIV, use of siRNA to target genes in several other viruses is being explored. Some of the work accomplished is summarized in Table 1.3.

So far, limited work has been published on in vivo use of siRNA to treat viral infections. In a study by McCaffrey et al[139] (Table 1.3), normal and SCID mice were injected using a technique called "hydrodynamic transfection," which employs injection of large volume of oligonucleotides in tail vein. Mice were injected with plasmids encoding the HBV genome with or without U6 promoter based plasmids encoding siRNA to HBV. Their results show that HBV specific siRNA significantly reduced viral mRNA and protein expression. This study provided a "proof of principle" for the applicability of siRNA in treating viral diseases. Song et al[146] employed another promising approach with potential applicability to treat viral or other forms of hepatitis. They demonstrated that in vivo hydrodynamic tail vein injection of Fas siRNA protected mice from Fas agonist (ConA, Jo2 monoclonal antibody) induced fulminant hepatitis. Mice were protected from fulminant hepatitis even if the injection of Fas siRNA was delayed 24 hours after induction of hepato-toxicity.[146] siRNA against caspase-8 rescued mice, even when siRNA was administered in the setting of liver failure.[147] In summary, studies performed thus far demonstrate that siRNA technology has a therapeutic potential in viral induced diseases.

TABLE 1.3 siRNA to Treat Viral Diseases

Virus	siRNA target	Cell Type	Findings	Ref
HIV-1	rev	293	4 log inhibition of HIV-1 DNA	125
	vif	Magi, Lymphocytes	Inhibition of early and late steps in HIV replication	127
	CD4, Gag, nef	Magi-CCR5, HeLa-CD4, H9, others	Inhibition of multiple steps in HIV replicative cycle	126
	Tat, Rev	293T, Jurkat, T-cells	Inhibition of gene expression and replication	128
	Gag	U87–$CD4^+$-$CXCR4^+$ T celllymphoblasts	Inhibition of HIV replication	129
	Tat, RT, p65	Magi	Inhibition of viral proteins and replication	133
	CXCR4,CCR5	U87–$CD4^+$	Blocking of acute infection by HIV-1	130
	CCR5	T-cells	3– to 7–fold reduction in infection by CCR5 tropic HIV-1 strain	131
	CCR5, p24	Macrophages	Reduction in HIV infection, combination abolished infection	132
	LEDGF/p75	HeLa	Inhibition of nuclear localization of HIV integrase	134
Polio	Capsid, Polymerase	HeLa	Protection from infection by siRNA pre-transfection, inhibition and clearing of virus	135
Hepatitis C	NS3,NS5	Huh-7 (S1179I)	Inhibition of replication	136
	5' core region	Huh-7.5	Clearance of replicating HCV from infected cells	114
	Various	Huh-7	Inhibition of virus specific protein expression Protection of naïve cells from HCV replicon RNA	113
	5_UTR	Huh-7 (5–2)	85% inhibition of replication as assessed by reporter gene	137

Hepatitis B	Core, x-ORF	Huh7, HepG2.2.15	Reduction in HBV sequence specific transcripts Reduction in viral replicative forms	138
	Multiple	Huh-7, in vivo	Reduced level of HBV genomes, In vivo experiments-reduced replicated HBV and decreased serum HBsAg	139
	Core	Hep AD38 & 79	Profound inhibition of viral replication	140
	Core	HepG	~90% inhibition of HBsAg and HBeAg	141
Hepatitis-D	Multiple	Huh-7	Inhibition of HDV genome replication with siRNA to HDV mRNA	142
Influenza	Nucleocapsid, PA	MDCK	Inhibition of viral RNA accumulation, replication	143
Rotavirus	VP4	MA104	Inhibition of VP4 synthesis. Poorly infectious progeny	144
RSV	Anti-P, anti-F	A549	With anti-P >10 fold reduction in viral progeny, inhibition of cytopathic effect, with anti-F absence of syntia formation	145

siRNA for the Treatment of Other Diseases

RNAi technology may hold promise as a therapeutic tool for other diseases aside from cancer and viral infections. Fas/Fas ligand-mediated hepatocyte apoptosis plays a major role in liver injury by auto-immune, alcohol, hepato-toxic drugs and transplant rejection. The strategy employed by Song et al[146] and discussed above may have therapeutic potential in many of these conditions.

Another avenue for siRNA based therapy is in the treatment of dominantly inherited diseases, such as the neurodegenerative disorders, where the protein encoded by the mutant allele plays a pathogenic role.[148] In these disorders, elimination of the mutant protein should ameliorate disease manifestations as demonstrated by Yamamoto et al[149] in a mouse model of Huntington disease. This novel approach using siRNA to silence these mutant alleles is a particularly exciting development, since presently there are no effective therapeutic modalities available for this disease. Xia et al[150] demonstrated the feasibility of this approach in neural PC12 cells expressing enhanced green fluorescent protein (eGFP) and expanded glutamine of 80 repeats (eGFP-Q80). The cells accumulated abnormal protein aggregates six days after transfection. This accumulation of protein aggregates was significantly reduced if cells were treated with adenoviral based siRNA to GFP. This same group has expanded the work and has recently reported silencing of mutant Machado-Joseph disease/spino-cerebellar ataxia type 3 allele and missense Tau mutation V337M responsible for fronto-temporal dementia.[151] Mutant Zn superoxide dismutase (SOD) causes amyotrophic lateral sclerosis. Though mutant allele differs from wild type with single nucleotide mismatch, Ding et al[152] reported effective silencing of the mutant gene using siRNA. In summary, RNAi technology holds great promise for the treatment of neuro-generative disorders caused by gain of function dominant mutations. Further progress will depend upon efficient in vivo delivery systems.

In Vivo Delivery of siRNA

Methods presently used to deliver siRNA include (1) synthetic dsRNA, (2) bacterial plasmid based, and (3) viral (adeno, lenti) techniques, with the latter two encoding shRNA with similar efficacy as synthetic dsRNA. Several studies have shown that the effect of transfected synthetic siRNA lasts from one to three weeks. Vector based systems theoretically can provide long-term silencing if the vector continues to express shRNA and is integrated into the host genome. The disease state will determine whether investigators should use short- or long-term gene down-regulation. So far most of the studies using RNAi have been performed in cell culture system. However, use of siRNA as a therapeutic tool will require efficient in vivo delivery methods. Limited success has been achieved in this direction as discussed below.

RNAi phenomenon by transfection of synthetic and vector based dsRNA in mouse oocytes, pre-implantation embryos and undifferentiated mouse embryonic stem cells was demonstrated even before discovery of siRNA and widespread applicability of RNAi technique to mammalian culture systems.[8,153,154] Since then, several studies have been performed demonstrating efficacy of siRNA in vivo in mice and rats. Lewis et al[155] achieved systemic silencing of a reporter gene by injecting siRNA into the mice tail vein. They employed a method in which nucleotides are injected in a large volume (1/10th of mouse wt) rapidly. This so-called "hydrodynamic" method has been employed by other investigators to silence endogenous or viral genes.[146,147,156] These studies clearly demonstrated that siRNA is taken up by the target tissues and leads to effective silencing of the target genes. However, humans will not tolerate a rapid systemic administration of such a large volume (~50% of blood volume) and alternate methods to deliver siRNA will need to be developed if it is to be used in humans.

Several other delivery systems have been employed by investigators to deliver siRNA in vivo. Sorensen et al intravenously injected mice with cationic plasmid-containing liposomes encoding the green fluorescent protein with its cognate siRNA and showed inhibition of gene expression in several organs.[157] In our studies, delivery of siRNA in 0.5 mL was effective in inhibiting target gene in xenogenic tumors.[76,89] Mohmmed et al injected mice with siRNA directed against *Plasmodium bergheri* in 200 μL phosphate buffered saline (PBS) after challenging the mice with the parasite.[166] They were able to demonstrate uptake of siRNA by the intracellular parasite. Recently, Kobayashi et al[158] studied in vivo kinetics of RNAi using vector based siRNA. Their results show dose a dependent inhibition of the reporter gene and further validated the efficacy of the hydrodynamic method of delivery. Interestingly, they also found silencing of the reporter after intramuscular injection of the siRNA vector.[158]

A potential applicability of siRNA may be in topical use or delivery to target tissues directly. Hommel et al[159] were able to knock down the dopamine synthase gene by introducing adeno-virus based siRNA into the mouse midbrain with stereotactic surgery. Matsuda and Cepko[160] demonstrate a technique, whereby plasmid based siRNA was transfected to retinal cells by direct sub-retinal injection followed by electroporation. In another study, Reich at al[161] successfully inhibited choroidal neovascularization in response to laser photocoagulation by sub-retinal injection of siRNA against murine vascular endothelial growth factor (mVEGF). These studies clearly demonstrate that the different approaches used by investigators to deliver siRNA are feasible and applicable to a variety of human diseases.

In plants the systemic spread of RNAi and inheritability is well established, but there is no clear evidence that this is the case in higher animals. Recent reports demonstrate a successful induction of RNAi by vector based siRNA into embryonic cells resulting in the creation of transgenic mice[162,163] with transmission of the genotype to the progeny. These approaches have immediate application for the creation of transgenic animals to study gene function, particularly in conditions where traditional gene knock-down experiments are lethal at the embryonic stage. However, the potential exists to use a similar approach for the treatment of humans with dominantly inherited disorders caused by gain of function mutations.

siRNA AS A MEANS TO DEVELOP TARGETED DRUGS

Knowledge of the pathways involved in carcinogenesis has facilitated the development of molecules that will block these pathways and induce cell arrest, differentiation or apoptosis. A prime example has been the use of STI-571 (Gleevec®) for patients with Philadelphia chromosome-positive chronic myelogenous leukemia (CML). Today we can test whether blocking a specific pathway with siRNA will have a functional consequence to the malignant cell. Moreover, investigators can block several targets either simultaneously or sequentially and be able to determine whether this approach will result in a detrimental effect on the survival of the malignant cell. In the near future these antisense approaches with siRNA will accelerate the discovery of new targets and the best way to sequence the agents for the treatment of human malignancies. Several groups are working on using siRNA for high throughput screening of potential drug targets.

CONCLUSION AND FUTURE PROSPECTS

Discovery of RNAi has been a dazzling development for the research community.[164] Combining the output from several different powerful techniques at hand such as the genome sequence database, microarray, proteomics and RNAi will lead to a more comprehensive understanding of normal and pathological cell behavior at a faster pace. Several groups are already working to integrate these technologies and studies using these technologies should lead to the identification of novel pathways and targets for pharmacological intervention to treat various diseases.

It is early to postulate whether RNAi plays a physiological role in higher eukaryotes, such as maintaining genomic stability by transposon silencing. Identification of several miRNA species in higher animals does provide a hint towards this role. In future studies, it may be possible to uncover genetic basis of disease(s) due to these regulatory RNAs and genes encoding these miRNAs.

A major emphasis by investigators has been on the use of siRNA directly as a "drug." This early excitement with RNAi mimics that seen with the discovery of antisense technology. However, as pointed out earlier, siRNAs differ in many ways from conventional antisense molecules and appear more promising. Use of naked synthetic siRNA molecules or vector-based systems will depend upon the desired effect on the disease being treated (that is, short- or long-term gene knock-down). The proof of principle for utility of siRNA as a drug has been demonstrated in many animal model systems. Now dedicated studies are needed to find and compare the different delivery methods in humans. This will involve looking at methods attempting systemic, loco-regional and topical delivery techniques. Several vector-based methods have been developed to generate RNAi in cells transfected or infected with viral based vectors. These all appear to be effective to a similar extent in in vitro and limited in vivo studies. However, its use in humans would require addressing various safety concerns. The pharmaceutical industry is actively involved with the academic institutions in developing siRNA as a research and therapeutic tool and soon we will see clinical trials with siRNA for the treatment of cancer and other diseases.

REFERENCES

1. Fire A, Xu S, Montgomery MK, et al. Potent and specific genetic interference by double-stranded RNA in Caenorhabditis elegans. Nature 1998;391:806–811.
2. Elbashir SM, Harborth J, Lendeckel W, et al. Duplexes of 21–nucleotide RNAs mediate RNA interference in cultured mammalian cells. Nature 2001;411:494–498.
3. Napoli C, Lemieux C, Jorgensen R. Introduction of a chimeric chalcone synthase gene into petunia results in reversible co-suppression of homologous genes in trans. Plant Cell 1990;2:279–289.
4. Palauqui JC, Vaucheret H. Transgenes are dispensable for the RNA degradation step of cosuppression. Proc Natl Acad Sci USA 1998;95:9675–9680.
5. Voinnet O, Vain P, Angell S, Baulcombe DC. Systemic spread of sequence-specific transgene RNA degradation in plants is initiated by localized introduction of ectopic promoterless DNA. Cell 1998;95:177–187.
6. Etemad-Moghadam B, Guo S, Kemphues KJ. Asymmetrically distributed PAR-3 protein contributes to cell polarity and spindle alignment in early *C. elegans* embryos. Cell 1995;83:743–752.
7. Wianny F, Zernicka-Goetz M. Specific interference with gene function by double-stranded RNA in early mouse development. Nat Cell Biol 2000;2:70–75.
8. Svoboda P, Stein P, Hayashi H, Schultz RM. Selective reduction of dormant maternal mRNAs in mouse oocytes by RNA interference. Development. 2000;127:4147–4156.
9. Caplen NJ, Fleenor J, Fire A, Morgan RA. dsRNA-mediated gene silencing in cultured *Drosophila* cells: a tissue culture model for the analysis of RNA interference. Gene 2000;252: 95–105.
10. Ui-Tei K, Zenno S, Miyata Y, Saigo K. Sensitive assay of RNA interference in *Drosophila* and Chinese hamster cultured cells using firefly luciferase gene as target. FEBS Lett 2000;479:79–82.
11. Hammond SM, Bernstein E, Beach D, Hannon GJ. An RNA-directed nuclease mediates post-transcriptional gene silencing in *Drosophila* cells. Nature 2000;404:293–296.
12. Ketting RF, Fischer SE, Bernstein E, et al. Dicer functions in RNA interference and in synthesis of small RNA involved in developmental timing in *C. elegans*. Genes Dev 2001;15:2654–2269.
13. Elbashir SM, Martinez J, Patkaniowska A, et al. Functional anatomy of siRNAs for mediating efficient RNAi in Drosophila melanogaster embryo lysate. EMBO J 2001;20:6877–6888.
14. Hutvagner G, McLachlan J, Pasquinelli AE, et al. A cellular function for the RNA-interference enzyme Dicer in the maturation of the let-7 small temporal RNA. Science 2001;293:834–838.

15. Lagos-Quintana M, Rauhut R, Lendeckel W, Tuschl T. Identification of novel genes coding for small expressed RNAs. Science 2001;294:853–858.
16. Lau NC, Lim LP, Weinstein EG, Bartel DP. An abundant class of tiny RNAs with probable regulatory roles in *Caenorhabditis elegans*. Science 2001;294:858–862.
17. Lee RC, Ambros V. An extensive class of small RNAs in *Caenorhabditis elegans*. Science 2001;294:862–864.
18. Hutvagner G, Zamore PD. A microRNA in a multiple-turnover RNAi enzyme complex. Science 2002;297:2056–2060.
19. Tabara H, Yigit E, Siomi H, Mello CC. The dsRNA binding protein RDE-4 interacts with RDE-1, DCR-1, and a DExH-box helicase to direct RNAi in *C. elegans*. Cell 2002;109:861–871.
20. Knight SW, Bass BL. A role for the RNase III enzyme DCR-1 in RNA interference and germ line development in *Caenorhabditis elegans*. Science 2001;293:2269–2271.
21. Nykanen A, Haley B, Zamore PD. ATP requirements and small interfering RNA structure in the RNA interference pathway. Cell 2001;107:309–321.
22. Sijen T, Fleenor J, Simmer F, et al. On the role of RNA amplification in dsRNA-triggered gene silencing. Cell 2001;107:465–476.
23. Nishikura K. A short primer on RNAi: RNA-directed RNA polymerase acts as a key catalyst. Cell 2001;107:415–418.
24. Lipardi C, Wei Q, Paterson BM. RNAi as random degradative PCR: siRNA primers convert mRNA into dsRNAs that are degraded to generate new siRNAs. Cell 2001;107:297–307.
25. Minoshima H, Suyama E, Kawasaki H, Taira K. [RNAi-mediated specific gene silencing and its application to medical treatments of viral infectious disease]. Uirusu 2003; 53:7–14. (in Japanese)
26. Hammond SM, Boettcher S, Caudy AA, et al. Argonaute2, a link between genetic and biochemical analyses of RNAi. Science 2001;293:1146–1150.
27. Williams RW, Rubin GM. ARGONAUTE1 is required for efficient RNA interference in Drosophila embryos. Proc Natl Acad Sci USA 2002;99:6889–6894.
28. Dudley NR, Goldstein B. RNA interference: silencing in the cytoplasm and nucleus. Curr Opin Mol Ther 2003;5:113–117.
29. Dudley NR, Labbe JC, Goldstein B. Using RNA interference to identify genes required for RNA interference. Proc Natl Acad Sci USA 2002;99:4191–4196.
30. Volpe TA, Kidner C, Hall IM, et al. Regulation of heterochromatic silencing and histone H3 lysine-9 methylation by RNAi. Science 2002;297:1833–1837.
31. Wassenegger M. Gene silencing. Int Rev Cytol 2002;219:61–113.
32. Mette MF, Aufsatz W, van der Winden J et al. Transcriptional silencing and promoter methylation triggered by double-stranded RNA. EMBO J 2000;19:5194–5201.
33. Domeier ME, Morse DP, Knight SW, et al. A link between RNA interference and nonsense-mediated decay in *Caenorhabditis elegans*. Science 2000;289:1928–1931.
34. Winston WM, Molodowitch C, Hunter CP. Systemic RNAi in *C. elegans* requires the putative transmembrane protein SID-1. Science 2002;295:2456–2459.
35. Klahre U, Crete P, Leuenberger SA, et al. High molecular weight RNAs and small interfering RNAs induce systemic posttranscriptional gene silencing in plants. Proc Natl Acad Sci USA 2002;99:11981–1196.
36. Chi JT, Chang HY, Wang NN, et al. Genomewide view of gene silencing by small interfering RNAs. Proc Natl Acad Sci USA 2003;100:6343–6346.
37. Bridge AJ, Pebernard S, Ducraux A, et al. Induction of an interferon response by RNAi vectors in mammalian cells. Nat Genet 2003;34:263–264.
38. Sledz CA, Holko M, de Veer MJ, et al. Activation of the interferon system by short-interfering RNAs. Nat Cell Biol 2003;5:834–839.

39. Jackson AL, Bartz SR, Schelter J, et al. Expression profiling reveals off-target gene regulation by RNAi. Nat Biotechnol 2003;21:635–637.

40. Braasch DA, Jensen S, Liu Y, et al. RNA interference in mammalian cells by chemically-modified RNA. Biochemistry 2003;42:7967–7975.

41. Schwarz DS, Hutvagner G, Haley B, Zamore PD. Evidence that siRNAs function as guides, not primers, in the *Drosophila* and human RNAi pathways. Mol Cell 2002;10:537–548.

42. Chiu YL, Rana TM. RNAi in human cells: basic structural and functional features of small interfering RNA. Mol Cell 2002;10:549–561.

43. Franch T, Petersen M, Wagner EG, et al. Antisense RNA regulation in prokaryotes: rapid RNA/RNA interaction facilitated by a general U-turn loop structure. J Mol Biol 1999;294: 1115–1125.

44. Vickers TA, Koo S, Bennett CF, et al. Efficient reduction of target RNAs by small interfering RNA and RNase H-dependent antisense agents. A comparative analysis. J Biol Chem 2003;278: 7108–7118.

45. Grunweller A, Wyszko E, Bieber B, et al. Comparison of different antisense strategies in mammalian cells using locked nucleic acids, 2′-O-methyl RNA, phosphorothioates and small interfering RNA. Nucleic Acids Res 2003;31:3185–3193.

46. Xu Y, Zhang HY, Thormeyer D, et al. Effective small interfering RNAs and phosphorothioate antisense DNAs have different preferences for target sites in the luciferase mRNAs. Biochem Biophys Res Commun 2003;306:712–717.

47. Lindbo JA, Silva-Rosales L, Proebsting WM, Dougherty WG. Induction of a highly specific antiviral state in transgenic plants: implications for regulation of gene expression and virus resistance. Plant Cell 1993;5:1749–1759.

48. Gonczy P, Echeverri C, Oegema K, et al. Functional genomic analysis of cell division in *C. elegans* using RNAi of genes on chromosome III. Nature 2000;408:331–336.

49. Fraser AG, Kamath RS, Zipperlen P, et al. Functional genomic analysis of *C. elegans* chromosome I by systematic RNA interference. Nature 2000;408:325–330.

50. Kamath RS, Ahringer J. Genome-wide RNAi screening in *Caenorhabditis elegans*. Methods 2003;30:313–321.

51. Ashrafi K, Chang FY, Watts JL, et al. Genome-wide RNAi analysis of Caenorhabditis elegans fat regulatory genes. Nature 2003;421:268–272.

52. Frankish H. Consortium uses RNAi to uncover genes' function. Lancet 2003;361:584.

53. Hannon GJ. RNA interference. Nature 2002;418:244–251.

54. Mousses S, Caplen NJ, Cornelison R, et al. RNAi microarray analysis in cultured mammalian cells. Genome Res 2003;13:2341–2347.

55. Kumar R, Conklin DS, Mittal V. High-throughput selection of effective RNAi probes for gene silencing. Genome Res 2003;13:2333–2340.

56. Aza-Blanc P, Cooper CL, Wagner K, et al. Identification of modulators of TRAIL-induced apoptosis via RNAi-based phenotypic screening. Mol Cell 2003;12:627–637.

57. Takasugi N, Tomita T, Hayashi I, et al. The role of presenilin cofactors in the gamma-secretase complex. Nature 2003;422:438–441.

58. Barnes JW, Tischkau SA, Barnes JA, et al. Requirement of mammalian Timeless for circadian rhythmicity. Science 2003;302:439–442.

59. Arakawa Y, Bito H, Furuyashiki T, et al. Control of axon elongation via an SDF-1alpha/Rho/ mDia pathway in cultured cerebellar granule neurons. J Cell Biol 2003;161:381–391.

60. Gaudilliere B, Shi Y, Bonni A. RNA interference reveals a requirement for myocyte enhancer factor 2A in activity-dependent neuronal survival. J Biol Chem 2002;277:46442–46446.

61. Anantharam A, Lewis A, Panaghie G, et al. RNA interference reveals that endogenous *Xenopus* MinK-related peptides govern mammalian K+ channel function in oocyte expression studies. J Biol Chem 2003;278:11739–11745.

62. McCrossan ZA, Lewis A, Panaghie G, et al. MinK-related peptide 2 modulates Kv2.1 and Kv3.1 potassium channels in mammalian brain. J Neurosci 2003;23:8077–8091.

63. Takemaru K, Yamaguchi S, Lee YS, et al. Chibby, a nuclear beta-catenin-associated antagonist of the Wnt/Wingless pathway. Nature 2003;422:905–909.

64. Kanamori M, Sandy P, Marzinotto S, et al. The PDZ protein tax-interacting protein-1 inhibits beta-catenin transcriptional activity and growth of colorectal cancer cells. J Biol Chem 2003;278:38758–3864.

65. Yamazaki H, Yanagawa S. Axin and the axin/arrow-binding protein DCAP mediate glucose-glycogen metabolism. Biochem Biophys Res Commun 2003;304:229–235.

66. Du K, Herzig S, Kulkarni RN, Montminy M. TRB3: a tribbles homolog that inhibits Akt/PKB activation by insulin in liver. Science 2003;300:1574–1577.

67. Yu JY, Taylor J, DeRuiter SL, et al. Simultaneous inhibition of GSK3alpha and GSK3beta using hairpin siRNA expression vectors. Mol Ther 2003;7:228–236.

68. Zhang F, Phiel CJ, Spece L, et al. Inhibitory phosphorylation of glycogen synthase kinase-3 (GSK-3) in response to lithium. Evidence for autoregulation of GSK-3. J Biol Chem 2003;278:33067–33077.

69. Czauderna F, Fechtner M, Aygun H, et al. Functional studies of the PI(3)-kinase signalling pathway employing synthetic and expressed siRNA. Nucleic Acids Res 2003;31:670–682.

70. Wang YJ, Wang J, Sun HQ, et al. Phosphatidylinositol 4 phosphate regulates targeting of clathrin adaptor AP-1 complexes to the Golgi. Cell 2003;114:299–310.

71. Pettus BJ, Bielawska A, Spiegel S, et al. Ceramide kinase mediates cytokine- and calcium ionophore-induced arachidonic acid release. J Biol Chem 2003;278:38206–38213.

72. Brummelkamp TR, Bernards R, Agami R. Stable suppression of tumorigenicity by virus-mediated RNA interference. Cancer Cell 2002;2:243–247.

73. Yin JQ, Gao J, Shao R, et al. siRNA agents inhibit oncogene expression and attenuate human tumor cell growth. J Exp Ther Oncol 2003;3:194–204.

74. Hingorani SR, Jacobetz MA, Robertson GP, et al. Suppression of BRAF(V599E) in human melanoma abrogates transformation. Cancer Res 2003;63:5198–5202.

75. Cioca DP, Aoki Y, Kiyosawa K. RNA interference is a functional pathway with therapeutic potential in human myeloid leukemia cell lines. Cancer Gene Ther 2003;10:125–133.

76. Verma UN, Surabhi RM, Schmaltieg A, et al. Small interfering RNAs directed against beta-catenin inhibit the in vitro and in vivo growth of colon cancer cells. Clin Cancer Res 2003;9:1291–1300.

77. Nagy P, Arndt-Jovin DJ, Jovin TM. Small interfering RNAs suppress the expression of endogenous and GFP-fused epidermal growth factor receptor (erbB1) and induce apoptosis in erbB1–overexpressing cells. Exp Cell Res 2003;285:39–49.

78. Chung BI, Malkowicz SB, Nguyen TB, et al. Expression of the proto-oncogene Axl in renal cell carcinoma. DNA Cell Biol 2003;22:533–540.

79. Bohula EA, Salisbury AJ, Sohail M, et al. The efficacy of small interfering RNAs targeted to the type 1 insulin-like growth factor receptor (IGF1R) is influenced by secondary structure in the IGF1R transcript. J Biol Chem 2003;278:15991–15997.

80. Harvey AJ, Crompton MR. Use of RNA interference to validate Brk as a novel therapeutic target in breast cancer: Brk promotes breast carcinoma cell proliferation. Oncogene 2003;22:5006–5010.

81. Heinonen JE, Smith CIE, Nore BF. Silencing of Bruton's tyrosine kinase (Btk) using short interfering RNA duplexes (siRNA). FEBS Lett 2002;527:274–278.

82. Wilda M, Fuchs U, Wossmann W, Borkhardt A. Killing of leukemic cells with a BCR/ABL fusion gene by RNA interference (RNAi). Oncogene 2002;21:5716–5724.

83. Scherr M, Battmer K, Winkler T, et al. Specific inhibition of bcr-abl gene expression by small interfering RNA. Blood 2003;101:1566–1569.

84. Wohlbold L, van der Kuip H, Miething C, et al. Inhibition of bcr-abl gene expression by small interfering RNA sensitizes for imatinib mesylate (STI571). Blood 2003;102:2236–2239.

85. Damm-Welk C, Fuchs U, Wossmann W, Borkhardt A. Targeting oncogenic fusion genes in leukemias and lymphomas by RNA interference. Semin Cancer Biol 2003;13:283–292.

86. Duxbury MS, Ito H, Benoit E, et al. RNA interference targeting focal adhesion kinase enhances pancreatic adenocarcinoma gemcitabine chemosensitivity*1. Biochem Biophys Res Commun 2003;311:786–792.

87. Spankuch-Schmitt B, Bereiter-Hahn J, Kaufmann M, Strebhardt K. Effect of RNA silencing of polo-like kinase-1 (PLK1) on apoptosis and spindle formation in human cancer cells. J Natl Cancer Inst 2002;94:1863–1877.

88. Chen Y, Stamatoyannopoulos G, Song C-Z. Down-regulation of CXCR4 by inducible small interfering RNA inhibits breast cancer cell invasion in vitro. Cancer Res 2003;63:4801–4804.

89. Williams NS, Gaynor RB, Scoggin S, et al. Identification and validation of genes involved in the pathogenesis of colorectal cancer using cDNA microarrays and RNA interference. Clin Cancer Res 2003;9:931–946.

90. Heidenreich O, Krauter J, Riehle H, et al. AML1/MTG8 oncogene suppression by small interfering RNAs supports myeloid differentiation of t(8;21)-positive leukemic cells. Blood 2003;101:3157–3163.

91. Ramos-Nino ME, Scapoli L, Martinelli M, et al. Microarray analysis and RNA silencing link fra-1 to cd44 and c-met expression in mesothelioma. Cancer Res 2003;63:3539–3545.

92. Hedvat CV, Yao J, Sokolic RA, Nimer SD. Myeloid ELF1-like factor is a potent activator of interleukin-8 expression in hematopoietic cells. J Biol Chem 2004;279:6395–6400.

93. Futami T, Miyagishi M, Seki M, Taira K. Induction of apoptosis in HeLa cells with siRNA expression vector targeted against bcl-2. Nucleic Acids Res 2002;2[suppl]:251–252.

94. Lin SL, Chuong CM, Ying SY. A novel mRNA-cDNA interference phenomenon for silencing bcl-2 expression in human LNCaP cells. Biochem Biophys Res Commun 2001;281:639–644.

95. Jiang M, Milner J. Bcl-2 constitutively suppresses p53–dependent apoptosis in colorectal cancer cells. Genes Dev 2003;17:832–837.

96. Shirane M, Nakayama KI. Inherent calcineurin inhibitor FKBP38 targets Bcl-2 to mitochondria and inhibits apoptosis. Nat Cell Biol 2003;5:28–37.

97. Crnkovic-Mertens I, Hoppe-Seyler F, Butz K. Induction of apoptosis in tumor cells by siRNA-mediated silencing of the livin/ML-IAP/KIAP gene. Oncogene 2003;22:8330–8336.

98. Grzmil M, Thelen P, Hemmerlein B, et al. Bax inhibitor-1 is overexpressed in prostate cancer and its specific down-regulation by RNA interference leads to cell death in human prostate carcinoma cells. Am J Pathol 2003;163:543–552.

99. Zhang L, Yang N, Mohamed-Hadley A, et al. Vector-based RNAi, a novel tool for isoform-specific knock-down of VEGF and anti-angiogenesis gene therapy of cancer. Biochem Biophys Res Commun 2003;303:1169–1178.

100. Sun B, Nishihira J, Suzuki M, et al. Induction of macrophage migration inhibitory factor by lysophosphatidic acid: relevance to tumor growth and angiogenesis. Int J Mol Med 2003;12: 633–641.

101. Bergamaschi D, Samuels Y, O'Neil NJ, et al. iASPP oncoprotein is a key inhibitor of p53 conserved from worm to human. Nat Genet 2003;33:162–167.

102. Zhang L, Fogg DK, Waisman DM. RNA Interference-mediated silencing of the S100A10 gene attenuates plasmin generation and invasiveness of Colo 222 colorectal cancer cells. J Biol Chem 2004;279:2053–2062.

103. Muller S, Kunkel P, Lamszus K, et al. A role for receptor tyrosine phosphatase zeta in glioma cell migration. Oncogene 2003;22:6661–6668.

104. De Schrijver E, Brusselmans K, Heyns W, et al. RNA interference-mediated silencing of the fatty acid synthase gene attenuates growth and induces morphological changes and apoptosis of LNCaP prostate cancer cells. Cancer Res 2003;63:3799–3804.

105. Riss D, Jin L, Qian X, et al. Differential expression of galectin-3 in pituitary tumors. Cancer Res 2003;63:2251–2255.

106. Rahman MM, Miyamoto H, Lardy H, Chang C. Inactivation of androgen receptor coregulator ARA55 inhibits androgen receptor activity and agonist effect of antiandrogens in prostate cancer cells. Proc Natl Acad Sci USA 2003;100:5124–5129.

107. Li K, Lin SY, Brunicardi FC, Seu P. Use of RNA interference to target cyclin E-overexpressing hepatocellular carcinoma. Cancer Res 2003;63:3593–3597.

108. Jiang M, Milner J. Selective silencing of viral gene expression in HPV-positive human cervical carcinoma cells treated with siRNA, a primer of RNA interference. Oncogene 2002;21:6041–6048.

109. Hall AH, Alexander KA. RNA interference of human papillomavirus type 18 E6 and E7 induces senescence in HeLa cells. J Virol 2003;77:6066–6069.

110. An J, Sun Y, Rettig MB. Transcriptional coactivation of c-Jun by the KSHV-encoded LANA. Blood 2004;103:222–228.

111. An J, Sun Y, Sun R, Rettig MB. Kaposi's sarcoma-associated herpesvirus encoded vFLIP induces cellular IL-6 expression: the role of the NF-kappaB and JNK/AP1 pathways. Oncogene 2003;22:3371–3385.

112. Sen A, Steele R, Ghosh AK, et al. Inhibition of hepatitis C virus protein expression by RNA interference. Virus Res 2003;96:27–35.

113. Wilson JA, Jayasena S, Khvorova A, et al. RNA interference blocks gene expression and RNA synthesis from hepatitis C replicons propagated in human liver cells. Proc Natl Acad Sci USA 2003;100:2783–2788.

114. Randall G, Grakoui A, Rice CM. Clearance of replicating hepatitis C virus replicon RNAs in cell culture by small interfering RNAs. Proc Natl Acad Sci USA 2003;100:235–240.

115. Hamasaki K, Nakao K, Matsumoto K, et al. Short interfering RNA-directed inhibition of hepatitis B virus replication. FEBS Lett. 2003;543:51–54.

116. Wu H, Hait WN, Yang JM. Small interfering RNA-induced suppression of MDR1 (P-glycoprotein) restores sensitivity to multidrug-resistant cancer cells. Cancer Res 2003;63:1515–1519.

117. Nieth C, Priebsch A, Stege A, Lage H. Modulation of the classical multidrug resistance (MDR) phenotype by RNA interference (RNAi). FEBS Lett 2003;545:144–150.

118. Collis SJ, Swartz MJ, Nelson WG, DeWeese TL. Enhanced radiation and chemotherapy-mediated cell killing of human cancer cells by small inhibitory RNA silencing of DNA repair factors. Cancer Res 2003;63:1550–1554.

119. Peng Y, Zhang Q, Nagasawa H, et al. Silencing expression of the catalytic subunit of DNA-dependent protein kinase by small interfering RNA sensitizes human cells for radiation-induced chromosome damage, cell killing, and mutation. Cancer Res 2002;62:6400–6404.

120. Campbell MA, Fitzgerald HA, Ronald PC. Engineering pathogen resistance in crop plants. Transgenic Res 2002;11:599–613.

121. Goldbach R, Bucher E, Prins M. Resistance mechanisms to plant viruses: an overview. Virus Res 2003;92:207–212.

122. Lindenbach BD, Rice CM. RNAi targeting an animal virus: news from the front. Mol Cell 2002;9:925–927.

123. Silva JM, Hammond SM, Hannon GJ. RNA interference: a promising approach to antiviral therapy? Trends Mol Med 2002;8:505–508.

124. Kitabwalla M, Ruprecht RM. RNA interference—a new weapon against HIV and beyond. N Engl J Med 2002;347:1364–1367.

125. Lee NS, Dohjima T, Bauer G, et al. Expression of small interfering RNAs targeted against HIV-1 rev transcripts in human cells. Nat Biotechnol 2002;20:500–505.

126. Novina CD, Murray MF, Dykxhoorn DM, et al. siRNA-directed inhibition of HIV-1 infection. Nat Med 2002;8:681–686.

127. Jacque JM, Triques K, Stevenson M. Modulation of HIV-1 replication by RNA interference. Nature 2002;418:435–438.

128. Coburn GA, Cullen BR. Potent and specific inhibition of human immunodeficiency virus type 1 replication by RNA interference. J Virol 2002;76:9225–9231.

129. Capodici J, Kariko K, Weissman D. Inhibition of HIV-1 infection by small interfering RNA-mediated RNA interference. J Immunol 2002;169:5196–5201.

130. Martinez MA, Gutierrez A, Armand-Ugon M, et al. Suppression of chemokine receptor expression by RNA interference allows for inhibition of HIV-1 replication. Aids 2002;16: 2385–2390.

131. Qin XF, An DS, Chen IS, Baltimore D. Inhibiting HIV-1 infection in human T cells by lentiviral-mediated delivery of small interfering RNA against CCR5. Proc Natl Acad Sci USA 2003; 100:183–188.

132. Song E, Lee SK, Dykxhoorn DM, et al. Sustained small interfering RNA-mediated human immunodeficiency virus type 1 inhibition in primary macrophages. J Virol 2003;77:7174–7181.

133. Surabhi RM, Gaynor RB. RNA interference directed against viral and cellular targets inhibits human immunodeficiency Virus Type 1 replication. J Virol 2002;76:12963–12973.

134. Maertens G, Cherepanov P, Pluymers W, et al. LEDGF/p75 is essential for nuclear and chromosomal targeting of HIV-1 integrase in human cells. J Biol Chem 2003;278:33528–33539.

135. Gitlin L, Karelsky S, Andino R. Short interfering RNA confers intracellular antiviral immunity in human cells. Nature 2002;418:430–434.

136. Kapadia SB, Brideau-Andersen A, Chisari FV. Interference of hepatitis C virus RNA replication by short interfering RNAs. Proc Natl Acad Sci USA 2003;100[suppl 4]:2014–2018.

137. Seo MY, Abrignani S, Houghton M, Han JH. Small interfering RNA-mediated inhibition of hepatitis C virus replication in the human hepatoma cell line Huh-7. J Virol 2003;77:810–812.

138. Shlomai A, Shaul Y. Inhibition of hepatitis B virus expression and replication by RNA interference*1. Hepatology 2003;37[suppl 4]:764–770.

139. McCaffrey AP, Nakai H, Pandey K, et al. Inhibition of hepatitis B virus in mice by RNA interference. Nat Biotechnol 2003;21:639–644.

140. Ying C, De Clercq E, Neyts J. Selective inhibition of hepatitis B virus replication by RNA interference. Biochem Biophys Res Commun 2003;309:482–484.

141. Tang N, Huang AL, Zhang BQ, et al. [Potent and specific inhibition of hepatitis B virus antigen expression by RNA interference]. Zhonghua Yi Xue Za Zhi 2003;83:1309–1312. (in Chinese)

142. Chang J, Taylor JM. Susceptibility of human hepatitis delta virus RNAs to small interfering RNA action. J Virol 2003;77:9728–9731.

143. Ge Q, McManus MT, Nguyen T, et al. RNA interference of influenza virus production by directly targeting mRNA for degradation and indirectly inhibiting all viral RNA transcription. Proc Natl Acad Sci USA 2003;100[suppl 5]:2718–2723.

144. Dector MA, Romero P, Lopez S, Arias CF. Rotavirus gene silencing by small interfering RNAs. EMBO Rep 2002;3:1175–1180.

145. Bitko V, Barik S. Phenotypic silencing of cytoplasmic genes using sequence-specific double-stranded short interfering RNA and its application in the reverse genetics of wild type negative-strand RNA viruses. BMC Microbiology [Electronic Resource]. 2001;1[suppl 1]:34.

146. Song E, Lee SK, Wang J, et al. RNA interference targeting Fas protects mice from fulminant hepatitis. Nat Med 2003;9:347–351.

147. Zender L, Hutker S, Liedtke C, et al. Caspase 8 small interfering RNA prevents acute liver failure in mice. PNAS 2003;100:7797–7802.

148. Zoghbi HY, Orr HT. Glutamine repeats and neurodegeneration. Annu Rev Neurosci 2000;23: 217–247.

149. Yamamoto A, Lucas JJ, Hen R. Reversal of neuropathology and motor dysfunction in a conditional model of Huntington's disease. Cell 2000;101:57–66.

150. Xia H, Mao Q, Paulson HL, Davidson BL. siRNA-mediated gene silencing in vitro and in vivo. Nat Biotechnol 2002;20:1006–1010.

151. Miller VM, Xia H, Marrs GL, et al. Allele-specific silencing of dominant disease genes. Proc Natl Acad Sci USA 2003;100:7195–7200.

152. Ding H, Schwarz DS, Keene A, et al. Selective silencing by RNAi of a dominant allele that causes amyotrophic lateral sclerosis. Aging Cell 2003;2:209–217.

153. Yang S, Tutton S, Pierce E, Yoon K. Specific double-stranded RNA interference in undifferentiated mouse embryonic stem cells. Mol Cell Biol 2001;21:7807–7816.

154. Svoboda P, Stein P, Schultz RM. RNAi in mouse oocytes and preimplantation embryos: effectiveness of hairpin dsRNA. Biochem Biophys Res Commun 2001;287:1099–1104.

155. Lewis DL, Hagstrom JE, Loomis AG, et al. Efficient delivery of siRNA for inhibition of gene expression in postnatal mice. Nat Genet 2002;32:107–108.

156. Giladi H, Ketzinel-Gilad M, Rivkin L, et al. Small interfering RNA inhibits hepatitis B virus replication in mice. Mol Ther 2003;8:769–776.

157. Sorensen DR, Leirdal M, Sioud M. Gene silencing by systemic delivery of synthetic siRNAs in adult mice. J Mol Biol 2003;327:761–766.

158. Kobayashi N, Matsui Y, Kawase A, et al. Vector-based in vivo RNA interference: dose- and time-dependent suppression of transgene expression. J Pharmacol Exp Ther 2004;308:688–693.

159. Hommel JD, Sears RM, Georgescu D, et al. Local gene knockdown in the brain using viral-mediated RNA interference. Nat Med 2003;9:1539–1544.

160. Matsuda T, Cepko CL. Electroporation and RNA interference in the rodent retina in vivo and in vitro. Proc Natl Acad Sci USA 2004;101:16–22.

161. Reich SJ, Fosnot J, Kuroki A, et al. Small interfering RNA (siRNA) targeting VEGF effectively inhibits ocular neovascularization in a mouse model. Mol Vis 2003;9:210–216.

162. Stein P, Svoboda P, Schultz RM. Transgenic RNAi in mouse oocytes: a simple and fast approach to study gene function. Dev Biol 2003;256:187–193.

163. Carmell MA, Zhang L, Conklin DS, et al. Germline transmission of RNAi in mice. Nat Struct Biol 2003;10:91–92.

164. Garber K. Better blocker: RNA interference dazzles research community. J Natl Cancer Inst 2003;95:500–502.

165. Guo J, Verna UN, Gaynor RB et al. Enhanced chemosensitivity to Irinotecan by RNA interference mediated down-regulation of the NF-κB p65 subunit. Clin Cancer Res (in press).

166. Mohmmed A, Dasaradhi PV, Bhatnagar RK et al. In vivo gene silencing in *Plasmodium berghei*—a mouse malaria model. Biochem Biophys Res Commun 2003;309:506–511.

Chapter 2

Microarray Analysis of Sarcomas

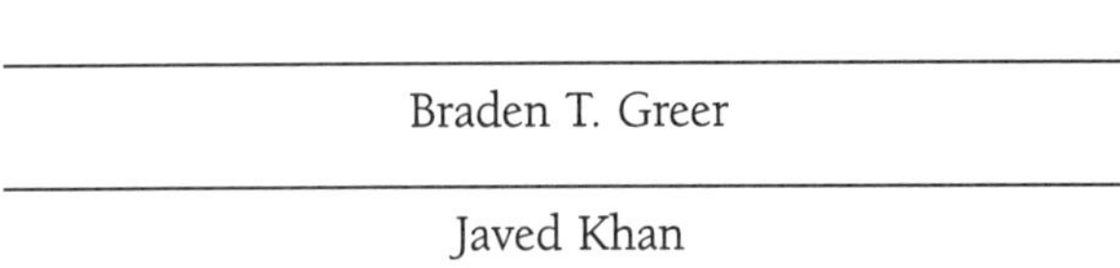

Braden T. Greer

Javed Khan

Sarcomas are highly malignant connective tissue neoplasms that are derived from mesodermal cells. They encompass a wide variety of tumors of disparate tissues of origin and include those that arise from bone, muscle, blood vessel, cartilage, and well over 100 different types have been described (Table 2.1). Sarcomas demonstrate a diversity of biological behavior, response to therapy and the presence of specific molecular features such as translocations. Classification systems have been difficult for pathologists due in part to the rarity of the tumors as well as lack of a full understanding of the process that confers the malignant properties to these tumors. Genetically, sarcomas can be divided into two broad categories. The first are those that contain specific translocations that involve genes that play a role in the development of the tissue of origin of that tumor and are akin to those found in many lymphoma/leukemias (Table 2.2). The fusion chimeric genes are hypothesized to contribute to or initiate the malignant process, although definitive proof for this in the majority of sarcomas has been lacking. These sarcomas have relatively simple karyotypes. The other category of sarcomas tend to show genomic instability and have complex karyotypes.

Currently, clinical management of soft tissue sarcomas is based on the tumor grade, which is utilized in many of the major tumor staging systems. The best

TABLE 2.1 Major Histological Categories of Sarcomas

Fibrous & Myofibroblastic
Fibrohistocytic
Lipomatous
Smooth Muscle
Skeletal Muscle
Vascular
Perivascular
Synovial
Neural
Osseous and cartilaginous
Miscellaneous

grading system include those of the National Cancer Institute (NCI)[1] and the French Sarcoma Group,[2] and are based on differentiation, mitotic rate and necrosis. Even so, this type of grading is extremely subjective. Unfortunately, more quantitative measurements of grade such as proliferation index, DNA flow cytometry, p53 status, etc., have not produced reliable and reproducible results and, thus, have not demonstrated improvement over conventional morphological assessment. Hence, these sarcomas are currently diagnosed and graded by histological features, morphology, and expression of certain proteins as detected by immunohistochemistry. Additionally, specific translocations (Table 2.2) as detected by reverse transcription-polymerase chain reaction (RT-PCR) or fluorescence in situ hybridization (FISH) are currently used as diagnostic markers.

In principle, the biological behaviors and underlying genomic or genetic alterations are ultimately reflected by the patterns of gene expression within each cancer. Therefore, the DNA microarray technology that allows the parallel expression analysis of tens of thousands of genes simultaneously offers a potential method for developing a more precise taxonomy of sarcomas and may overcome the lack of diagnostic rigor, for many of these sarcomas, and potentially enable prognostic prediction that could be used to guide therapy.

GENE EXPRESSION PROFILING OF SARCOMAS

We initially investigated if cancers of a specific diagnostic category had a gene expression signature specific for that cancer using alveolar rhabdomyosarcoma (ARMS) as a model because these tumors are known to be relatively uniform genetically.[3] At that time it was unclear as to whether the intrinsic genomic instability of tumors would lead to such extensive random fluctuations in global gene expression that identifying a unique signature would be difficult or impossible.

TABLE 2.2 Diagnostic Specific Translocations in Sarcomas

Sarcoma	Translocation	Fusion Genes
Alveolar rhabdomyosarcoma	t(2;13)(q35;q14) t(1;13)(p36;q14)	*PAX3-FOXO1A* *PAX7- FOXO1A*
Alveolar soft-part sarcoma	t(X;17)(p11.2;q25)	*ASPL-TFE3*
Clear-cell sarcoma (malignant melanoma of soft parts)	t(12;22)(q13;q12)	*ATF1-EWS*
Congenital fibrosarcoma and mesoblastic nephroma	t(12;15)(p13;q25)	*ETV6-NTRK3*
Dermatofibrosarcoma protuberans and giant-cell fibroblastoma	t(17;22)(q22;q13)	*COL1A1-PDGFB*
Desmoplastic round-cell tumor	t(11;22)(p13;q12)	*WT1-EWS*
Endometrial stromal sarcoma	t(7;17)(p15;q21)	*JAZF1-JJAZ1*
Ewing sarcoma and peripheral primitive neuroectodermal tumors	t(11;22)(q24;q12) t(21;22)(q22;q12) t(7;22)(p22;q12) t(17;22)(q12;q12) t(2;22)(q33;q12)	*EWS-FLI1* *EWS-ERG* *EWS-ETV1* *EWS-E1AF* *FEV-EWS*
Inflammatory myofibroblastic tumor	t(2;19)(p23;p13.1) t(1;2)(q22-23;p23)	*ALK-TPM4* *TPM3-ALK*
Myxoid chondrosarcoma, extraskeletal	t(9;22)(q22;q12) t(9;17)(q22;q11) t(9;15)(q22;q21)	*EWS-CHN(TEC)* *RBP56-CHN(TEC)* *TEC-TCF12*
Myxoid liposarcoma	t(12;16)(q13;p11) t(12;22)(q13;q12)	*TLS(FUS)-CHOP* *EWS-CHOP*
Synovial sarcoma	t(X;18)(p11;q11) t(X;18)(p11;q11) t(X;18)(p11;q11)	*SYT-SSX1* *SYT-SSX2* *SYT-SSX4*

Sixty percent of ARMS tumors have a translocation t(2;13)(q35;q14), resulting in fusion of the 5′ end of the *PAX3* gene with the 3′ end of *FOXO1A* to produce a novel fusion transcription factor, PAX3-FOXO1A.[4]

By using simple Pearson's correlation analysis (Fig. 2.1A) it became apparent that ARMS cell lines exhibited expression profiles that are more similar to ARMS than non-ARMS. The similarity in the gene expression pattern for all the cell lines in this study can be visualized by the tendency of points to fall near the diagonal and quantified by the Pearson correlation coefficient (Fig. 2.1A). Next, we used the Pearson correlation coefficients to perform a multidimensional scaling (MDS)

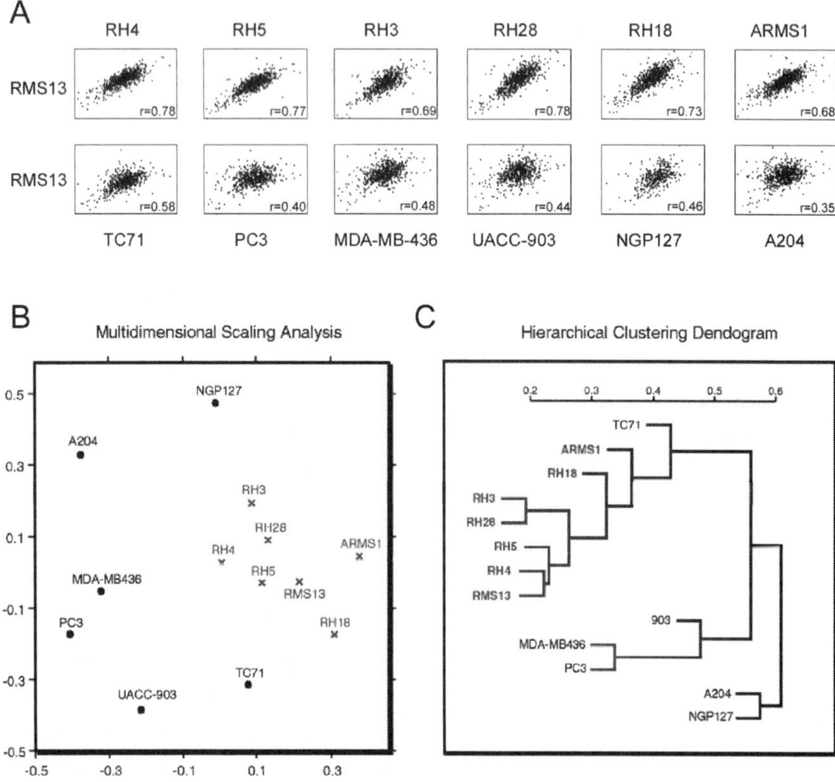

FIGURE 2.1 Statistical analysis of all genes on array filtered for green and red intensities of ⩾2000 fluorescence units. (A) Twelve representational scatter plots of rhabdomyosarcoma-13 (RMS13) versus the six other alveolar rhabdomyosarcoma (ARMS) and six non-ARMS cell lines. Each scatter plot shows the values of the $\log_{10}$ (tumor/control) ratio values filtered for intensities of >2000 fluorescence unit for both control (green) and tumor (red) channels for each pair of experiments. The Pearson rank correlation coefficient of each pair is indicated. (B) Positions of the cell lines in two-dimensional Euclidean distances were determined using the method of multidimensional scaling to make the distance between cell lines correspond as closely as possible to 1 minus the Pearson correlation coefficient of the log ratio values. The x and y scales are arbitrary. Cell lines falling close to one another in the plot had high correlation values. Using this method, we found that the ARMS cell lines cluster together and the non-ARMS tumors fall at the periphery of the plot. (C) The hierarchical clustering dendrogram indicates the order in which the 13 cell lines were combined to form clusters. The calculation of the dendrogram uses 1 minus the Pearson correlation coefficient of log ratios as the dissimilarity measure. The scale represents the distance between merged clusters, and cell lines that were most similar were combined first. Using this method, we found that the seven ARMS cell lines again clustered together. Figure adapted from Khan et al.[3]

analysis, which represents the relationships among all cell lines. The coordinates for each cell line are calculated such that the distances between points reflect the Pearson correlations of the logarithms of expression ratios between the cell lines. Through MDS we observed the non-ARMS tumors at the periphery of the plot, with the ARMS tumors falling in a defined cluster (Fig. 2.1B). This result also can be displayed as a hierarchical clustering dendrogram inferred from the MDS (Fig. 2.1C). Although the microarrays used in this study contain only a small sample of the genome, evidence of a pattern common to ARMS is clearly apparent. Additionally, we found that one of the genes that was highly expressed in ARMS was *FOXO1A*, which was noteworthy in that the probe that detected this gene (3-prime end of the *FOXO1A* gene) also will detect the *PAX3-FOXO1A*; hence, one can speculate that this translocation could have been discovered, had it not been already, as a result of DNA microarray experiments since there would have been clues as to the involvement of *FOXO1A* in ARMS.

We then asked if it was possible to identify gene expression signatures for cancers of more than two diagnostic categories and whether these signatures can be used to diagnose unknown cancers. We used the small round blue cell tumors (SRBCT) as a model.[5] The SRBCTs of childhood, which include neuroblastoma (NB), rhabdomyosarcoma (RMS), non-Hodgkin's lymphoma (NHL), and the Ewing's family of tumors (EWS), are so named because of their similar appearance on routine histology.[6] However, accurate diagnosis of the SRBCT is essential, because the treatment options, response to therapy, and prognosis vary widely depending on the diagnosis. As their name implies, these cancers are difficult to distinguish by light microscopy, and currently no single test can precisely distinguish these cancers. In clinical practice, several techniques are utilized for diagnosis, including immunohistochemistry,[7] cytogenetics, interphase FISH,[8] and RT-PCR.[9] Immunohistochemistry allows the detection of protein expression, but it can only examine a single protein at a time. For instance, Ewing's sarcoma is diagnosed by evidence of MIC2 expression[10] and lack of expression of the leukocyte common antigen CD45 (excluding lymphoma), muscle specific actin, or myogenin (excluding RMS).[11] However, reliance on detection of MIC2 alone can lead to incorrect diagnosis as MIC2 expression does occur occasionally in other tumor types including RMS and NHL.[6] Molecular techniques such as RT-PCR are used increasingly for diagnostic confirmation following the discovery of tumor specific translocations such as *EWS-FLI1*; t(11;22)(q24;q12) in EWS, and the *PAX3-FKHR*; t(2;13)(q35;q14) in alveolar rhabdomyosarcoma (ARMS), and can be utilized for many of the sarcomas listed in Table 2.2. However, molecular markers do not always provide a definitive diagnosis, as on occasion there is failure to detect the classical translocations, either due to technical difficulties or the presence of variant translocations.

We speculated that artificial neural networks (ANNs) could provide an excellent solution to this diagnosis/classification problem. ANNs are computer-based algorithms, modeled on the structure and behavior of neurons in the human brain, which can be trained to recognize and categorize complex patterns.[12] Pattern recognition is achieved by adjusting parameters of the ANN by a process of error minimization through learning from experience. They can be calibrated using any type of input data, such as gene expression levels generated by DNA microarrays, and the output can be grouped into any given number of categories. ANNs have been applied recently to clinical problems such as diagnosing myocardial infarcts[13] and arrhythmias from electrocardiograms,[14] and for interpreting radiographs and magnetic resonance images.[15] We calibrated ANN models (Fig. 2.2A) on the expression profiles of a training set of 63 SRBCTs across four diagnostic categories. A potential difficulty with ANN-based pattern recognition models is the ability to elucidate causal links from the output to the original input data. To solve this problem and to identify the most significant genes, we calculated the sensitivity of the classification to a change in the expression level of each gene. This generated a list of genes, which were ranked by their significance to the classification. Using this list, we established for our samples that the top 96 genes reduced the number of misclassifications to zero (Fig. 2.2C), thus opening the potential for cost effective fabrication of SRBCT subarrays for diagnostic use. When we tested the ANN models calibrated using the 96 genes on 25 blinded samples, all 20 samples of SRBCT were classified correctly and the five non-SRBCT samples were rejected (Fig. 2.3). These results were visualized using multidimensional scaling and hierarchical clustering (Fig. 2.4). This supports the potential use of these methods in future clinical practice as an adjunct to routine histological diagnosis.

As expected, our method identified genes related to tumor histogenesis, but included genes that may not normally be expressed in the corresponding mature tissue. Of the 14 genes that have not previously been reported to be highly expressed in EWS, four (*TUBB5, ANXA1, NOE1* and *GSTM5*) were neural specific genes, lending more credence to the proposed neural histogenesis of EWS. Twenty genes were highly expressed only in RMS, including eight specific for muscle tissue and five (*FGFR4*, *IGF2*, *MYL4*, *ITGA7*, and *IGFBP5*) related to myogenesis. Among the latter, *IGF2*, *MYL4* and *IGFBP5* expression has been reported in RMS, and only *ITGA7* and *IGFBP5* were found to be expressed in our two normal muscle samples. Of the genes specifically expressed in a cancer type, 41 had not been previously reported, including seven ESTs with no current known function. All of these warrant further study and may provide new insights into the biology of these cancers. For example, *FGFR4*, a tyrosine kinase receptor that is expressed during myogenesis and prevents terminal differentiation in myocytes, was found to be highly expressed only in RMS and not in normal muscle. The relatively strong differential expression of *FGFR4* in RMS was confirmed by immunostaining of tissue microarrays. Although the high expression of *FGFR4* in most cases of RMS suggests that it may be relevant to the biology of this tumor, it also is expressed in some other cancers and normal tissues. This

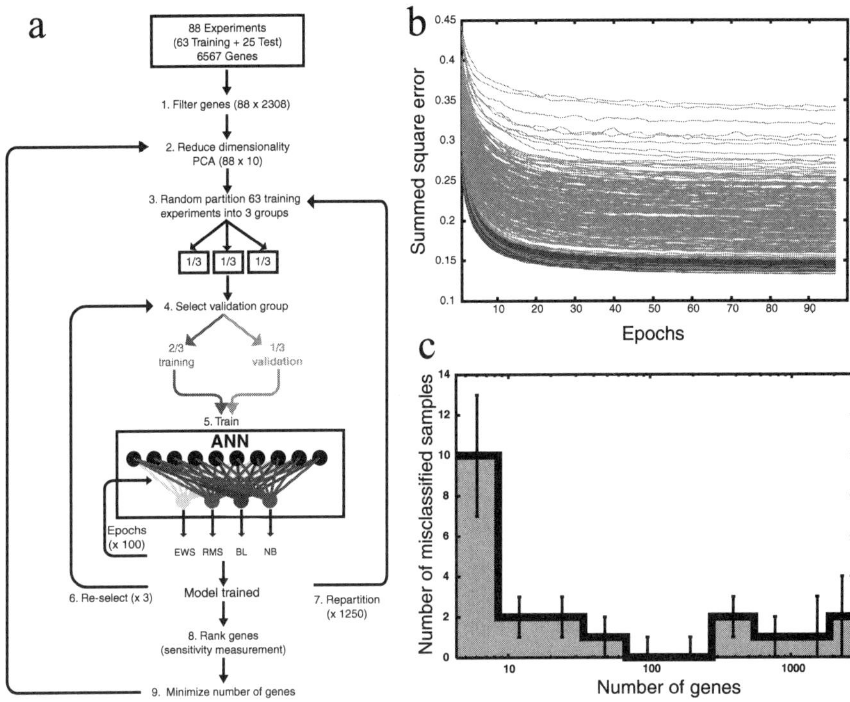

FIGURE 2.2 (A) Artificial neural network workflow diagram. The 88 experiments were quality filtered (1) and the dimension of the dataset further reduced from 2308 to 10 by principal components analysis (PCA) (2). Next, the 63 training samples were randomly partitioned into three groups (3) and one of the three groups was selected for validation (4). The network was trained for 100 epochs using the two remaining groups (5). The samples in the validation group were tested and a different group was selected for validation (6). This process (steps 4 to 6) was repeated until each group was used for validation exactly one time. Then the data were repartitioned into three new random groups (3) and steps 4 to 6 repeated again. In total, the data were repartitioned 1250 times, thus generating 3750 trained models. After this procedure, the genes were ranked using the sensitivity measurement (8), and increasing numbers of the top ranking genes were used for training (steps 2 to 6); the gene set that produced the minimal number of errors (9) was used to calibrate the computer-based algorithms (ANNs) for testing the 25 blinded samples. (B) Training error results from step 5 of panel A. A plot of the classification error with increasing training epochs. The light gray lines represent the error of the validation samples and the darker lines represent the classification error of the training samples. The consistent decrease in error over increasing epochs implies that over fitting of the data did not occur. (C) Gene minimization results from step 9 of panel A. This is a plot of the average number of misclassifications when increasing numbers of genes were used. The number of misclassifications minimized at 96 and 192 genes. The top ranking 96 genes were used to calibrate the neural networks for subsequent training and testing of the 25 blinded test samples. Figure adapted from Khan et al.[5]

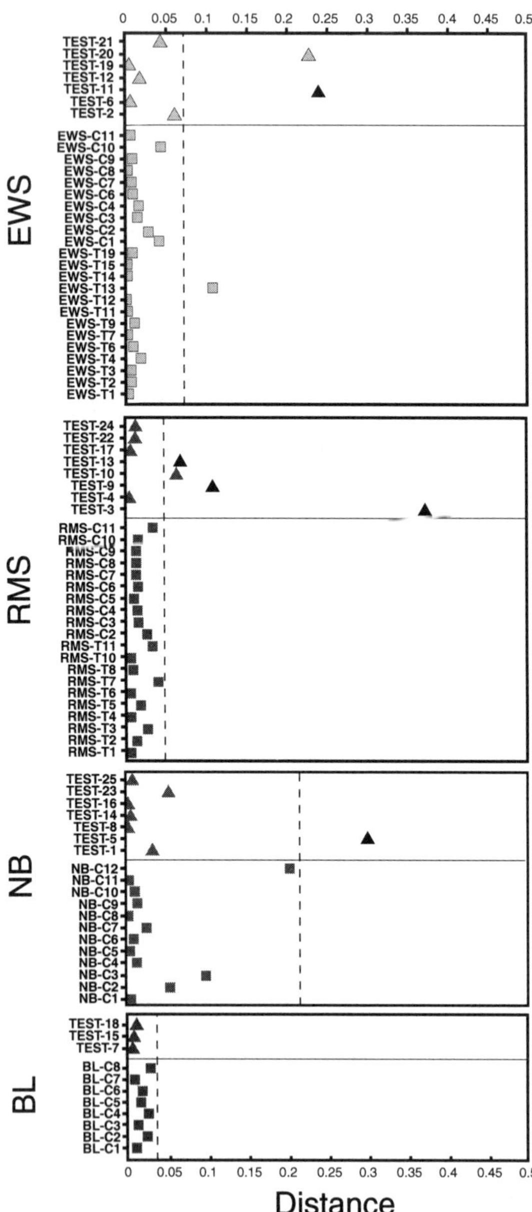

FIGURE 2.3 Classification and diagnosis of the small round blue cell tumor (SRBCT) samples. The x-axis is the Euclidean distance between an ideal computer-based algorithm (ANN) output vote and the observed average vote. The vertical dotted line represents the empirical 95 percentile boundary beyond which diagnosis is not confident. Testing samples are represented by triangles, and training samples are shown as squares. Black triangles are the non-SRBCT samples not associated with any of the diagnostic categories. Two testing samples are correctly diagnosed but lie outside the 95 percentile boundary (Test20-EWS; and Test10-RMS). Only one training sample (EWS-T13) lies outside the 95 percentile boundary. All five non-SRBCT samples lie outside the 95 percentile boundary as they should. Figure adapted from Khan et al.[5]

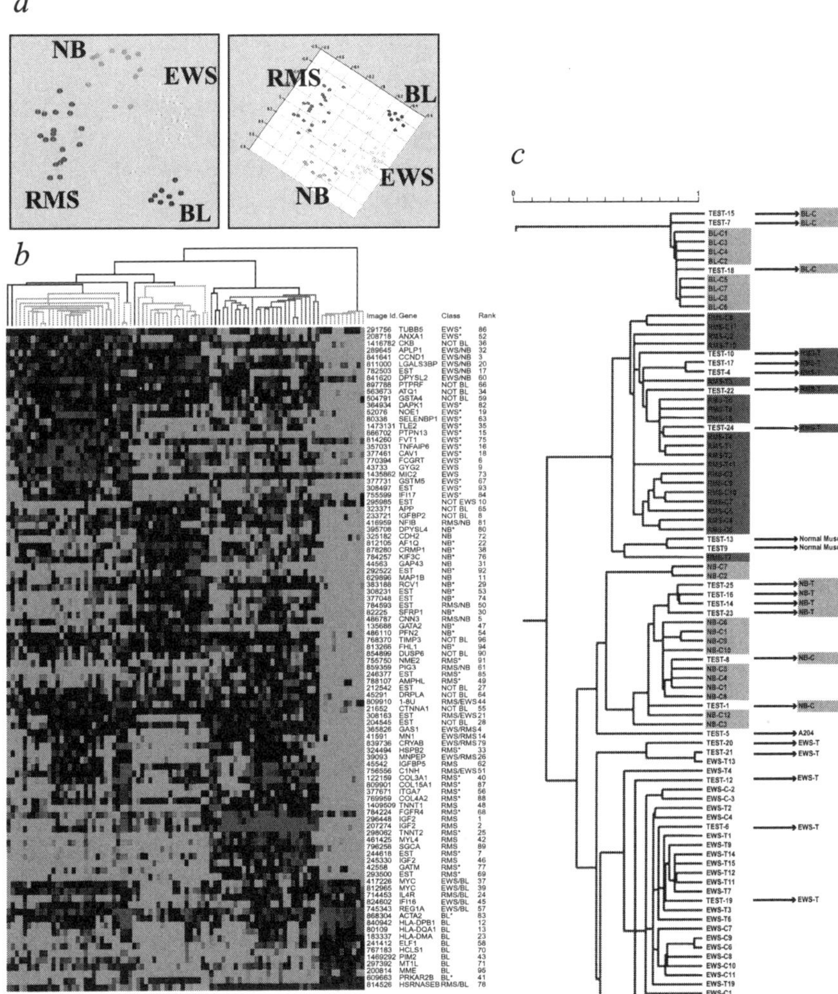

FIGURE 2.4 Multidimensional scaling analysis (MDS) and hierarchical clustering using the top 96 discriminating genes. (A) Two views of the multidimensional scaling results depicting the difference in gene expression of the four SRBCT classes. (B) Hierarchical clustering and heatmap of genes and samples with dendrogram colored according to clinical diagnosis. (C) Enlargement of the sample dendrogram in panel B. All 63 training samples were correctly clustered within their diagnostic categories. Figure adapted from Khan et al.[5] (See p.1 of color insert.)

suggests that, while *FGFR4* expression in RMS may be of biological and therapeutic interest, it is unlikely to be applicable as a sole differential diagnostic marker for these tumors.

Since this study, several gene expression profiling studies have been reported in other sarcomas including studies profiling synovial sarcomas (SS).[16,17] Nagayama et al reported on the expression profiles of 13 SS cases and 34 other spindle-cell sarcomas.[17] Hierarchical clustering analysis grouped SS and malignant peripheral nerve sheath tumors into the same category, and these two types of tumors shared expression patterns of numerous genes relating to neural differentiation. Several genes were up-regulated in almost all SS cases, and the presumed functions of known genes among them were related to migration or differentiation of neural crest cells, suggesting the possibility of neuroectodermal origin of SS. Moreover, they were able to divide SS cases into two putative subclasses.

Fritz et al[18] profiled 16 dedifferentiated and pleomorphic liposarcomas by comparative genomic hybridization (CGH) to genomic microarrays (Matrix-CGH), cDNA-derived microarrays for expression profiling, and by quantitative PCR. They discovered that Matrix-CGH revealed copy number gains of numerous oncogenes (e.g., *CCND1, MDM2, GLI, CDK4, MYB, ESR1,* and *AIB1*), several of which correlate with high levels of transcript from the respective gene. In addition, a number of genes were found differentially expressed in dedifferentiated and pleomorphic liposarcomas. They concluded that, for the distinction of these types of liposarcomas, genomic profiling appears to be more advantageous than RNA expression analysis.

Nielsen et al[19] performed DNA microarray analysis on a series of 41 soft-tissue tumors to identify new diagnostic markers. They found that synovial sarcomas, gastrointestinal stromal tumors (GIST), neural tumors, and a subset of the leiomyosarcomas, showed distinct gene-expression patterns (Fig. 2.5). In contrast, other tumor categories, that is, malignant fibrous histiocytoma, liposarcoma, and the remaining leiomyosarcomas, shared molecular profiles that were not predicted by histological features or immunohistochemistry. Of special note is that both Nielsen et al and Allander et al[20] (who also profiled GIST) identified *KIT*, known to be mutated in GIST, as one of the most highly expressed genes in this tumor. There were several gene sets that distinguished the different sarcomas, raising the intriguing possibility that several of the "top" differentially expressed genes may harbor dominantly acting mutations and be involved in the etiology of these cancers. However, many uncharacterized genes also contributed to the distinction between the tumor types. Since large numbers of uncharacterized genes contributed to distinctions between the tumors, some of these could be useful markers for diagnosis, have prognostic significance, or prove possible targets for treatment.

Sjorgren et al[21] profiled extraskeletal myxoid chondrosarcomas (EMCs), which are characterized by recurrent chromosome translocations resulting in fusions of the nuclear receptor TEC to various NH(2)-terminal partners. cDNA mi-

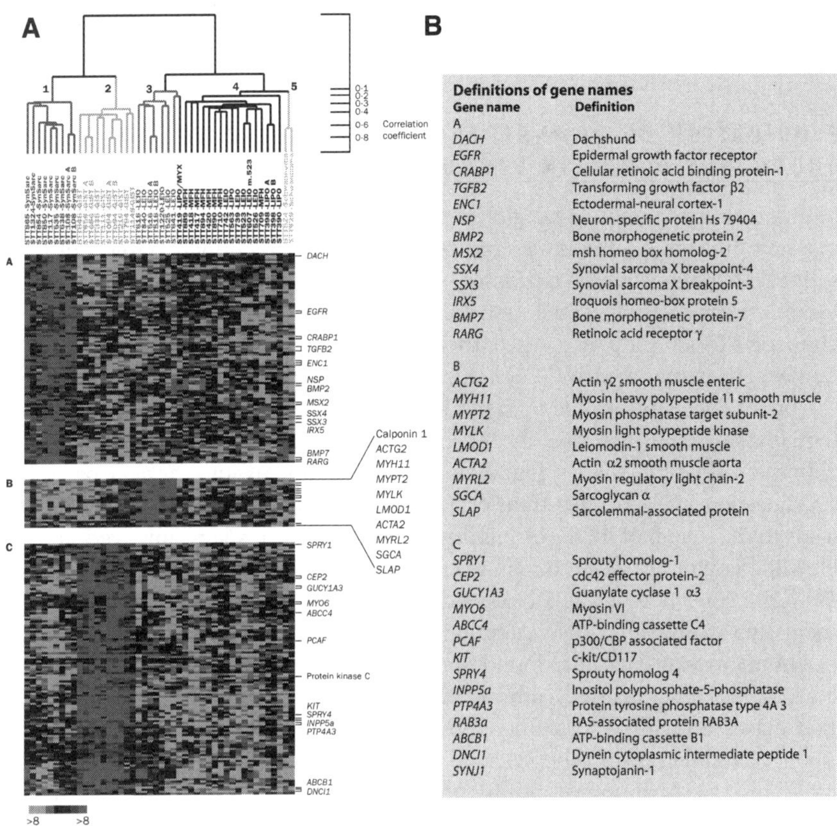

Definitions of gene names

Gene name	Definition
A	
DACH	Dachshund
EGFR	Epidermal growth factor receptor
CRABP1	Cellular retinoic acid binding protein-1
TGFB2	Transforming growth factor β2
ENC1	Ectodermal-neural cortex-1
NSP	Neuron-specific protein Hs 79404
BMP2	Bone morphogenetic protein 2
MSX2	msh homeo box homolog-2
SSX4	Synovial sarcoma X breakpoint-4
SSX3	Synovial sarcoma X breakpoint-3
IRX5	Iroquois homeo-box protein 5
BMP7	Bone morphogenetic protein-7
RARG	Retinoic acid receptor γ
B	
ACTG2	Actin γ2 smooth muscle enteric
MYH11	Myosin heavy polypeptide 11 smooth muscle
MYPT2	Myosin phosphatase target subunit-2
MYLK	Myosin light polypeptide kinase
LMOD1	Leiomodin-1 smooth muscle
ACTA2	Actin α2 smooth muscle aorta
MYRL2	Myosin regulatory light chain-2
SGCA	Sarcoglycan α
SLAP	Sarcolemmal-associated protein
C	
SPRY1	Sprouty homolog-1
CEP2	cdc42 effector protein-2
GUCY1A3	Guanylate cyclase 1 α3
MYO6	Myosin VI
ABCC4	ATP-binding cassette C4
PCAF	p300/CBP associated factor
KIT	c-kit/CD117
SPRY4	Sprouty homolog 4
INPP5a	Inositol polyphosphate-5-phosphatase
PTP4A3	Protein tyrosine phosphatase type 4A 3
RAB3a	RAS-associated protein RAB3A
ABCB1	ATP-binding cassette B1
DNCI1	Dynein cytoplasmic intermediate peptide 1
SYNJ1	Synaptojanin-1

FIGURE 2.5 Clustering and differential gene expression of synovial sarcoma (sample cluster 1, genes A), leimyosarcoma (sample cluster 3, genes B) and GIST (sample cluster 3, genes C). Figure adapted from Nielson et al.[19] (See p. 2 of color insert.)

croarray analysis of the gene expression patterns of two EMCs and a myxoid liposarcoma reference tumor revealed a remarkably distinct and uniform expression profile in both EMCs despite the fact that they had different histologies and expressed different fusion transcripts. The most differentially expressed gene in both tumors was *CHI3L1*, which encodes a secreted glycoprotein (YKL-40) previously implicated in various pathological conditions of extracellular matrix degradation as well as in cancer. These findings suggest that EMC exhibits a tumor-specific gene expression profile, including overexpression of several cancer-related genes as well as genes implicated in chondrogenesis and neural-neuroendocrine differentiation, thus distinguishing it from other soft tissue sarcomas.

ELUCIDATION OF DOWNSTREAM TARGETS OF CHIMERIC FUSION ONCOGENES FOUND IN SARCOMAS

Monitoring the temporal and global changes in gene expression using DNA microarray profiling methods also has been effective in identifying targets of transcription factors (TFs). An example is the investigation of the molecular effects of tumor specific chromosome translocations that encode chimeric TFs. These chimeric TFs are thought to exert their oncogenic effects through the dysregulation of gene expression, and DNA microarrays provide an opportunity to observe the broad effects of oncogenic transcription factors on gene expression and potentially elucidate their role in oncogenesis. An example is the *PAX3-FOXO1A* chimeric oncogene that is found in the ARMS, and results from a particular translocation, t(2;13). This translocation is found in the majority of ARMS, and leads to the fusion of the DNA binding domain of *PAX3*, a gene involved in muscle differentiation, with the transactivation domain of *FOXO1A*. The *PAX3-FOXO1A* gene retains the DNA binding specificity of *PAX3* and might act by increasing expression of genes containing *PAX3* binding sites. Utilizing murine cDNA microarrays, we have found that the *PAX3-FOXO1A* gene triggers cells into a myogenic differentiation pathway producing a population of rhabdomyoblasts that may eventually lead to the development of fully malignant muscle cancer upon accumulation of other genetic aberrations.[22] Since this report, DNA microarrays have been used to profile the downstream effect of a growing number of oncogenes and tumor suppressor genes.[23–25]

In other sarcomas, Xie et al[26] investigated the downstream targets of *SYT-SSX* using DNA microarrays. They used antisense oligonucleotides to block the expression of the *SYT-SSX* fusion gene in synovial sarcoma cells and compared *SYT-SSX* inhibited cells with cells that were not inhibited. They found that the DNA repair gene *XRCC4* and the DNA mismatch repair gene *MSH2* were down-regulated, whereas the gene encoding for the serine/threonine protein kinase *PRK* (also known as *CNK*), and the macrophage inhibitory cytokine *MICI* (also known as *PLAB*) were up-regulated after the inhibition of *SYT-SSX*. In comparison, expression of the *XRCC4* gene exhibited the strongest alteration. Consistently, the protein expression of *XRCC4* was found to be decreased after *SYT-SSX* inhibition, whereas there were no detectable changes for the other gene products.

Nishimori and colleagues[27] reported the *Id2* (inhibitor of DNA binding 2) gene as a novel target of transcriptional activation by *EWS-FLI1* and *EWS-ERG*, two fusion proteins that characterize the Ewing's family tumors (EFTs). To identify downstream targets of these *EWS-ETS* fusion proteins, they introduced *EWS-ETS* fusion constructs into a human fibrosarcoma cell line by retroviral transduction. cDNA microarray analysis revealed that *Id2* expression was up-regulated by introducing the *EWS-ETS* fusion gene but not by the normal full-length

ETS gene. An *Id2* promoter-luciferase reporter assay showed that transactivation by *EWS-ETS* involves the minimal *Id2* promoter and may function in cooperation with *c-Myc* within the full-length regulatory region. A chromatin immunoprecipitation assay revealed direct interaction between the *Id2* promoter and *EWS-FLI1* fusion protein in vivo. Significantly higher expression of *Id2* and *c-Myc* was observed in all six EFT cell lines examined compared to six other sarcoma cell lines. Moreover, high levels of *Id2* expression were observed also in five of the six primary tumors examined. They concluded that their data suggest that the oncogenic effect of *EWS-ETS* may be mediated in part by up-regulating *Id2* expression.

MICROARRAYS AND METASTATIC GENES IN SARCOMAS

Not only can microarrays be utilized to develop a molecular taxonomy of sarcomas and investigate the downstream effects of fusion oncogenes, they also can be used to investigate the differences between high and low metastatic sarcomas. Khanna and colleagues[28] investigated metastatic osteosarcoma as a model. Despite advances in the management of osteosarcoma (OSA) and other solid tumors, the development of metastases continues to be the most significant problem and cause of death for cancer patients. In an attempt to define genetic determinants of pulmonary metastasis, they applied cDNA microarrays to a recently described murine model of OSA that is characterized by orthotopic tumor growth, a period of minimal residual disease, spontaneous pulmonary metastasis, and cell line variants that differ in metastatic potential. Microarray data analysis identified 53 genes (of 3166 unique cDNAs) that were differentially expressed between the primary tumors of the more aggressive (K7M2) and less aggressive (K12) OSA models. By review of the literature, these differentially expressed genes were assigned to six non-mutually exclusive metastasis-associated categories (proliferation and apoptosis, motility and cytoskeleton, invasion, immune surveillance, adherence, and angiogenesis). Functional studies to evaluate K7M2 and K12 for differences in each of these metastasis-associated processes revealed enhanced motility, adherence, and angiogenesis in the more aggressive K7M2 model. Ten of the 53 differentially expressed genes that were assigned to the motility and cytoskeleton, adherence, and angiogenesis categories were considered as most likely to define differences in the metastatic behavior of the two models. *Ezrin*, a gene not described previously in OSA, with functions in motility, invasion, and adherence, was overexpressed threefold in K7M2 compared with K12 by microarray. The potential relevance of *ezrin* in OSA was suggested by its expression in five of five human OSA cell lines. This work represented a rational approach to the evaluation of microarray data and will be useful to identify genes that may be causally associated with metastasis.

Subsequent to that study, Yu et al[29] investigated the genes involved in the metastatic process. Patients presenting with metastatic rhabdomyosarcoma (RMS), the most common soft-tissue sarcoma in children, continue to have a very poor clinical prognosis due in large part to our rudimentary knowledge of molecular events that dictate metastatic potential. cDNA microarray analysis of primary RMS cell lines derived from hepatocyte growth factor/scatter factor-transgenic, *Ink4a/Arf*-deficient mice identified a signature of genes whose expression was significantly different between highly and poorly metastatic cells (Fig. 3.6). Subsequent in vivo functional studies revealed that the actin filament-plasma membrane crosslinker *ezrin* (as in the work of Khanna et al) and the homeodomain-containing transcription factor *Six1* had essential roles in determining the metastatic fate of RMS cells. Notably, *ezrin* and *Six1* expression levels

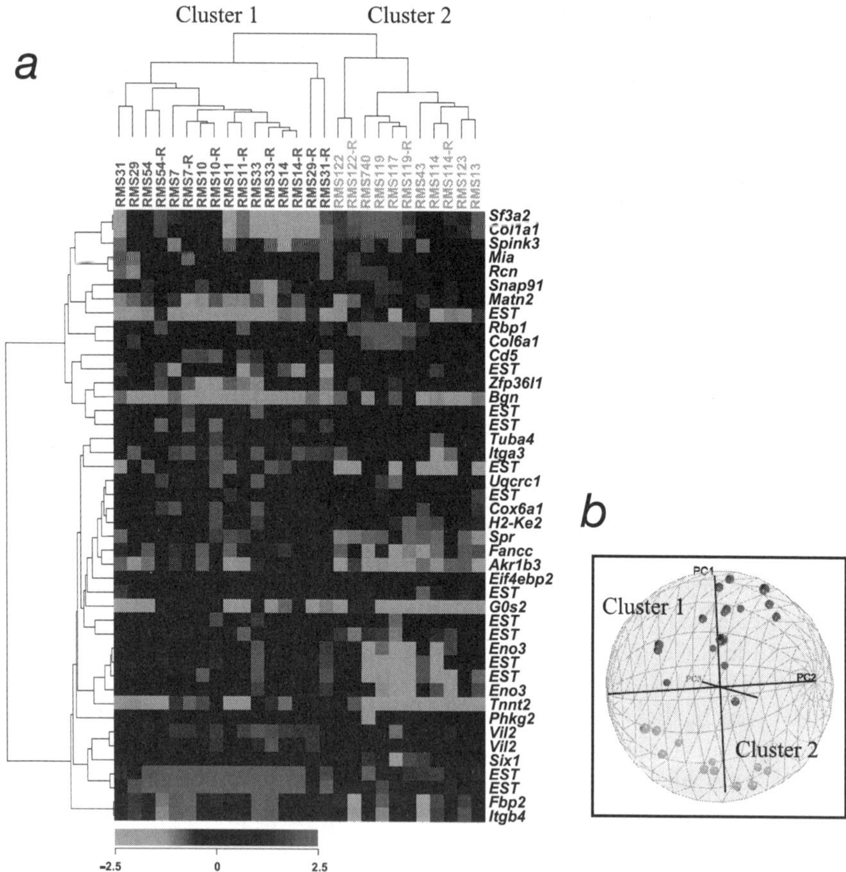

FIGURE 2.6 Utilization of DNA microarrays to identify genes involved in the metastatic process. (A) Hierarchical clustering using the genes that were differentially expressed between highly metastatic (sample cluster 1) and poorly metastatic (sample cluster 2) RMS cell lines. (B) Principal components analysis of the samples and genes from panel A shows that the samples separate widely according to the metastatic potential. Figure adapted from Yu et al.[29] (See p. 3 of color insert.)

were highly correlated with RMS clinical stage. The identification of *ezrin* as a metastatic gene in another cancer, and of *ezrin* and *Six1* as critical regulators of metastasis provides new mechanistic and therapeutic insights into this pediatric cancer.

CONCLUSIONS

1. Sarcomas are a diverse group of relatively rare malignancies that are derived from bone, muscle, cartilage, and other connective tissue and more than 100 different diagnostic types have been described on the basis of standard pathological investigations.
2. Most sarcomas have abnormalities in the RB, *p53*, and/or specific growth-factor signaling pathways.[30] In several sarcoma types, specific genetic alterations lead to activation of specific tyrosine kinase growth-factor receptors, and these have been treated successfully with drugs that selectively inhibit the activated kinase receptor.
3. DNA microarrays are able to identify gene expression profiles for sarcomas and will define a more specific molecular taxonomy of these cancers.
4. Gene expression profiles can detect downstream effects of fusion oncogenes that are expressed as a result of specific translocations. Correlation of gene expression profiles with these specific translocations and other sarcoma-specific mutations will elucidate more precisely the mechanism of tumorigenesis in these cancers.
5. Gene expression profiling has identified genes involved in a more aggressive phenotype, such as genes involved in the metastatic process.
6. However, before we can usher in the golden age of molecular taxonomies using microarrays there are several obstacles that need to be overcome. Firstly, there is a need for standard operating procedures for sample acquisition by most surgeons and pathologists that are in the cutting edge of patient care. A wide variety of artifactual changes can be introduced by differences in sample handling procedures such as delays in freezing to allowing samples to thaw during transport. Secondly, it is important to have "good" clinical information regarding each sample, which is crucial to perform correlative studies. Thirdly, since there is a diversity of platforms in which microarrays are performed (Affymetrix, cDNA, Oligoarrays, Compugen, Operon, Agilent, Amersham/Motorola, etc.), it is difficult for investigators to compare their results with others. Therefore, further research needs to be undertaken such that the results from these platforms can be compared. Additionally, there is a need for standard methodologies for microarray experiments (direct and indirect labeling, amplification, various controls, etc.). As more and more diagnostic or prognostic signature studies are performed and published using small arrays and relatively small numbers of patients, questions remain as to whether these "diagnostic & prognostic" signature genes are the best ones. By the very evolving nature of the data released by the

Human Genome Project, more and more genes are being discovered as well as their splice variants, so that many of the currently utilized microarrays are incomplete. Therefore, are we ready to take these to the clinic to determine therapy? Should we wait for the best set of genes? How do we define the best? What is the best platform to use?

7. Therefore, it is the opinion of the authors that all samples of tumors on treatment protocols should have gene expression profiling performed, using standard operating procedures and standard platforms. Additionally, prospective studies correlating gene expression data with prognosis, chemo- and radiosensitivities are needed. This will require coordinated efforts with central laboratories that perform these microarrays because of the rarity of these tumors.
8. Finally, it is hoped that the diagnostic/prognostic/translocation-specific gene expression signatures identified by microarrays will not only help in the management of these tumors, but also will identify new molecular targets for therapy.

REFERENCES

1. Costa J, Wesley RA, Glatstein E, Rosenberg SA. The grading of soft tissue sarcomas. Results of a clinicohistopathologic correlation in a series of 163 cases. Cancer 1984;53:530–541.
2. Trojani M, Contesso G, Coindre JM, et al. Soft-tissue sarcomas of adults; study of pathological prognostic variables and definition of a histopathological grading system. Int J Cancer 1984;33:37–42.
3. Khan J, Simon R, Bittner M, et al. Gene expression profiling of alveolar rhabdomyosarcoma with cDNA microarrays. Cancer Res 1998; 58:5009–5013.
4. Galili N, Davis RJ, Fredericks WJ, et al. Fusion of a fork head domain gene to PAX3 in the solid tumor alveolar rhabdomyosarcoma. Nat Genet 1993; 5:230–235.
5. Khan J, Wei JS, Ringner M, et al. Classification and diagnostic prediction of cancers using gene expression profiling and artificial neural networks. Nat Med 2001;7:673–679.
6. Triche TJ. Pathology and molecular diagnosis of pediatric malignancies. In Pizzo PA, Poplack DG, eds. Principles and Practice of Pediatric Oncology. Philadelphia, PA: Lippincott-Raven, 1997.
7. Triche TJ, Askin FB. Neuroblastoma and the differential diagnosis of small-, round-, blue- cell tumors. Hum Pathol 1983;14:569–595.
8. Taylor C, Patel K, Jones T, et al. Diagnosis of Ewing's sarcoma and peripheral neuroectodermal tumor based on the detection of t(11;22) using fluorescence in situ hybridisation. Br J Cancer 1993;67:128–133.
9. McManus AP, Gusterson BA, Pinkerton CR, Shipley JM. The molecular pathology of small round-cell tumors—relevance to diagnosis, prognosis, and classification. J Pathol 1996;178: 116–121.
10. Kovar H, Dworzak M, Strehl S, et al. Overexpression of the pseudoautosomal gene MIC2 in Ewing's sarcoma and peripheral primitive neuroectodermal tumor. Oncogene 1990; 5:1067—1070.
11. Kumar S, Perlman E, Harris CA, et al. Myogenin is a specific marker for rhabdomyosarcoma: an immunohistochemical study in paraffin-embedded tissues. Mod Pathol 2000;13:988–993.

12. Bishop CM. Neural Networks for Pattern Recognition. Oxford, UK: Clarendon Press, 1995.

13. Heden B, Ohlin H, Rittner R, Edenbrandt L. Acute myocardial infarction detected in the 12-lead ECG by artificial neural networks. Circulation 1997;96:1798–1802.

14. Silipo R, Gori M, Taddei A, et al. Classification of arrhythmic events in ambulatory electrocardiogram, using artificial neural networks. Comput Biomed Res 1995;28:305–318.

15. Abdolmaleki P, Buadu LD, Murayama S, et al. Neural network analysis of breast cancer from MRI findings. Radiat Med 1997;15:283–293.

16. Allander SV, Illei PB, Chen Y, et al. Expression profiling of synovial sarcoma by cDNA microarrays: association of ERBB2, IGFBP2, and ELF3 with epithelial differentiation. Am J Pathol 2002;161:1587–1595.

17. Nagayama S, Katagiri T, Tsunoda T, et al. Genome-wide analysis of gene expression in synovial sarcomas using a cDNA microarray. Cancer Res 2002;62:5859–5866.

18. Fritz B, Schubert F, Wrobel G, et al. Microarray-based copy number and expression profiling in dedifferentiated and pleomorphic liposarcoma. Cancer Res 2002;62:2993–2998.

19. Nielsen TO, West RB, Linn SC, et al. Molecular characterisation of soft tissue tumors: a gene expression study. Lancet 2002;359:1301–1307.

20. Allander SV, Nupponen NN, Ringner M, et al. Gastrointestinal stromal tumors with KIT mutations exhibit a remarkably homogeneous gene expression profile. Cancer Res 2001;61:8624–8628.

21. Sjogren H, Meis-Kindblom JM, Orndal C, et al. Studies on the molecular pathogenesis of extraskeletal myxoid chondrosarcoma-cytogenetic, molecular genetic, and cDNA microarray analyses. Am J Pathol 2003;162:781–792.

22. Khan J, Bittner ML, Saal LH, et al. cDNA microarrays detect activation of a myogenic transcription program by the PAX3-FKHR fusion oncogene. Proc Natl Acad Sci USA 1999;96: 13264–13269.

23. O'Hagan RC, Schreiber-Agus N, Chen K, et al. Gene-target recognition among members of the myc superfamily and implications for oncogenesis. Nat Genet 2000;24:113–119.

24. Ren B, Cam H, Takahashi Y, et al. E2F integrates cell cycle progression with DNA repair, replication, and G(2)/M checkpoints. Genes Dev 2002;16:245–256.

25. Dorsam ST, Ferrell CM, Dorsam GP, et al. The transcriptome of the leukemogenic homeoprotein HOXA9 in human hematopoietic cells. Blood 2004;103:1674–1684.

26. Xie Y, Tornkvist M, Aalto Y, et al. Gene expression profile by blocking the SYT-SSX fusion gene in synovial sarcoma cells. Identification of XRCC4 as a putative SYT-SSX target gene. Oncogene 2003;22:7628–7631.

27. Nishimori H, Sasaki Y, Yoshida K, et al. The Id2 gene is a novel target of transcriptional activation by EWS-ETS fusion proteins in Ewing family tumors. Oncogene 2002;21:8302–8309.

28. Khanna C, Khan J, Nguyen P, et al. Metastasis-associated differences in gene expression in a murine model of osteosarcoma. Cancer Res 2001;61:3750–3759.

29. Yu Y, Khan J, Khanna C, et al. Expression profiling identifies the cytoskeletal organizer Ezrin and the developmental homeoprotein Six1 as key metastatic regulators. Nat Med 2004;10: 175–181.

30. Helman LJ, Meltzer P. Mechanisms of sarcoma development. Nat Rev Cancer 2003;3:685–694.

Chapter 3

ErbB/HER Family of Growth Factor Receptors

Noa Ben-Baruch

Yosef Yarden

Fifty years ago, Rita Levy-Montalcini and Stanley Cohen discovered the first growth factors, namely, the nerve growth factor (NGF) and the epidermal growth factor (EGF), through studies of the sympathetic nervous system of the chick and the salivary gland of the mouse. These discoveries opened the way for understanding how extracellular peptides regulate cellular responses (collectively called signal transduction). The identity and architecture of the plasma membrane receptors for EGF and related polypeptide growth factors have been resolved by Axel Ullrich and co-workers (reviewed[1]), and the multiple signaling pathways they instigate were uncovered through molecular cloning.[2] Almost concurrently, the physiological roles of both the receptors and their ligands were elucidated through genetic manipulation of mice, which led to comprehensive understanding of the physiology of EGF-receptors[3] (see references therein). Cells respond to EGF and related growth factors primarily by accelerating the rate of their division, an observation that attracted the attention of cancer researchers. The importance of auto-stimulatory loops, involving self-produced growth factors (autocrine stimulation) was delineated by George Todaro and Michael Sporn.[4] On the other hand, carcinogen-induced mutations that unleash the oncogenic potential of a rodent molecule related to the EGF-receptor, HER2/Neu, were discovered by Robert Weinberg.[5] Importantly, similar mutations do not exist in the human orthologue, called ErbB-2/HER2, but studies by Denis Slamon and others detected its frequent overexpression in subsets of human carcinomas.[6] Understandably, attempts to pharmacologically inhibit growth factor actions expanded with the emergence of their many links to cancer. Mark Greene demonstrated that monoclonal antibodies to Neu can inhibit tumor growth in rodents,[7] and almost two decades later a humanized antibody, Herceptin/Trastuzumab, has been approved for treatment of Neu/ErbB-2-positive metastasizing breast cancers.[8] Likewise, Alexander Levitzki and coworkers developed low molecular weight kinase inhibitors of ErbB molecules,[9] which led to the recent approval of such a drug, named Iressa/Gefitinib, for the treatment of lung cancer.

The present review highlights the most recent advances in our understanding of ErbB/HER receptors, and their significance to cancer detection and therapy. Following an introduction to the structure and biochemical functions of the ErbB signaling network, we describe several molecular concepts that are currently emerging from basic research laboratories. This will be followed by the current view of the physiological function of the ErbB network, as learned by using genetically manipulated animals. The significance of ErbB proteins and their ligands to cancer development, detection and prognosis will precede a final chapter on the therapeutic implications of ErbB signaling.

THE ErBB SIGNALING NETWORK: NEW CONCEPTS AND OPEN QUESTIONS

Although an EGF-like motif is present in many cell adhesion and other proteins, only eleven known molecules bind to ErbB proteins through an EGF-like motif, which contains six canonical cysteines. These are: EGF, transforming growth factor-α (TGF-α), betacellulin, heparin-binding EGF (HB-EGF), epiregulin, amphiregulin, epigen, and four neuregulins. The ligands are synthesized as transmembrane precursors that undergo cleavage to generate soluble growth factors capable of receptor recognition.[10] The receptors are transmembrane glycoproteins with a large extracellular domain, which contains two cysteine-rich motifs: a single transmembrane domain and a large cytoplasmic portion that harbors an enzymatic tyrosine kinase activity. There are four distinct ErbB molecules. Whereas ErbB-1 (EGFR/HER1), ErbB-3, and ErbB-4 each bind several ligands, ErbB-2 binds no known ligand with high affinity.[11] And unlike ErbB-1, ErbB-2, and ErbB-4, ErbB-3 displays no catalytic activity.[12] Almost invariably, ligand binding to the ectodomain of a receptor tyrosine kinase is followed by activation of the intracellular kinase, which phosphorylates itself as well as a distinct set of signaling molecules. Hence, both the ligand-less ErbB-2 molecule and the kinase-defective ErbB-3 are unable to signal when singly present.

How ErbB-2 and ErbB-3 participate in signaling by EGF-like ligands? Early studies have shown that the kinase function of the monomeric form of ErbB-1 is inactive, but EGF binding promotes receptor dimerization and kinase activation.[13,14] ErbB-2 emerged as the preferred partner of the ligand-occupied ErbB molecules (heterodimerization),[15,16] which explains why its presence enhances signaling by all EGF-like growth factors. Similarly, when ErbB-3 is recruited into heterodimers containing an active kinase it can enhance signaling. These observations established the notion that signaling by EGF-like ligands is funneled through a layered signaling network consisting of eleven ligands and eight homo- and heterodimeric receptor complexes. The latter engage distinct sets of enzymes, or adaptor molecules, to their autophosphorylated tyrosine residues.[17] Most adaptors recruit enzymes, either protein kinases, phosphatases, lipases, or guanosine 5′-triphosphate (GTP)-exchange proteins, which initiate a pleiotropic response (Fig. 3.1). Besides activation of small GTP-binding proteins like Ras and

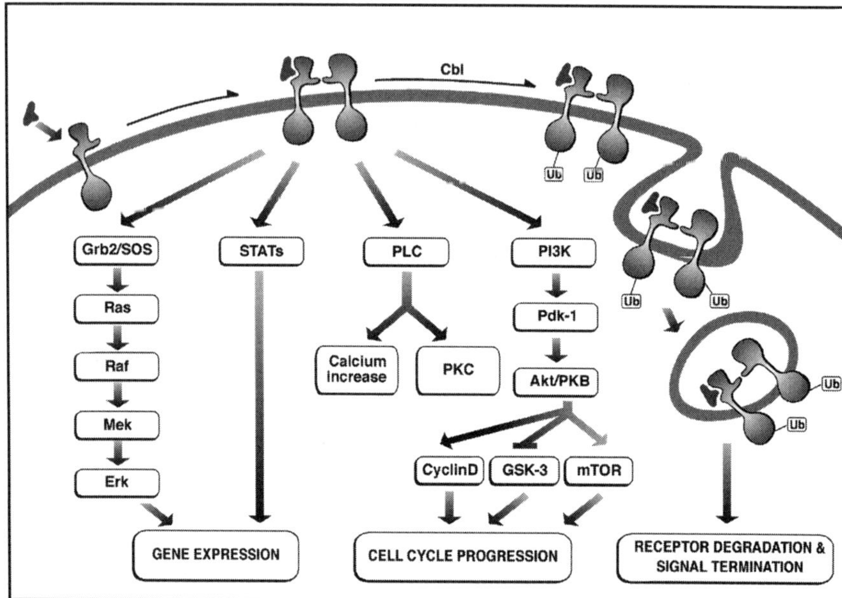

FIGURE 3.1 Signaling pathways activated by ErbB proteins. Ligand binding to an ErbB protein is followed by rapid receptor dimerization and autophosphorylation. Tyrosine-phosphorylated receptor's residues recruit signaling molecules, which initiate linear cascades such as the Ras/Erk and the PI3K/PKB pathways. Similarly, STAT proteins are phosphorylated and translocated to the nucleus to regulate gene expression, and activation of phospholipase C (PLC) instigates activation of protein kinase C (PKC) as well as an increase in intracellular calcium ion concentrations. Several other pathways are not represented. Ligand-induced c-Cbl mediated, ubiquitylation of active receptors are the major processes that terminate signaling. Ubiquitin- (Ub-) decorated receptors are sorted for internalization through clathrin-coated pits of the plasma membrane, and this is followed by further sorting at the level of the multivesicular endocytic compartment. The final fate of internalized receptors is degradation in the lysosome, but a recycling pathway allows escape and repeated engagement in signaling pathways.

Rho, ErbB signals are mediated by several linear kinase cascades, primarily the Erk pathway and the Akt/PKB route, to enable cell division and escape from apoptosis.

Mechanism of Ligand-induced Receptor Dimerization

The extracellular domain of ErbB-1 comprises four sub-domains. Domains II and VI (also called CR1 and CR2) are cysteine-rich, whereas domains I and III are cysteine-free and directly interact with the ligand.[18] Earlier studies demonstrated that EGF forms a 2:2 complex with the soluble receptor's ectodomain.[19] Although it was shown that another ligand, NRG-1, recognizes ErbB-3 through two sites located at both ends of the growth factor molecule,[20] the exact mechanism that couples ligand binding to receptor dimerization remained unknown because no ErbB molecule could be crystallized until very recently. The three-dimensional structures of unactivated ErbB-1[21] and ErbB-3,[22] as well as of the activated form of ErbB-1,[23,24] resolved a surprisingly complex mode of receptor activation (Fig. 3.2). Accordingly, the unactivated state of ErbB proteins is auto-inhibited because domains II and IV are held together by several hydrogen bonds. Conceivably, ligand binding to domain I induces a domain rearrangement that relieves a tethered portion of domain II (termed the "dimerization arm"), which is responsible for the majority of receptor-receptor interactions in the dimer. Within the dimer

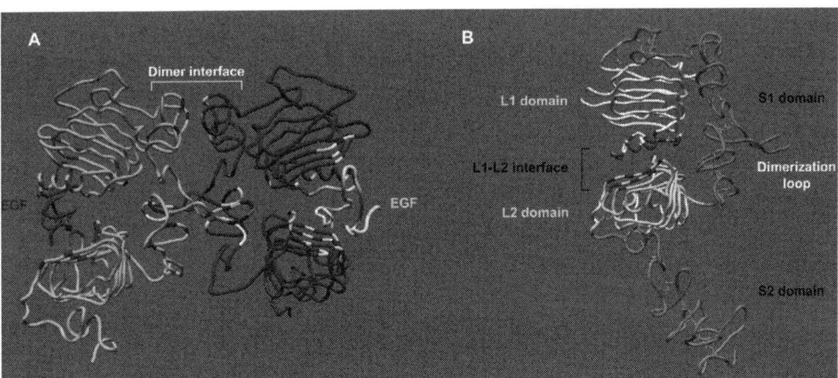

FIGURE 3.2 Three-dimensional structures of ErbB proteins. (**A**) A dimer of the extracellular domain of ErbB-1 is shown in a complex with EGF. Note the 'back-to-back' orientation of the receptors, bivalent ligand binding to the L1 and L2 sub-domains, and the large dimer interface. (**B**) A monomeric ErbB-2 (extracellular domain) is shown and the four sub-domains indicated. Note that in analogy to ErbB-1, the structure of ErbB-2 leaves no space for EGF binding, but the S1 sub-domain is pre-extended. Gaps in the S1 and L1 domains indicate unknown folding. The L1-L2 interface is indicated, as are intramolecular cyesteine bridges.

each ligand bivalently binds to a single receptor (through domains I and III), and the receptors are oriented in a "back-to-back" orientation, stabilized by intercalation of each dimerization arm into the other receptor. Because bivalent binding of a ligand to domains I and III entails disruption of domain II/IV interactions and dramatic intramolecular movements, it is likely that the ligand binds to a small population of performed receptor dimers. Evidence for preformed inactive dimers has been reported.[25]

Determining the structure of the extracellular domain of ErbB-2 raised additional questions but also solved important issues. Several lines of evidence led to the proposition that no EGF-like ligand can bind to ErbB-2 with high affinity.[11] Instead, by forming heterodimers with ErbB-1, ErbB-3 and ErbB-4, ErbB-2 can enhance and prolong signal transduction.[26] The recently resolved structure of the ectodomain of ErbB-2 supports this prediction.[27,28] ErbB-2 folds into a structure similar to the structure of a ligand-bound ErbB-1: unlike the unactivated structures of ErbB-1 and ErbB-3, domains I and III of ErbB-2 are juxtaposed and the dimerization arm is already extended (Fig. 3.2). Hence, even in the absence of a stimulatory ligand ErbB-2 exists in an active conformation, poised to interact with other ErbB receptors. Two additional features revealed by the crystals of ErbB-2 are the absence of a ligand-binding site, and the inability of ErbB-2 to form homodimers due to electrostatic repulsion.

Why ErbB-2 is Oncogenic When Overexpressed

The above-described structural evidence along with biochemical studies[29] suggest that ErbB-2 homodimers do not exist under physiological conditions. Consistent with the possibility that the relatively high transforming potential of ErbB-2 is due to heterodimer formation, rather than homodimerization, cell transformation by ErbB-3 and ErbB-4 requires the presence of ErbB-2, or ErbB-1,[30] and mitogenic signals emanating from ErbB-2-containing heterodimers are stronger than signals generated by other receptor complexes. A combination of diverse biochemical attributes underlies the mitogenic superiority of ErbB-2. First, ErbB-2 over-expression decelerates the rate of dissociation of several growth factors from their respective ErbB receptors.[31,32]. Second, ErbB-2 engages a set of adaptors that allow effective coupling to the Ras-MAPK pathway. When combined with ErbB-3, a receptor carrying multiple docking sites for the phosphatidylinositol 3 kinase (PI3K),[33] the ErbB-2/ErbB-3 heterodimer robustly couples to both MAPK and Akt, pathways leading to enhanced proliferation and escape from apoptosis (reviewed[34]). Last, unlike ErbB-1, ErbB-2 avoids several negatively acting machineries, including Ras-GAP[35] and receptor degradation.[36,37] In conclusion, overexpression of ErbB-2 to the extent observed in some subsets of human tumors is expected to profoundly sensitize cells to most, if not all, stromal and autocrine EGF family ligands.

Negative Regulation of ErbB Signaling

The ability of ErbB-2 to escape negatively acting pathways focused the attention on the machinery that normally terminates growth factor signaling (reviewed[38]). These pathways can be grouped into early-induced mechanisms and late machinery, the components of which are newly synthesized upon growth factor stimulation. An example is the receptor-associated late transducer (RALT/Mig-6), a feedback inhibitor of ErbB-2 mitogenic and transforming signals.[39] RALT transcription is controlled by the Ras-MAPK pathway, and it undergoes proteasomal degradation, which terminates its negative action. Similar features underlie regulation of another feedback regulator called Sprouty-2.[40] However, unlike RALT, Sprouty regulates EGF signaling through interlinked positive and negative feedback loops.[41,42] One effector of Sprouty is c-Cbl, an E3 ubiquitin ligase that targets internalized growth factor receptors to lysosomal degradation.[43] Ligand-induced endocytosis of growth factor receptors is considered a major mechanism that terminates signal transduction (reviewed[44]). Unlike ErbB-1, which is rapidly recruited to clathrin-coated regions of the plasma membrane, and internalizes into early endosomes, ErbB-2 is internalization-defective. Another step of regulation occurs at the multivesicular body (MVB) when receptors destined for lysosomal degradation are trapped in internal vesicles that accumulate hydrolytic enzymes. Sorting at the MVB as well as at the plasma membrane is controlled by Cbl-mediated ubiquitylation of cargo proteins,[44] and consistent with their distinct intracellular itineraries, ErbB-1 is more potently coupled to c-Cbl than does ErbB-2.[45,46] In fact, the small fraction of ErbB-2 molecules that internalizes into early endosomes is preferentially recycled back to the cell surface, unlike ErbB-1 molecules, which continue their journey through the MVB to lysosomes.[47,48] Apparently, ErbB molecules richly decorated by monomeric ubiquitins[49,50] are recognized by a large set of endocytic adaptors like Hrs and Epsin, which contain an ubiquitin-interacting motif (UIM).[51,52] Nevertheless, the mechanisms that differentially regulate intracellular trafficking of distinct ErbB proteins remain largely unknown.

Regulation of ErbB-4 by Proteolysis

The neuregulin receptors ErbB-3 and ErbB-4 are regulated by mechanisms distinct from those controlling ErbB-1. For example, proteasomal degradation of ErbB-3 is deregulated by a dedicated E3 ubiquitin ligase,[53] and this receptor constitutively recycles following internalization.[48,54] ErbB-4 displays a unique mechanism of regulation (reviewed[55]). Its internalization is relatively slow and instead, a proteolytic mechanism seems to dominate ErbB-4 desensitization. Ligand- and protein kinase C-regulated shedding of the ectodomain of ErbB-4 terminates signaling.[56] The relevant proteolytic enzyme has been identified as the tumor necrosis factor-alpha converting enzyme (TACE), a transmembrane metalloproteinase.[57] Shedding generates an 80-kD fragment, comprising the transmembrane and cytoplamic domains. A second membrane-localized protease activity, γ-secretase, subsequently cleaves within the transmembrane domain and liberates an 80-kD fragment.[58,59] Apparently, the fragment translocates to the nucleus, but its biochemical function remains unknown.

RECENT LESSONS FROM GENETICALLY MANIPULATED ANIMALS

Genetic manipulations of mouse embryos revealed essential functions of the ErbB network. In general, inactivation of ErbB receptors results in more severe and extensive developmental defects than targeting of individual ligands. In addition, the genetic background impacts severity of some phenotypes, suggesting yet unknown links between ErbB and other regulators. Whereas inactivation of ErbB-1 impairs epithelial development in many organs.[3,60–62] ErbB-2 and ErbB-4 together control development of the cardiac trabecula (reviewed[63]), and ErbB-3 plays an essential role in development of sympathetic ganglia and the heart.[64,65] The relatively limited penetrance of mutations that inactivate specific ligands is exemplified by the mild phenotypes of TGF-α ablation, which are confined to the skin and eye.[66,67] Likewise, considerable redundancy and cooperation in the action of ErbB ligands are exemplified by the mildly defective valvulogenesis displayed by HB-EGF null mice, and lack of phenotype of betacellulin-targeted animals.[68] Examples include formation and maintenance of the neuromuscular junction[69] and differentiation of Schwann cells.[70]

Genetically modified animals reflect two important attributes of the ErbB signaling network. First, determination of some cell lineages by inductive, paracrine ligand-to-ErbB interactions depend on formation of heterodimeric, rather than homodimeric complexes. For example, heterodimers comprising ErbB-2 and ErbB-4 are driven by NRG-1 and control heart trabecula development, but this ligand controls Schwann cell development through activation of a complex between ErbB-2 and ErbB-3.[70] Second, the notion that transmembrane precursors of EGF-like ligands must undergo proteolysis to become available for their receptors is strikingly supported by the phenotype of TACE/ADAM17 null mice. TACE is an integral membrane metalloprotease originally implicated in processing of the tumor necrosis factor. TACE null animals display a spectrum of defects reminiscent of those observed in ErbB-1$^{-/-}$ or TGF-α null mice, and several biochemical lines of evidence attribute to TACE a role in processing of several precursors of EGF-like ligands.[71]

ErbB Signaling in Animal Models of Oncogenesis

Consistent with the frequently observed overexpression of various ErbB receptors in sporadic breast cancer, evidence from transgenic animals strongly implicate ErbB signaling in oncogenesis of the mammary gland. The current paradigm assumes that steroid hormones acting upon the fatty mammary mesenchyme induce production of paracrine ErbB ligands. Consequently, the secreted ligands regulate ErbB proteins expressed in the epithelium of nascent ducts. Indeed, all four ErbB proteins and multiple EGF-like ligands are expressed throughout mammary development and involution,[72] and mammary-specific expression of ErbB-1 or TGF-α results in frequent induction of mammary adenocarcinomas.[73,74] Similarly, mammary-specific expression of an activated ErbB-2 is associated with the appearance of metastatic mammary tumors.[75] Conceivably, certain EGF-like ligands and their respective ErbB receptors play essential roles in specific phases of mammary gland development, and tumor growth reflects hyperactivation in certain phases. In support of this notion, dominant negative forms of ErbB-2 and ErbB-4 can block lobuloalveolar development[76] and mammary terminal differentiation,[77] respectively, whereas co-expression of ErbB-2 and TGF-α accelerated mammary tumor progression.[78]

Importantly, transgenic mice carrying the erbB-2 proto-oncogene under the transcriptional control of a strong viral promoter/enhancer developed focal mammary tumors only after a long latency period, and most tumors expressed a spontaneous mutant.[79] The activating mutation results in constitutive dimerization of mutant ErbB-2 proteins. Slow onset of mammary tumors characterizes another transgenic model in which the endogenous promoter of erbB-2 drives expression of an activated ErbB-2 molecule.[80] Remarkably, selective genomic amplification of the activated erbB-2 allele was associated with tumor progression, implying that like human breast cancers, genetic alterations of the *erbB-2* gene are essential for tumor development. In conclusion, ErbB receptors and their ligands play pivotal roles in mammary gland development, and cancer may arise when ligands like TGF-α or the ErbB-2 co-receptor are overexpressed. Predictably, ErbB signaling is involved in neoplastic transformation of additional epithelial organs, such as ovary and lung. However, elucidation of these possibilities is limited by the availability of animal model systems.

CLINICAL SIGNIFICANCE OF ErbB SIGNALING IN HUMAN CANCER

The oncogenic potential of ErbB receptors in experimental models prompted investigation into their roles in cancer prognosis, prediction of response to various therapeutic modalities, and interactions with other receptors in a variety of human malignancies. The expression patterns of ErbB-1 and ErbB-2, and to a lesser extent that of ErbB-3 and 4, in various tumors has been extensively studied (reviewed[81,82]). Several methods are used to determine expression status of the *erbB* genes.[83] Gene amplification is determined by in situ hybridization (FISH or CISH), polymerase chain reaction (PCR), or Southern blotting. Overexpression can be detected by using reverse transcriptase PCR, Northern blotting, immunohistochemistry (IHC), Western blotting, or enzyme-linked immunosorbent assay (ELISA). Emerging promising techniques are coming from the testing of ErbB activity by determining the level of phosphorylated receptors or by testing the activation status of downstream effectors (e.g., Erk and Akt/PKB).[84] IHC and FISH are by far the most common techniques used to assess ErbB levels. Although IHC determination is frequently used, it is prone to multiple technical and observer pitfalls, making it problematic, especially when used in low volume laboratories. FISH has a higher concordance rate between low volume and high volume laboratories and is less prone to technical problems; however, this test is more expensive and requires special instrumentation, which is not usually available in pathology laboratories. In general, there is a high concordance between a negative IHC staining for ErbB-2 (score 0 or +1) and no gene amplification, as well as between positive IHC staining (+3) and the presence of gene amplification. A moderate IHC staining (+2) is associated in 70% of cases with no gene amplification. Hence, it requires the utilization of FISH for exact determination of ErbB-2 status.[85,86]

Tumors that overexpress ErbB-1 or ErbB-2 tend to be poorly differentiated with vascular invasion and a higher metastatic potential.[82,87] Breast cancer tumors that overexpress ErbB-2 are more likely to be of ductal rather than lobular origin, with high tumor grade, DNA aneuploidy, p53 mutations, topoisomerase IIa amplification, and an absence of steroid hormone receptors. Nevertheless, approximately 10% of tumors that overexpress ErbB-2 do express steroid hormone receptors.[88] Moreover, the expression level of ErbB-2 is inversely correlated with levels of steroid hormone receptors. Thus, patients with higher levels of ErbB-2 tend to have lower levels of steroid hormone receptors than patients with lower levels of ErbB-2.[88] This inverse correlation is in accordance with the observation that breast tumors with high levels of ErbB-2 are usually resistant to hormonal treatments, and it may underlie resistance to selective hormone receptor modulators, such as Tamoxifen.[89]

Mutant and Variant Forms of ErbB-1 and ErbB-2

In addition to wildtype ErbB-1, cancer cells also have been shown to express various mutated ErbB-1 molecules. The most common mutant, variously named EGFRvIII, de2-7 EGFR, or delta-EGFR, is one in which amino acids 6-273 (exons 2-7) of the extracellular domain are deleted. This in-frame deletion is common in glioblastomas and in several other types of cancer, including breast, ovarian, lung and medulloblastoma tumors.[90] The loss of part of the extracellular domain creates a novel, cancer cell-specific epitope, which has been used to raise tumor-specific antibodies and immunize tumor-bearing animals.[91] EGFRvIII is constitutively active, although it cannot bind EGF, and only minimally activated by ErbB-1 ligands.[92] While the prognostic significance of

EGFRvIII in carcinomas remains incompletely understood, the mutant confers radio-resistance that exceeds the cytoprotective activity of wildtype ErbB-1.[93]

Single nucleotide polymorphism (SNP) within the transmembrane domain of ErbB-2 has been detected and associated with an increased risk of breast cancer[94,95] and gastric carcinoma.[96] The polymorphic site involves codon 655, which encodes either an isoleucine (most normal subjects) or a valine, and the valine/valine genotype is rare. While an association with ethnic origins cannot be excluded, theoretical models predict that a valine at position 655 of the transmembrane domain can enhance a relatively unstable, but active, conformation of ErbB-2.[97]

Prognostic and Therapeutic Implications of ErbB Expression

ErbB-1 Overexpression of ErbB-1/EGFR has been implicated as a poor prognostic feature in various human malignancies including breast, head and neck, ovarian, bladder and esophageal cancer, but excluding non-small cell lung cancer.[98] Co-expression of ErbB-1 and its ligands have been observed in various tumors and implicated as a poor prognostic feature.[81] However, the routine use of ErbB-1 expression as a clinical tool regarding prognosis and therapy has not been established. Overexpression of ErbB-1 has been implicated in relative resistance to radiotherapy,[99] but a role in chemoresistance is less characterized.[100]

ErbB-2 A comprehensive recent review examined the data from 81 published studies covering over 27,000 breast cancer patients.[101] The expression of ErbB-2 was determined in most studies either by FISH for gene amplification, or by immunohistochemistry for protein overexpression. In 73 studies, which included over 25,000 patients, ErbB-2 overexpression was an adverse prognostic factor in a univariate (13 studies) or multivariate (52 studies) analyses. In eight studies covering about 2,000 patients no correlation was found between ErbB-2 expression and prognosis in breast cancer. As discussed above, the method of determination of ErbB-2 expression status is of paramount importance in establishing prognosis and response to therapy. All nine studies that used FISH or CISH found an adverse prognostic significance of *erbB-2* gene amplification, and in eight of the nine studies gene amplification was an independent factor, as determined by a multivariate analysis.

The prognostic significance of ErbB-2 expression in other tumors is not as well studied, but several reports suggest prognostic implications in pancreatic, ovarian, gastric and prostate cancer.[82,87] The routine testing of ErbB-2 expression as part of the histopathologic diagnosis of breast cancer is increasingly performed and is being used to help evaluate the patient's prognosis and aid in determining the best therapeutic options. Overexpression of ErbB-2 clearly correlated to resistance to endocrine therapy by Tamoxifen in patients with early and metastatic breast cancer (reviewed[102]). The bidirectional cross-talk between ErbB receptors and steroid hormone receptors has been implicated in primary and acquired resistance to hormonal therapy in breast cancer.[103] A recent study evaluated the benefit from Tamoxifen versus Letrozole, an aromatase inhibitor, as primary therapy for ER-positive patients with locally advanced breast cancer.[104] The results suggested that in ErbB-2 negative patients the response rate to both drugs was comparable; however, in patients with overexpression of ErbB-2, only Letrozole produced a meaningful response. This observation is in agreement with the extreme sensitivity to estrogen as a growth modulator in breast tumors that overexpress ErbB-2 and are steroid hormone receptor positive; aromatase inhibitors suppress estrogen levels to nearly undetectable amounts and are thus the better choice for this group of patients.

The correlation between ErbB-2 overexpression and anthracyline sensitivity in adjuvant therapy for early breast cancer was shown in several retrospective studies (reviewed[105]). Clinical trials that studied the added value of doxorubicin in the adjuvant setting of early breast cancer[106] concluded that patients with overexpression of ErbB-2 had significantly longer disease-free survival (DFS) when treated with a doxorubicin-containing regimen. Another study compared the addition of doxorubicin-containing chemotherapy to Tamoxifen versus Tamoxifen alone in postmenopausal node-positive ER-positive patients.[107] The results indicated a significant benefit only in women with ErbB-2-positive tumors. These results may be attributed to the relative resistance of ErbB-2-positive tumors to Tamoxifen, as discussed above. The differential benefit of non-anthracycline containing therapy and taxanes in ErbB-2 positive tumors is not as well defined.[108]

Soluble ErbB Proteins

Soluble forms of all ErbB proteins exist in body fluids, but their physiologic and clinical significance are currently unknown. A soluble ErbB-1 of 110 kD has been detected in normal sera, but its concentration is significantly lower in women with advanced stage ovarian cancer.[109] A naturally occurring secreted form of the human ErbB-3 receptor, p85 ErbB-3, is a potent negative regulator of ligand-stimulated ErbB-2 activation.[110] Likewise, the extracellular domain of ErbB-2 is naturally and slowly released through degradation of the transmembrane receptor. This form is detectable in the serum of patients with advanced breast cancer, and it neutralizes the activity of anti-ErbB-2 antibodies.[8] Recent analysis of breast tumors indicated that the soluble form of ErbB-2 is more frequently detected in metastatic lymph nodes than in primary tumors.[111] In summary, while the presence of soluble ErbB proteins may reduce the efficacy of immunotherapy, it also may negate the action of the respective growth factors. Hence, the clinical potential of soluble ErbB proteins as prognostic markers or pharmaceutical agents justifies future investigation.

CANCER THERAPY TARGETED AT ErbB SIGNALING

The ErbB network offers several advantages for development of cancer therapies. First, EGF-like ligands are among the most potent mitogens of epithelial cells, the precursors of carcinomas. Second, ErbB signaling is well understood: the three dimensional structures of most ligands and receptors are available and downstream signaling pathways are relatively well characterized. Third, the receptors face the extracellular environment, and therefore they are accessible to treatments that do not penetrate the cell. Last, the catalytic tyrosine kinase activity of ErbB receptors is essential for signaling, and its inhibition is readily achieved due the relatively deep nucleotide-binding pocket. Two drugs that specifically target ErbB signaling have been approved for clinical practice. These are Herceptin/Trastuzumab, a humanized monoclonal antibody (mAb) approved for treatment of women with metastatic breast cancer whose tumors overexpress ErbB-2, and the small molecule ErbB-1 blocker, Gefitinib (ZD1839, Iressa), the use of which is limited to patients with non-small cell lung cancer (NSCLC) previously treated with chemotherapy. Several other compounds are in various phases of development and they can be grouped into four categories: mAbs, tyrosine kinase inhibitors, chaperone antagonists, and various other strategies, including gene therapy and aptamers. Figure 3.3 presents the major molecules targeted by ErbB related therapeutic strategies, along with examples of specific compounds and drugs.

Immuotherapy Directed at ErbB Receptors

The ability of anti-ErbB-1 mAbs to block EGF signaling[112] and mimic in part the action of a ligand[113] marked the beginning of ErbB-directed immunotherapy. Likewise, antibodies to rodent[114] and human ErbB-2[115] exhibited anti-proliferative responses when tested in cultures and in animals bearing ErbB-2-driven tumors. To avoid development of a human anti-mouse (HAMA) antibody response, chimerization or humanization of rodent antibody molecules is necessary. Thus, chimeric (e.g., IMC-225) and humanized (e.g., hR3 and EMD-72000) forms of anti-ErbB-1 antibodies were developed as well as a fully human antibody called ABX-EGF. Similarly, one of the murine mAbs to ErbB-2 has been humanized. The humanized immunoglobulin G1 antibody, Herceptin/Trastuzumab, contains as few as 5% rodent residues.[116] In second/third line Herceptin monotherapy of 222 women with advanced ErbB-2-positive metastatic cancer there were 8 complete responses and 26 partial responses, which represents an overall response rate of 15%.[117] Moreover, the median response duration was significantly better than achieved with patient's previous chemotherapy regimen. An important lesson learned in this and other trials is that the higher level of ErbB-2 overexpression, the greater the benefit generated by the antibody. The value of Herceptin as first

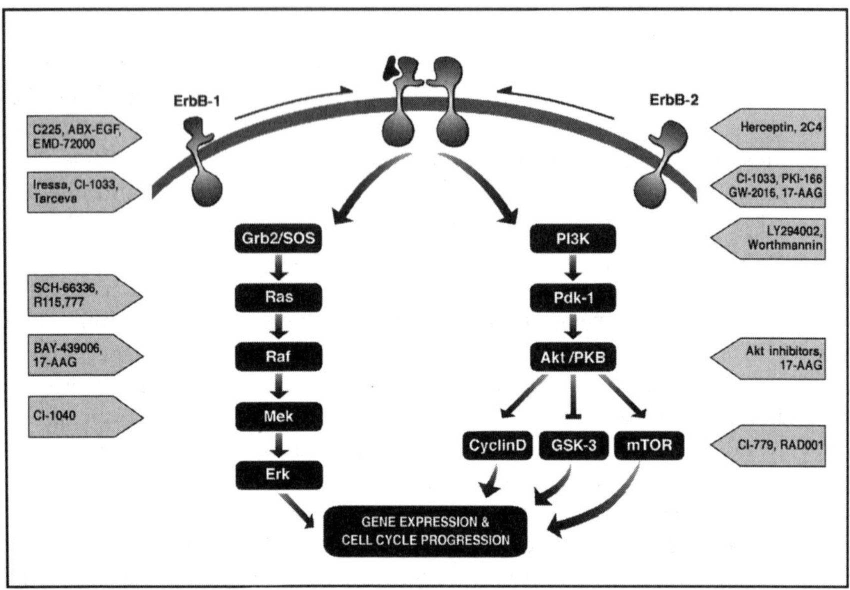

FIGURE 3.3 Potential drugs that intercept ErbB signaling. An ErbB-1/ErbB-2 heterodimer is presented, along with two major signaling pathways (see Fig. 4.1). Compounds that target specific components of the signaling pathways, including ErbB-1 and ErbB-2, are indicated. Note that 17-AAG, a drug that targets Hsp90, accelerates proteolysis of several components of the ErbB network. See text for details.

line therapy in patients with ErbB-2 positive metastatic breast cancer was demonstrated by Vogel et al[118] with a 35% response rate in patients with high expression (+3) of ErbB-2. The therapeutic efficacy of Herceptin has been demonstrated also in a pivotal phase III trial, which combined the antibody with chemotherapy as first line therapy for metastatic breast cancer.[119] When compared to chemotherapy alone, the overall response rate increased from 32 to 50%, and time to disease progression increased from 4.6 to 7.4 months. Overall survival was increased by 9 months in the subgroup of high expressors (+3) of ErbB-2, treated with chemotherapy plus Herceptin, as compared to chemotherapy alone. The clinical benefit of combining Herceptin with paclitaxel and anthracyclins was notable. However, the combination of Herceptin with anthracycline also was associated with cardiotoxicity, which limits the use of this combination.[120] Last, evidence from model experimental systems indicate that Herceptin is effective when combined with various other chemotherapeutic agents, including vinorelbine, docectaxel and cisplatin.[121]

Several anti-ErbB-1 antibodies are currently in phase II and III clinical trials, including the C225 human-mouse chimeric molecule. C225 prevents ligand-induced receptor activation and downstream signaling, which results in cell cycle arrest, promotion of apoptosis, and inhibition of angiogenesis. When tested on cultured cells, the antibody enhances the anti-tumor effects of chemotherapy and radiation therapy.[122,123] In patients, single-agent activity has been observed against a variety of tumor types, including colon carcinoma, head and neck cancer, ovarian carcinoma, and renal cell carcinoma (reviewed[124,125]). Although the antibody was well tolerated with only mild toxicities, which were limited to skin rash and diarrhea, responses were seen in only a minority of the patients treated. In some clinical trials, anti-EGFR agents enhanced the effects of conventional chemotherapy and radiation therapy. For example, when combined with radiation therapy, C225 treatment of patients with locally advanced head and neck cancers produced objective responses in 15 of 15 patients,[126] and in a phase III study conducted on head and neck cancer patients the combination of IMC-C225 and cisplatin achieved an objective response rate of 23%.[127] As with anti-ErbB-2 antibodies, the mechanism of immunotherapy is incompletely understood. Several mechanisms have been proposed to account for the anti-tumor activities of therapeutic antibodies, including blockade of signaling pathways and activation of apoptosis. Perhaps the best established mechanism is engagement of Fc-gamma receptors on effector cells.[128] Herceptin engages both stimulatory and inhibitory antibody receptors on myeloid cells, thus modulating their cytotoxic potential. Nevertheless, antibodies that lack the Fc portion still retain anti-tumor activity in animals, suggesting involvement of non-immunological mechanisms. According to one possibility, which was raised by analyzing the anti-tumor activity of a series of anti-ErbB-2 antibodies, endocytic removal of the receptor from the cell surface reduces its availability for heterodimer formation, and thereby inhibits tumor growth.[129] Consistent with this paradigm, combinations of antibodies directed to different epitopes of ErbB-2 blocked tumor growth and enhanced receptor degradation more effectively than each antibody alone.[130]

Analysis of anti-ErbB-1 antibodies indicated that inhibition of ligand binding is not an essential feature of a tumor-inhibitory antibody.[131] In addition, such a mechanism does not exist in the case of the ligand-less receptor, ErbB-2. On the other hand, a specific sub-class of anti-ErbB-2 antibodies was found to inhibit heterodimerization of ErbB-2,[132] in line with the existence of a dimerization arm in the structure of ErbB-2.[28] An anti-ErbB-2 antibody (called 2C4) that inhibits heterodimerization is currently in clinical trials.[133] It is hoped that 2C4 will inhibit growth of tumors that express ErbB-2 at low to moderate levels. However, it is currently unclear if such tumors are driven by the ErbB network. It is reasonable to assume that tumors that carry no mutated, or otherwise genetically altered, ErbB receptor are not driven by the ErbB network. However, like in the case of the estrogen receptor, survival of some tumor cells may depend on the availability of EGF-like ligands, and therefore targeting the receptors may still block tumor growth. This question is relevant to the issue of patient selection and development of resistance to ErbB-targeted therapies.

Along with 2C4, a few other immunologic agents are under clinical development. These include Herceptin-DM-1, a covalent conjugate of Herceptin and mytansinoid, a highly potent microtubule toxin. Due to receptor-mediated endocytosis, the conjugate delivers the toxin only into the cytoplasm of ErbB-2-expressing cells. MDX-H210 is a bispecific antibody directed against both ErbB-2 and the Fc gamma receptor, which mediates macrophage-induced lysis of ErbB-2-overexpressing tumor cells.[134] The anti-tumor efficacy of the fully human anti-ErbB-1 antibody ABX-EGF was evaluated in renal cancer patients. Despite mild toxicities and no allergic reactions to the human antibody, responses were partial or minor.[135] Another promising type of antibody is represented by the 806 monoclonal antibody, which recognizes EGFRvIII, a deletion mutant expressed in brain and epithelial tumors. Interestingly, 806 decorates not only cells expressing the deletion mutant, but also a subset of ErbB-1-overexpressing tumors.[136] The therapeutic potential of 806 and other antibodies to the mutant form of ErbB-1 will require further investigation.

Tyrosine Kinase Inhibitors

The kinase domain of ErbB-1 is bilobular with a deep pocket that accommodates a nucleotide triphosphate molecule.[137] Although antagonists of the substrate-binding site are potentially able to block kinase activity, and they may be more selective than compounds that bind to the nucleotide-binding site, so far only adenosine 5′-triphosphate (ATP)-competitive inhibitors have been developed for clinical applications. Remarkably, and contrary to predictions, specific inhibitors can be synthesized, which discriminate between highly homologous kinase domains such as the catalytic portions of ErbB-1 and ErbB-2.[138] In addition, the structures of the most effective inhibitors converge on specific patterns (Fig. 3.4), which likely reflect the anatomy of the ErbB target site. The IC50 values of such compounds may be as low as sub-nanomolar. Compounds like Iressa (gefitinib, ZD-1839), PKI-166 and Tarceva (Erlonitib, OSI-774) were designed to selectively inhibit ErbB-1, whereas other compounds were designed to inhibit two or more ErbB receptors (e.g., GW-2016, PKI166). The irreversible pan-ErbB inhibitor CI-1033 has been developed in an attempt to prolong target suppression, and also broaden specificity to all ErbB proteins.[139] The inhibitor makes use of a cysteine residue uniquely present within the kinase domain of ErbB proteins, and radiolabeling studies confirmed its high specificity.

When tested on cultured cells and in tumor-bearing animals, tyrosine kinase inhibitors elicit apoptosis, and in the case of Iressa the underlying mechanism involves inhibition of phosphorylation of the proapoptotic protein BAD.[140] Other studies suggest that Iressa inhibits tumor cell proliferation and angiogenesis, and shows synergy with standard cancer therapies.[141] Iressa is an orally available drug, that generates moderate objective response rates (6% to 20%) in multiple solid tumors including lung, colorectal, head and neck, and ovarian carcinomas. Extensive experience is available in NSCLC with response rates of 11% to 18%

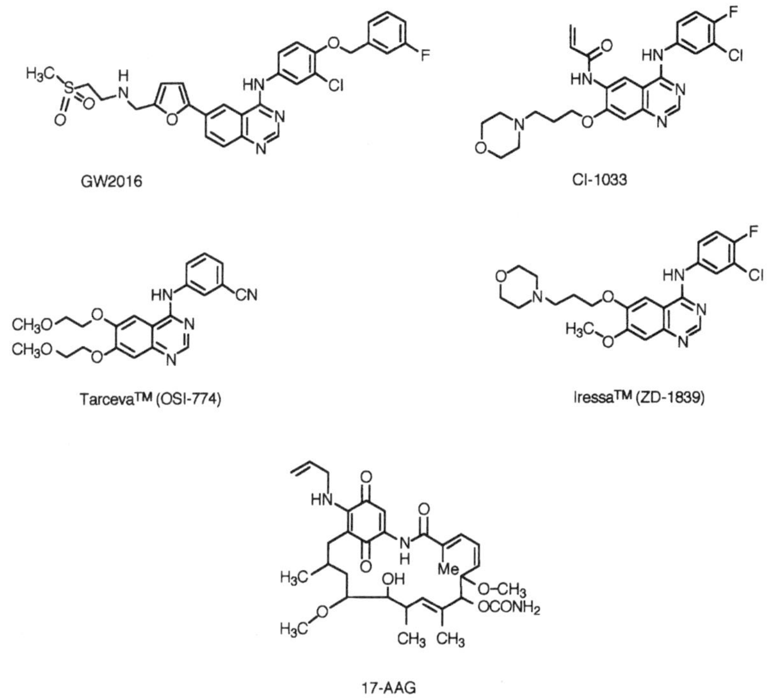

GW2016

CI-1033

Tarceva™ (OSI-774)

Iressa™ (ZD-1839)

17-AAG

FIGURE 3.4 Chemical structures of several low molecular weight inhibitors of ErbB proteins. The general chaperone inhibitor, 17-AAG, is shown along with the indicated tyrosine kinase inhibitors, which are currently in clinical development.

in two phase II trials of patients previously treated with platinum-based chemotherapy (reviewed[142]). Of note are two aspects: (1) patients with bronchoalveolar carcinoma have a higher response rate than other types of NSCLC, and (2) non-smokers seem to also have higher response rates to Iressa. These results led to the approval in 2003 of Iressa for the treatment of advanced NSCLC previously treated with chemotherapy. Surprisingly, the addition of Iressa to chemotherapy (paclitaxel/carboplatin or gemcitabine/cisplatin) provided no additional benefit over chemotherapy alone in patient survival, or time to disease progression, in two phase III trials that examined over 2000 previously untreated NSCLC patients.[143,144] These negative results limit clinical application of Iressa, and they may be due to either trial design or to biological factors. For example, patients enrolled on the phase III trials were not selected on the basis of ErbB-1 expression or activation status in tumors. Alternatively, there might be negative interactions between Iressa and cytotoxic drugs, although this possibility is not supported in preclinical models.[141]

Chaperone Inhibitors

The frequent escape of tumors from chemotherapy and radiotherapy is mediated by a physiologic stress response, which involves heat shock protein 90 (Hsp90).[145] Hence, blocking this escape pathway may sensitize cancer cells to cytotoxic treatments. Hsp90 chaperones a selected set of signaling proteins essential for the rapid growth of cancer cells. The set of Hsp90 clients comprises transcription factors and protein kinases, including several receptor tyrosine kinases like Met and ErbB-2. The amino terminal ATP/ADP binding pocket of Hsp90 is the target of several natural and synthetic compounds (e.g., geldanamycin [GA], radicicol, and 17-allylaminogeldanamycin [17AAG]). Upon binding to Hsp90, the blockers transform the chaperone into a form that accelerates ubiquitylation and proteasomal degradation of all client proteins. The kinase domain of ErbB-2 is recognized by Hsp90,[146] which binds to a motif within the amino-terminal lobe of the kinase.[147] Although Hsp90 blockers induce extensive degradation of ErbB-2, while sparing other ErbB proteins, future clinical application will necessitate target selectivity since many other Hsp90 clients are destabilized by drugs such as geldanamycin. One way to circumvent the problem is by using dimers of geldanamyicin.[148] Alternatively, selective client destruction may be achieved by using an irreversible kinase inhibitor. The inhibitor binds ErbB-2 rather specifically, which disrupts the association with Hsp90, and leads to proteasomal degradation of ErbB-2.[149] Hsp90 blockers such as 17-AAG, a drug currently in phase I clinical trials, hold promise especially in the context of chemotherapy. Low doses of Hsp90 inhibitors sensitize leukemic cells to doxorubicin,[150] and a combination of geldanamycin and Taxol effectively inhibited carcinoma cells.[151] Because several downstream effectors of ErbB-2 serve as Hsp90 clients (e.g., Akt and Raf1), chaperone blockers may be especially effective on ErbB-2-overexpressing tumors. However, inhibition of Hsp90 is associated with toxicity to the liver and other organs, which blurs the true clinical potential of chaperone antagonists.

Other Approaches to Pharmacological Interception of ErbB Signaling

The efficacy of drugs targeting specific ErbB proteins may be enhanced in the presence of agents that specifically block downstream signaling pathways. In the context of ErbB, the most critical cascades are the MAPK and Akt pathways. Ras regulates both pathways and therefore small molecule Ras blockers are attractive from a clinical perspective.[152] Several low molecular weight farnesyl transferase inhibitors, which prevent association of Ras with the plasma membrane, reached clinical stages of evaluation. Likewise, specific antisense phosphortioate oligodeoxyribonucleotides that block expression of specific Ras proteins are in clinical tests. Along the same pathway (Fig. 3.3), kinase inhibitors targeting Raf (e.g., BAY439006), Mek (e.g., CI-1040) and phosphatidylinositol 3-kinase (e.g., LY294002) are in various stages of clinical development.

Several other strategies are under development. The ability of an adenoviral gene product to downregulate ErbB-2 has been exploited by using gene therapy.[153] Antisense strategies that block expression of erbB-2 or erbB-1, RNA aptamers that target the dimeric state of ErbB proteins,[154] and inhibitors of histone deacetylation and the 26S proteasome are therapeutic strategies relevant to ErbB signaling. Various bispecific antibodies targeting an ErbB protein and an immune cell surface protein as well as conjugates of neuregulins with toxins, or drugs, have been reported, and some agents are in clinical testing. Last, active immunization against ErbB receptors by generating endogenous antibodies and T cells may result in long-lived immunity and therapeutic benefit. ErbB-2-specific vaccines have been tested in human clinical trials and early results demonstrate that significant levels of HER-2/neu immunity can be generated upon vaccination.[155]

PERSPECTIVES AND FUTURE DIRECTIONS

Prognostic and therapeutic strategies directed at ErbB proteins provide an exemplification of the important interface between basic and clinical research. Deeper understanding of the molecular mechanisms underlying ligand binding to, and consequent activation of ErbB proteins will likely emerge from the current flood of ErbB structural information. Likewise, a fuller list of effector molecules that interact with activated forms of ErbB proteins will lead to better understanding of the ErbB circuit. When combined with reliable animal models, this type of information may translate into the identification of effective drug combinations. Both conventional cytotoxic drugs as well as the more selective anti-signaling agents are candidates for combination therapy.

Predictably, combination chemistry and recombinant DNA technology will improve efficacy of low molecule inhibitors and biologicals (e.g., antibodies and soluble forms of ErbB proteins) that intercept ErbB signaling. Nevertheless, many questions remain open and the challenges are overwhelming. Above all, it remains to be seen if blocking the non-mutated and non-overexpressed forms of ErbB proteins has a significant therapeutic potential. This is especially relevant to ErbB-3 and ErbB-4, whose role in malignant transformation remains poorly characterized. Even with the better established targets, ErbB-2 and ErbB-1, several critical issues pertinent to therapy remain open. They include the presence of activating growth factors, level of receptor expression and activity status, and relationships to the presence of other ErbB proteins. These issues are relevant to the selection of patients most likely to benefit from a specific agent, selection of the most appropriate dose and schedule of drug administration, and identification of surrogates of patient outcome. In conclusion, work over the last three decades has clearly established ErbB signaling as a valid target for cancer therapy. As more molecules are being tested and approved, the arsenal of drugs that intercept ErbB signal transduction becomes wider and provide a more extensive basis for drug combinations.

Acknowledgments

We thank Bose S. Kochupurakkal and Anthony W. Burgess for insightful help. Y.Y. is the incumbent of the Harold and Zelda Goldenberg Professorial Chair in Molecular Cell Biology. Our laboratory is supported by research grants from the Willner Center for Vascular Biology, the National Cancer Institute (grant CA72981), The Israel Science Foundation, Cap-CURE, and the U.S. Army (grant DAMD 17-00-1-0499).

REFERENCES

1. Yarden Y, Ullrich A. Growth factor receptor tyrosine kinases. Ann Rev Biochem 1988;57:443–478.
2. Schlessinger J. Cell signaling by receptor tyrosine kinases. Cell 2000;103:211–225.
3. Sibilia M, Steinbach JP, Stingl L et al. A strain-independent postnatal neurodegeneration in mice lacking the EGF receptor. EMBO J 1998;17:719–731.
4. Sporn MB, Todaro GJ. Autocrine secretion and malignant transformation of cells. N Engl J Med 1980;308:878–880.
5. Schechter AL, Stern DF, Vaidyanathan L et al. The neu oncogene: an erb-B-related gene encoding a 185,000-Mr tumour antigen. Nature 1984;312:513–516.
6. Slamon DJ, Clark GM, Wong SG et al. Human breast cancer: correlation of relapse and survival with amplification of the HER-2/*neu* oncogene. Science 1987;235:177–182.
7. Drebin JA, Link VC, Stern DF et al. Down-modulation of an oncogene protein product and reversion of the transformed phenotype by monoclonal antibodies. Cell 1985;41:697–706.
8. Baselga J, Tripathy D, Mendelsohn J et al. Phase II study of weekly intravenous recombinant humanized anti-p185HER2 monoclonal antibody in patients with HER2/neu-overexpressing metastatic breast cancer. J Clin Oncol 1996;14:737–744.
9. Levitzki A. Tyrphostins: tyrosine kinase blockers as novel antiproliferative agents and dissectors of signal transduction. FASEB J 1992;6:3275–382.
10. Massague J, Pandiella A. Membrane-anchored growth factors. Ann Rev Biochem 1993;62:515–541.
11. Klapper LN, Glathe S, Vaisman N et al. The ErbB-2/HER2 oncoprotein of human carcinomas may function solely as a shared coreceptor for multiple stroma-derived growth factors. Proc Natl Acad Sci USA 1999;96:4995–5000.
12. Guy PM, Platko JV, Cantley LC et al. Insect cell-expressed p180erbB3 possesses an impaired tyrosine kinase activity. Proc Natl Acad Sci USA 1994;91:8132–8136.

13. Yarden Y, Schlessinger J. Self-phosphorylation of epidermal growth factor receptor: Evidence for a model of intermolecular allosteric activation. Biochemistry 1987;26:1434–1442.

14. Yarden Y, Schlessinger J. Epidermal growth factor induce rapid, reversible aggregation of purified epidermal growth factor receptor. Biochemistry 1987;26:1443–1445.

15. Tzahar E, Waterman H, Chen X et al. A hierarchical network of interreceptor interactions determines signal transduction by Neu differentiation factor/neuregulin and epidermal growth factor. Mol Cell Biol 1996;16:5276–5287.

16. Graus Porta D, Beerli RR, Daly JM, Hynes NE. ErbB-2, the preferred heterodimerization partner of all ErbB receptors, is a mediator of lateral signaling. EMBO J 1997;16:1647–1655.

17. Yarden Y, Sliwkowski MX. Untangling the ErbB signalling network. Nat Rev Mol Cell Biol 2001;2:127–137.

18. Lax I, Bellot F, Howk R et al. Functional analysis of the ligand binding site of EGF-receptor utilizing chicken/human receptor molecules. EMBO J 1989;8:421–427.

19. Lemmon MA, Bu Z, Ladbury JE et al. Two EGF molecules contribute additively to stabilization of the EGFR dimer. EMBO J 1997;16:281–294.

20. Tzahar, E, Pinkas Kramarski R, Moyer JD et al. Bivalence of EGF-like ligands drives the ErbB signaling network. EMBO J 1997;16:4938–4950.

21. Ferguson KM, Berger MB, Mendrola JM et al. EGF activates its receptor by removing interactions that autoinhibit ectodomain dimerization. Mol Cell 2003;11:507–517.

22. Cho HS, Leahy DJ. Structure of the extracellular region of HER3 reveals an interdomain tether. Science 2002;297:1330–1333.

23. Garrett, TP, McKern NM, Lou M et al. Crystal structure of a truncated epidermal growth factor receptor extracellular domain bound to transforming growth factor alpha. Cell 2002;110: 763–773.

24. Ogiso, H, Ishitani R, Nureki O et al. Crystal structure of the complex of human epidermal growth factor and receptor extracellular domains. Cell 2002;110:775–787.

25. Gadella TW, Jovin TM. Oligomerization of epidermal growth factor receptors on A431 cells studied by time-resolved fluorescence imaging microscopy. A stereochemical model for tyrosine kinase receptor activation. J Cell Biol 1995;129:1543–1558.

26. Olayioye MA, Neve RM, Lane HA, Hynes NE. The ErbB signaling network: receptor heterodimerization in development and cancer. EMBO J 2000;19:3159–3167.

27. Cho HS, Mason K, Ramyar KX et al. Structure of the extracellular region of HER2 alone and in complex with the Herceptin Fab. Nature 2003;421:756–760.

28. Garrett, TP, McKern NM, Lou M et al. The crystal structure of a truncated ErbB2 ectodomain reveals an active conformation, poised to interact with other ErbB receptors. Mol Cell 2003;11:495–505.

29. Cohen BD, Kiener PA, Green JM et al. The relationship between human epidermal growth-like factor receptor expression and cellular transformation in NIH3T3 cells. J Biol Chem 1996;271:30897–30903.

30. Zhang K, Sun J, Liu N et al. Transformation of NIH 3T3 cells by HER3 or HER4 receptors requires the presence of HER1 or HER2. J Biol Chem 1996;271:3884–3890.

31. Sliwkowski MX, Schaefer G, Akita RW et al. Coexpression of erbB2 and erbB3 proteins reconstitutes a high affinity receptor for heregulin. J Biol Chem 1994;269:14661–14665.

32. Karunagaran D, Tzahar E, Beerli RR et al. ErbB-2 is a common auxiliary subunit of NDF and EGF receptors: implications for breast cancer. EMBO J 1996;15:254–264.

33. Prigent SA, Gullick WJ. Identification of c-erbB-3 binding sites for phosphatidylinositol 3′-kinase and SHC using an EGF receptor/c-erbB-3 chimera. EMBO J 1994;13:2831–2841.

34. Citri A, Skaria KB, Yarden Y. The deaf and the dumb: the biology of ErbB-2 and ErbB-3. Exp Cell Res 2003;284:54–65.
35. Fedi P, Pierce JH, di Fiore PP, Kraus MH. Efficient coupling with phosphatidylinositol 3-kinase, but not phospholipase C gamma or GTPase-activating protein, distinguishes ErbB-3 signaling from that of other ErbB/EGFR family members. Mol Cell Biol 1994;14:492–500.
36. Baulida J, Kraus MH, Alimandi M et al. All ErbB receptors other than the epidermal growth factor receptor are endocytosis impaired. J Biol Chem 1996;271:5251–5257.
37. Pinkas-Kramarski R, Soussan L, Waterman H et al. Diversification of Neu differentiation factor and epidermal growth factor signaling by combinatorial receptor interactions. EMBO J 1996;15:2452–2467.
38. Dikic I, Giordano S. Negative receptor signalling. Curr Opin Cell Biol 2003;15:128–135.
39. Fiorentino L, Pertica C, Fiorini M et al. Inhibition of ErbB-2 mitogenic and transforming activity by RALT, a mitogen-induced signal transducer which binds to the ErbB-2 kinase domain. Mol Cell Biol 2000;20:7735–7750.
40. Guy GR, Wong ES, Yusoff P et al. Sprouty: how does the branch manager work? J Cell Sci 2003;116(Pt 15):3061–3068.
41. Hall AB, Jura N, DaSilva J et al. hSpry2 is targeted to the ubiquitin-dependent proteasome pathway by c-Cbl. Curr Biol 2003;13:308–314.
42. Rubin C, Litvak V, Medvedovsky H et al. Sprouty fine-tunes EGF signaling through interlinked positive and negative feedback loops. Curr Biol 2003;13:297–307.
43. Thien CB, Langdon WY. Cbl: many adaptations to regulate protein tyrosine kinases. Nat Rev Mol Cell Biol 2001;2:294–307.
44. Waterman H, Yarden Y. Molecular mechanisms underlying endocytosis and sorting of ErbB receptor tyrosine kinases. FEBS Lett 2001;490:142–152.
45. Levkowitz G, Klapper LN, Tzahar E et al. Coupling of the c-Cbl protooncogene product to ErbB-1/EGF-receptor but not to other ErbB proteins. Oncogene 1996;12:1117–1125.
46. Muthuswamy SK, Gilman M, Brugge JS. Controlled dimerization of ErbB receptors provides evidence for differential signaling by homo- and heterodimers. Mol Cell Biol 1999;19:6845–6857.
47. Lenferink AE, Pinkas Kramarski R, van de Poll ML et al. Differential endocytic routing of homo- and hetero-dimeric ErbB tyrosine kinases confers signaling superiority to receptor heterodimers. EMBO J 1998;17:3385–3397.
48. Worthylake R, Opresko LK, Wiley HS. ErbB-2 amplification inhibits down-regulation and induces constitutive activation of both ErbB-2 and epidermal growth factor receptors. J Biol Chem 1999;274:8865–8874.
49. Haglund, K, Sigismund S, Polo S et al. Multiple monoubiquitination of RTKs is sufficient for their endocytosis and degradation. Nat Cell Biol 2003;5:461–466.
50. Mosesson Y, Shtiegman K, Katz M et al. Endocytosis of receptor tyrosine kinases is driven by monoubiquitylation, not polyubiquitylation. J Biol Chem 2003;278:21323–21326.
51. Katz M, Shtiegman K, Tal-Or P et al. Ligand-independent degradation of epidermal growth factor receptor involves receptor ubiquitylation and Hgs, an adaptor whose ubiquitin-interacting motif targets ubiquitylation by Nedd4. Traffic 2002;3:740–751.
52. Polo S, Sigismund S, Faretta M et al. A single motif responsible for ubiquitin recognition and monoubiquitination in endocytic proteins. Nature 2002;416:451–455.
53. Qiu XB, Goldberg AL. Nrdp1/FLRF is a ubiquitin ligase promoting ubiquitination and degradation of the epidermal growth factor receptor family member, ErbB3. Proc Natl Acad Sci USA 2002;99:14843–14848.

54. Waterman H, Sabanai I, Geiger B, Yarden Y. Alternative intracellular routing of ErbB receptors may determine signaling potency. J Biol Chem 1998;273:13819–13827.

55. Carpenter G. ErbB-4: mechanism of action and biology. Exp Cell Res 2003;284:66–77.

56. Vecchi M, Carpenter G. Constitutive proteolysis of the ErbB-4 receptor tyrosine kinase by a unique, sequential mechanism. J Cell Biol 1997;139:995–1003.

57. Rio C, Buxbaum JD, Peschon JJ, Corfas G. Tumor necrosis factor-alpha-converting enzyme is required for cleavage of erbB4/HER4. J Biol Chem 2000;275:10379–10387.

58. Ni CY, Murphy MP, Golde TE, Carpenter G. gamma-Secretase cleavage and nuclear localization of ErbB-4 receptor tyrosine kinase. Science 2001;294:2179–2181.

59. Ni CY, Yuan H, Carpenter G. Role of the ErbB-4 carboxyterminus in gamma -secretase cleavage. J Biol Chem 2002;25:25.

60. Miettinen P, Berger J, Meneses J et al. Epithelial immaturity and multiorgan faliure in mice lacking epidermal growth factor receptor. Nature 1995;376:337–341.

61. Sibilia, M, Wagner EF. Strain-dependent epithelial defects in mice lacking the EGF receptor. Science 1995;269:234–238.

62. Threadgill DW, Dlugosz AA, Hansen LA et al. Targeted disruption of mouse EGF receptor: effect of genetic background on mutant phenotype. Science 1995;269:230–234.

63. Lemke G. Neuregulins in development. Mol Cell Neurosci 1996;7:247–262.

64. Erickson SL, O'Shea KS, Ghaboosi N et al. ErbB3 is required for normal cerebellar and cardiac development: a comparison with ErbB2-and heregulin-deficient mice. Development 1997; 124:4999–5011.

65. Britsch S, Li L, Kirchhoff S et al. The ErbB2 and ErbB3 receptors and their ligand, neuregulin-1, are essential for development of the sympathetic nervous system. Genes Dev 1998;12:1825–1836.

66. Luetteke NC, Qiu TH, Peiffer RL et al. TGFa deficiency results in hair follicles and eye abnormalities in targeted and Waved-1 mice. Cell 1993;73:263–278.

67. Mann G, Fowler K, Gabriel A et al. Mice with null mutations of the TGFα gene have abnormal skin architecture, wavy hair, and curly whiskers and often develop corneal inflammation. Cell 1993;73:249–261.

68. Jackson LF, Qiu TH, Sunnarborg SW et al. Defective valvulogenesis in HB-EGF and TACE-null mice is associated with aberrant BMP signaling. EMBO J 2003;22:2704–2716.

69. Burden SJ. Building the vertebrate neuromuscular synapse. J Neurobiol 2002;53:501–511.

70. Garratt AN, Britsch S, Birchmeier C. Neuregulin, a factor with many functions in the life of a Schwann cell. Bioessays 2000;22:987–996.

71. Lee DC, Sunnarborg SW, Hinkle CL et al. TACE/ADAM17 processing of EGFR ligands indicates a role as a physiological convertase. Ann N Y Acad Sci 2003;995:22–38.

72. Schroeder JA, Lee DC. Dynamic expression and activation of ERBB receptors in the developing mouse mammary gland. Cell Growth Differ 1998;9:451–464.

73. Sandgren EP, Luetteke NC, Palmiter RD et al. Overexpression of TGFa in transgenic mice: induction of epithelial hyperplasia, pancreatic metaplasia and carcinoma of the breast. Cell 1990;61:1121–1135.

74. Matsui M, Halter SA, Holt JT et al. Development of mammary hyperplasia and neoplasia in MMTV-TGFa transgenic mice. Cell 1991;61:1147–1155.

75. Bouchard L, Lamarre L, Tremblay PJ, Jolicoeur P. Stochastic appearance of mammary tumors in transgenic mice carrying the MMTV/c-*neu* oncogene. Cell 1989;57:931–936.

76. Jones FE, Stern DF. Expression of dominant-negative ErbB2 in the mammary gland of transgenic mice reveals a role in lobuloalveolar development and lactation. Oncogene 1999;18: 3481–3490.

77. Jones FE, Welte T, Fu XY, Stern DF. ErbB4 signaling in the mammary gland is required for lobuloalveolar development and Stat5 activation during lactation. J Cell Biol 1999;147:77–88.

78. Muller W, Artega C, Muthuswamy S et al. Synergistic interaction of the neu proto-oncogene product and transforming growth factor alpha in the mammary epithelium of transgenic mice. Mol Cell Biol 1996;16:5726–5736.

79. Siegel PM, Dankort DL, Hardy WR, Muller WJ. Novel activating mutations in the neu proto-oncogene involved in induction of mammary tumors. Mol Cell Biol 1994;14:7068–7077.

80. Andrechek ER, Muller WJ. Tyrosine kinase signalling in breast cancer: tyrosine kinase-mediated signal transduction in transgenic mouse models of human breast cancer. Breast Cancer Res 2000;2:211–216.

81. Salomon DS, Brandt R, Ciardiello F, Normanno N. Epidermal growth factor-related peptides and their receptors in human malignancies. Crit Rev Oncol Hematol 1995;19:183–232.

82. Klapper LN, Kirschbaum MH, Sela M, Yarden Y. Biochemical and clinical implications of the ErbB/HER signaling network of growth factor receptors. Adv Cancer Res 2000;77:25–79.

83. Di Leo, A, Dowsett M, Horten B, Penault-Llorca F. Current status of HER2 testing. Oncology 2002;63(suppl 1):25–32.

84. DiGiovanna MP, Chu P, Davison TL et al. Active signaling by HER-2/neu in a subpopulation of HER-2/neu-overexpressing ductal carcinoma in situ: clinicopathological correlates. Cancer Res 2002;62:6667–6673.

85. Hoang MP, Sahin AA, Ordonez NG, Sneige N. HER-2/neu gene amplification compared with HER-2/neu protein overexpression and interobserver reproducibility in invasive breast carcinoma. Am J Clin Pathol 2000;113:852–859.

86. Lebeau A, Deimling D, Kaltz C et al. Her-2/neu analysis in archival tissue samples of human breast cancer: comparison of immunohistochemistry and fluorescence in situ hybridization. J Clin Oncol 2001;19:354–363.

87. Hynes NE, Stern DF. The biology of erbB-2/neu/HER-2 and its role in cancer. Biochem Biophys Acta 1994;1198:165–184.

88. Konecny G, Pauletti G, Pegram M et al. Quantitative association between HER-2/neu and steroid hormone receptors in hormone receptor-positive primary breast cancer. J Natl Cancer Inst 2003;95:142–153.

89. Schiff R, Massarweh S, Shou J, Osborne CK. Breast cancer endocrine resistance: how growth factor signaling and estrogen receptor coregulators modulate response. Clin Cancer Res 2003; 9(1 Pt 2):447S–54S.

90. Moscatello DK, Holgado-Madruga M, Godwin AK et al. Frequent expression of a mutant epidermal growth factor receptor in multiple human tumors. Cancer Res 1995;55:5536–5539.

91. Heimberger AB, Crotty LE, Archer GE et al. Epidermal growth factor receptor VIII peptide vaccination is efficacious against established intracerebral tumors. Clin Cancer Res 2003;9:4247–4254.

92. Wong AJ, Ruppert JM, Bigner SH et al. Structural alterations of the epidermal growth factor receptor gene in human gliomas. Proc Natl Acad Sci USA 1992;89:2965–2969.

93. Lammering G, Hewit TH, Valerie K et al. EGFRvIII-mediated radioresistance through a strong cytoprotective response. Oncogene 2003;22:5545–5553.

94. Xie D, Shu XO, Deng Z et al. Population-based, case-control study of HER2 genetic polymorphism and breast cancer risk. J Natl Cancer Inst 2000;92:412–417.

95. McKean-Cowdin R, Kolonel LN, Press MF et al. Germ-line HER-2 variant and breast cancer risk by stage of disease. Cancer Res 2001;61:8393–8394.

96. Kuraoka K, Matsumura S, Hamai Y et al. A single nucleotide polymorphism in the transmembrane domain coding region of HER-2 is associated with development and malignant phenotype of gastric cancer. Int J Cancer 2003;107:593–596.

97. Fleishman SJ, Schlessinger J, Ben-Tal N. A putative molecular-activation switch in the transmembrane domain of erbB2. Proc Natl Acad Sci USA 2002;99:15937–15940.

98. Franklin WA, Veve R, Hirsch FR et al. Epidermal growth factor receptor family in lung cancer and premalignancy. Semin Oncol 2002;29(suppl 4):3–14.

99. Sartor CI. Biological modifiers as potential radiosensitizers: targeting the epidermal growth factor receptor family. Semin Oncol 2000;27(suppl 11):15–20; discussion 92–100.

100. Fischer-Colbrie J, Witt A, Heinzl H et al. EGFR and steroid receptors in ovarian carcinoma: comparison with prognostic parameters and outcome of patients. Anticancer Res 1997;17: 613–619.

101. Ross JS, Fletcher JA, Linette GP et al. The Her-2/neu gene and protein in breast cancer 2003: biomarker and target of therapy. Oncologist 2003;8:307–325.

102. Ring A, Dowsett M. Human epidermal growth factor receptor-2 and hormonal therapies: clinical implications. Clin Breast Cancer 2003;4(Suppl 1):S34–S41.

103. Johnston SR, Head J, Pancholi S et al. Integration of signal transduction inhibitors with endocrine therapy: an approach to overcoming hormone resistance in breast cancer. Clin Cancer Res 2003;9(1 Pt 2):524S–532S.

104. Ellis MJ, Coop A, Singh B et al. Letrozole is more effective neoadjuvant endocrine therapy than tamoxifen for ErbB-1- and/or ErbB-2-positive, estrogen receptor-positive primary breast cancer: evidence from a phase III randomized trial. J Clin Oncol 2001;19:3808–3816.

105. Ravdin PM. Is Her2 of value in identifying patients who particularly benefit from anthracyclines during adjuvant therapy? A qualified yes. J Natl Cancer Inst Monogr 2001:30:80–84.

106. Paik S, Park C. HER-2 and choice of adjuvant chemotherapy in breast cancer. Semin Oncol 2001;28:332–335.

107. Ravdin P, Green S, Albain K et al. Initial report of the SWOG biological correlative study of c-erbB-2 expression as a predictor of outcome in a trial comparing adjuvant CAF T with tamoxifen alone. Proc ASCO 1998;17:97a.

108. Sparano JA. Taxanes for breast cancer: an evidence-based review of randomized phase II and phase III trials. Clin Breast Cancer 2000;1:32–40; discussion 41–42.

109. Baron AT, Lafky JM, Boardman CH et al. Serum sErbB1 and epidermal growth factor levels as tumor biomarkers in women with stage III or IV epithelial ovarian cancer. Cancer Epidemiol Biomarkers Prev 1999;8:129–137.

110. Lee H, Akita RW, Sliwkowski MX, Maihle NJ. A naturally occurring secreted human ErbB3 receptor isoform inhibits heregulin-stimulated activation of ErbB2, ErbB3, and ErbB4. Cancer Res 2001;61:4467–4473.

111. Molina MA, Saez R, Ramsey EE et al. NH(2)-terminal truncated HER-2 protein but not full-length receptor is associated with nodal metastasis in human breast cancer. Clin Cancer Res 2002;8:347–353.

112. Masui H, Kawamoto T, Sato JD et al. Growth inhibition of human tumor cells in athymic mice by anti-epidermal growth factor receptor monoclonal antibodies. Cancer Res 1984;44:1002–1007.

113. Schreiber AB, Lax I, Yarden Y et al. Monoclonal antibodies against receptor for epidermal growth factor induce early and delayed effects of epidermal growth factor. Proc Natl Acad Sci USA 1981;78:7535–7539.

114. Drebin JA, Stern DF, Link VC et al. Monoclonal antibodies identify a cell-surface antigen associated with an activated cellular oncogene. Nature 1984; 312:579–588.

115. Hudziak RM, Lewis GD, Winget M et al. p185HER2 monoclonal antibody has antiproliferative effects in vitro and sensitizes human breast tumor cells to tumor necrosis factor. Mol Cell Biol 1989;9:1165–1172.

116. Carter P, Presta L, Gorman CM et al. Humanization of an anti-p185HER2 antibody for human cancer therapy. Proc Natl Acad Sci USA 1992;89:4285–4289.

117. Cobleigh MA, Vogel CL, Tripathy D et al. Multinational study of the efficacy and safety of humanized anti-HER2 monoclonal antibody in women who have HER2-overexpressing metastatic breast cancer that has progressed after chemotherapy for metastatic disease. J Clin Oncol 1999;17:2639–2648.

118. Vogel CL, Cobleigh MA, Tripathy D et al. Efficacy and safety of trastuzumab as a single agent in first-line treatment of HER2-overexpressing metastatic breast cancer. J Clin Oncol 2002;20:719–726.

119. Slamon DJ, Leyland-Jones B, Shak S et al. Use of chemotherapy plus a monoclonal antibody against HER2 for metastatic breast cancer that overexpresses HER2. N Engl J Med 2001;344 :783–792.

120. Slamon D, Pegram M. Rationale for trastuzumab (Herceptin) in adjuvant breast cancer trials. Semin Oncol 2001;28(suppl 3):13–19.

121. Pietras RJ, Pegram MD, Finn RS et al. Remission of human breast cancer xenografts on therapy with humanized monoclonal antibody to HER-2 receptor and DNA-reactive drugs. Oncogene 1998;17:2235–2249.

122. Harari PM, Huang SM. Radiation response modification following molecular inhibition of epidermal growth factor receptor signaling. Semin Radiat Oncol 2001;11:281–289.

123. Ciardiello F, Tortora G. Epidermal growth factor receptor (EGFR) as a target in cancer therapy: understanding the role of receptor expression and other molecular determinants that could influence the response to anti-EGFR drugs. Eur J Cancer 2003;39:1348–1354.

124. Grunwald V, Hidalgo M. Development of the epidermal growth factor receptor inhibitor Tarceva (OSI-774). Adv Exp Med Biol 2003;532:235–246.

125. Mendelsohn J, Baselga J. Status of epidermal growth factor receptor antagonists in the biology and treatment of cancer. J Clin Oncol 2003;21:2787–2799.

126. Bonner JA, Ezekiel MP, Robert F et al. Continued response following treatment with IMC-C225, an EGFr-MoAb, combined with RT in advanced head and neck malignancies. Proc ASCO 2000;19:5F.

127. Burtness B, Li Y, Fllod W et al. Phase III trial comparing cisplatin (C) + placebo (P) + anti-epidermal growth factor antibody (EGF-R) C225 in patients (pts) with metastatic/recurrent head and neck cancer (HNC). Proc ASCO 2002;21:901.

128. Clynes RA, Towers TL, Presta LG, Ravetch JV. Inhibitory Fc receptors modulate in vivo cytoxicity against tumor targets. Nat Med 2000;6:443–446.

129. Hurwitz E, Stancovski I, Sela M, Yarden Y. Suppression and promotion of tumor growth by monoclonal antibodies to ErbB-2 differentially correlate with cellular uptake. Proc Nat Acad Sci USA 1995;92:3353–3357.

130. Spiridon CI, Ghetie MA, Uhr J et al. Targeting multiple Her-2 epitopes with monoclonal antibodies results in improved antigrowth activity of a human breast cancer cell line in vitro and in vivo. Clin Cancer Res 2002;8:1720–1730.

131. Fan Z, Mendelsohn J. Therapeutic application of anti-growth factor receptor antibodies. Curr Opin Oncol 1998;10:67–73.

132. Klapper LN, Vaisman N, Hurwitz E et al. A subclass of tumor-inhibitory monoclonal antibodies to ErbB-2/HER2 blocks crosstalk with growth factor receptors. Oncogene 1997;14:2099–2109.

133. Albanell J, Codony J, Rovira A et al. Mechanism of action of anti-HER2 monoclonal antibodies: scientific update on trastuzumab and 2C4. Adv Exp Med Biol 2003;532:253–268.

134. Posey JA, Raspet R, Verma U et al. A pilot trial of GM-CSF and MDX-H210 in patients with erbB-2-positive advanced malignancies. J Immunother 1999;22:371–379.

135. Lynch DH, Yang XD. Therapeutic potential of ABX-EGF: a fully human anti-epidermal growth factor receptor monoclonal antibody for cancer treatment. Semin Oncol 2002;29(suppl 4): 47–50.

136. Jungbluth AA, Stockert E, Huang HJ et al. A monoclonal antibody recognizing human cancers with amplification/overexpression of the human epidermal growth factor receptor. Proc Natl Acad Sci USA 2003;100:639–644.

137. Stamos J, Sliwkowski MX, Eigenbrot C, Structure of the epidermal growth factor receptor kinase domain alone and in complex with a 4-anilinoquinazoline inhibitor. J Biol Chem 2002;277: 46265–46272.

138. Gazit A, Osherov N, Posner I et al. Tyrphostins. 2. Heterocyclic and alpha-substituted benzylidenemalononitrile tyrphostins as potent inhibitors of EGF receptor and *Erb*B2/neu tyrosine kinases. J Med Chem 1991;34:1896–1907.

139. Fry DW, Bridges AJ, Denny WA et al. Specific, irreversible inactivation of the epidermal growth factor receptor and erbB2, by a new class of tyrosine kinase inhibitor. Proc Natl Acad Sci USA 1998;95:12022–12027.

140. Gilmore AP, Valentijn AJ, Wang P et al. Activation of BAD by therapeutic inhibition of epidermal growth factor receptor and transactivation by insulin-like growth factor receptor. J Biol Chem 2002;277:27643–27650.

141. Ciardiello F, Caputo R, Bianco R et al. Antitumor effect and potentiation of cytotoxic drugs activity in human cancer cells by ZD-1839 (Iressa), an epidermal growth factor receptor-selective tyrosine kinase inhibitor. Clin Cancer Res 2000;6:2053–2063.

142. Dancey JE, Freidlin B. Targeting epidermal growth factor receptor—are we missing the mark? Lancet 2003;362:62–64.

143. Giaccone G, Johnson DH, Manegold C et al. A phase III clinical trial of ZD1839 ('Iressa') in combination with gemcitabine and cisplatin in chemotherapy naive patients with advanced non-small-cell lung cancer (INTACT1). Am Oncol 2002;13(suppl 5):2(abstract 40).

144. Johnson DH, Herbst RS, Giaccone G et al. ZD1839 ('Iressa') in combination with paclitaxel and carboplatin in chemotherapy-naive patients with advanced non-small-cell lung cancere (NSCLC): results from a phase III clinical trial (INTACT2). Am Oncol 2002;13(suppl 5):128 (abstract 4680).

145. Neckers L. Hsp90 inhibitors as novel cancer chemotherapeutic agents. Trends Mol Med 2002;8:S55–S61.

146. Xu W, Mimnaugh E, Rosser MF et al. Sensitivity of mature Erbb2 to geldanamycin is conferred by its kinase domain and is mediated by the chaperone protein Hsp90. J Biol Chem 2001;276: 3702–3708.

147. Tikhomirov O, Carpenter G. Identification of ErbB-2 kinase domain motifs required for geldanamycin-induced degradation. Cancer Res 2003;63:39–43.

148. Zheng FF, Kuduk SD, Chiosis G et al. Identification of a geldanamycin dimer that induces the selective degradation of HER-family tyrosine kinases. Cancer Res 2000;60:2090–2094.

149. Citri A, Alroy I, Lavi S et al. Drug-induced ubiquitylation and degradation of ErbB receptor tyrosine kinases: implications for cancer therapy. EMBO J 2002;21:2407–2417.

150. Blagosklonny MV, Fojo T, Bhalla KN et al. The Hsp90 inhibitor geldanamycin selectively sensitizes Bcr-Abl-expressing leukemia cells to cytotoxic chemotherapy. Leukemia 2001;15: 1537–1543.

151. Nguyen DM, Lorang D, Chen GA et al. Enhancement of paclitaxel-mediated cytotoxicity in lung cancer cells by 17-allylamino geldanamycin: in vitro and in vivo analysis. Ann Thorac Surg 2001;72:371–378; discussion 378–379.

152. Downward J. Targeting RAS signalling pathways in cancer therapy. Nat Rev Cancer 2003;3: 11–22.

153. Wang, SC, Zhang L, Hortobagyi GN, Hung MC. Targeting HER2: recent developments and future directions for breast cancer patients. Semin Oncol 2001;28(suppl 18):21–29.

154. Chen CH, Chernis GA, Hoang VQ, Landgraf R. Inhibition of heregulin signaling by an aptamer that preferentially binds to the oligomeric form of human epidermal growth factor receptor-3. Proc Natl Acad Sci USA 2003;100:9226–9231.

155. Bernhard H, Salazar L, Schiffman K et al. Vaccination against the HER-2/neu oncogenic protein. Endocr Relat Cancer 2002;9:33–44.

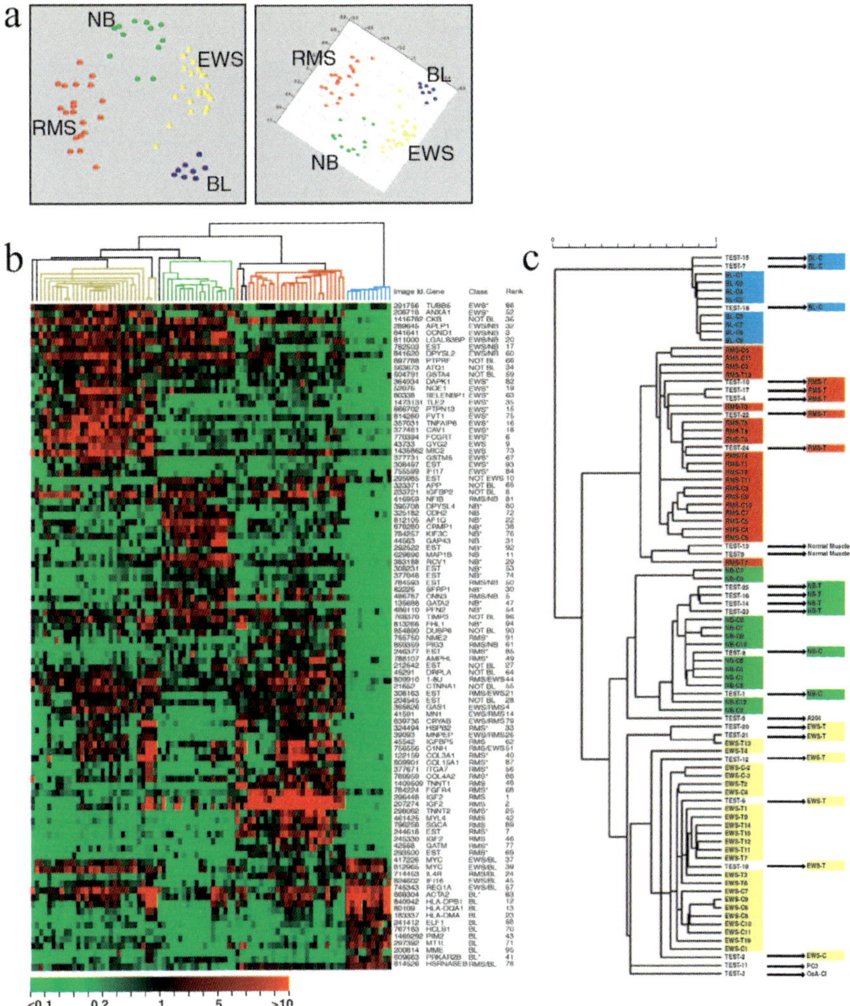

FIGURE 2.4

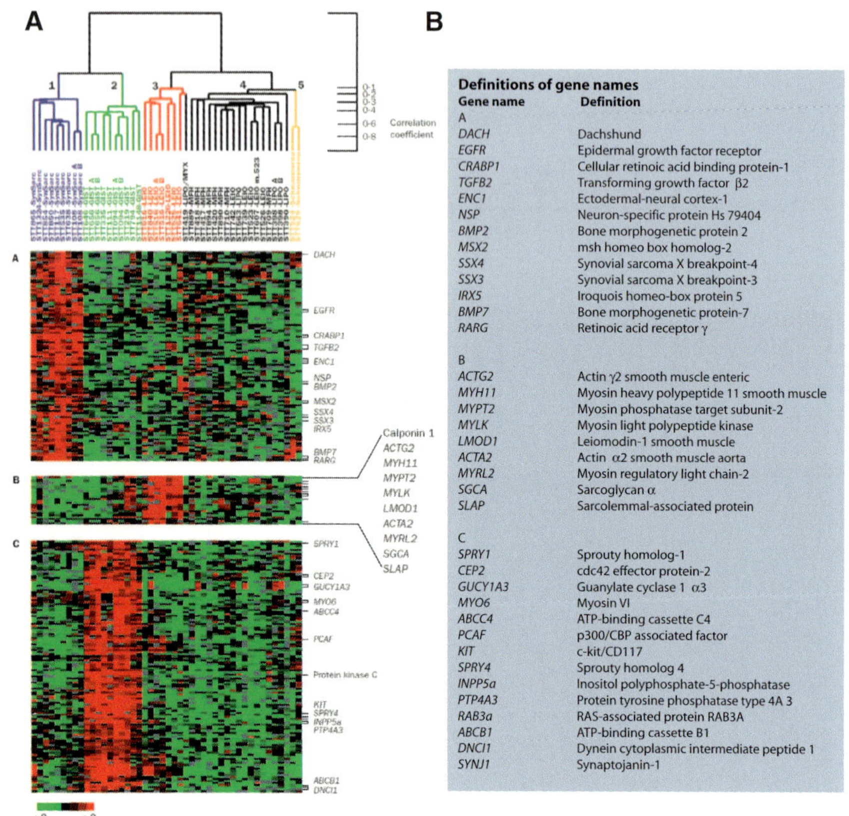

Definitions of gene names

Gene name	Definition
A	
DACH	Dachshund
EGFR	Epidermal growth factor receptor
CRABP1	Cellular retinoic acid binding protein-1
TGFB2	Transforming growth factor β2
ENC1	Ectodermal-neural cortex-1
NSP	Neuron-specific protein Hs 79404
BMP2	Bone morphogenetic protein 2
MSX2	msh homeo box homolog-2
SSX4	Synovial sarcoma X breakpoint-4
SSX3	Synovial sarcoma X breakpoint-3
IRX5	Iroquois homeo-box protein 5
BMP7	Bone morphogenetic protein-7
RARG	Retinoic acid receptor γ
B	
ACTG2	Actin γ2 smooth muscle enteric
MYH11	Myosin heavy polypeptide 11 smooth muscle
MYPT2	Myosin phosphatase target subunit-2
MYLK	Myosin light polypeptide kinase
LMOD1	Leiomodin-1 smooth muscle
ACTA2	Actin α2 smooth muscle aorta
MYRL2	Myosin regulatory light chain-2
SGCA	Sarcoglycan α
SLAP	Sarcolemmal-associated protein
C	
SPRY1	Sprouty homolog-1
CEP2	cdc42 effector protein-2
GUCY1A3	Guanylate cyclase 1 α3
MYO6	Myosin VI
ABCC4	ATP-binding cassette C4
PCAF	p300/CBP associated factor
KIT	c-kit/CD117
SPRY4	Sprouty homolog 4
INPP5a	Inositol polyphosphate-5-phosphatase
PTP4A3	Protein tyrosine phosphatase type 4A 3
RAB3a	RAS-associated protein RAB3A
ABCB1	ATP-binding cassette B1
DNCI1	Dynein cytoplasmic intermediate peptide 1
SYNJ1	Synaptojanin-1

FIGURE 2.5

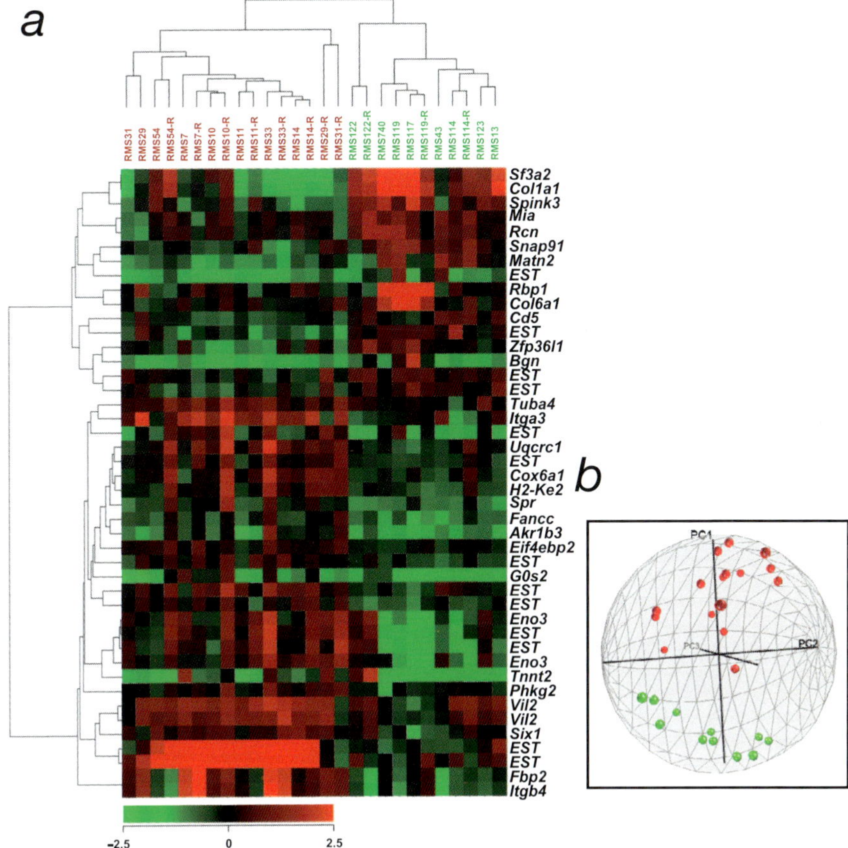
a
RMS31
RMS29
RMS54
RMS54-R
RMS7
RMS7-R
RMS10
RMS10-R
RMS11
RMS11-R
RMS33
RMS33-R
RMS14
RMS14-R
RMS29-R
RMS31-R
RMS122
RMS122-R
RMS740
RMS119
RMS117
RMS119-R
RMS43
RMS114
RMS114-R
RMS123
RMS13
Sf3a2
Col1a1
Spink3
Mia
Rcn
Snap91
Matn2
EST
Rbp1
Col6a1
Cd5
EST
Zfp36l1
Bgn
EST
EST
Tuba4
Itga3
EST
Uqcrc1
EST
Cox6a1
H2-Ke2
Spr
Fancc
Akr1b3
Eif4ebp2
EST
G0s2
EST
EST
Eno3
EST
EST
Eno3
Tnnt2
Phkg2
Vil2
Vil2
Six1
EST
EST
Fbp2
Itgb4
-2.5
0
2.5
b
PC1
PC2
PC3

FIGURE 2.6

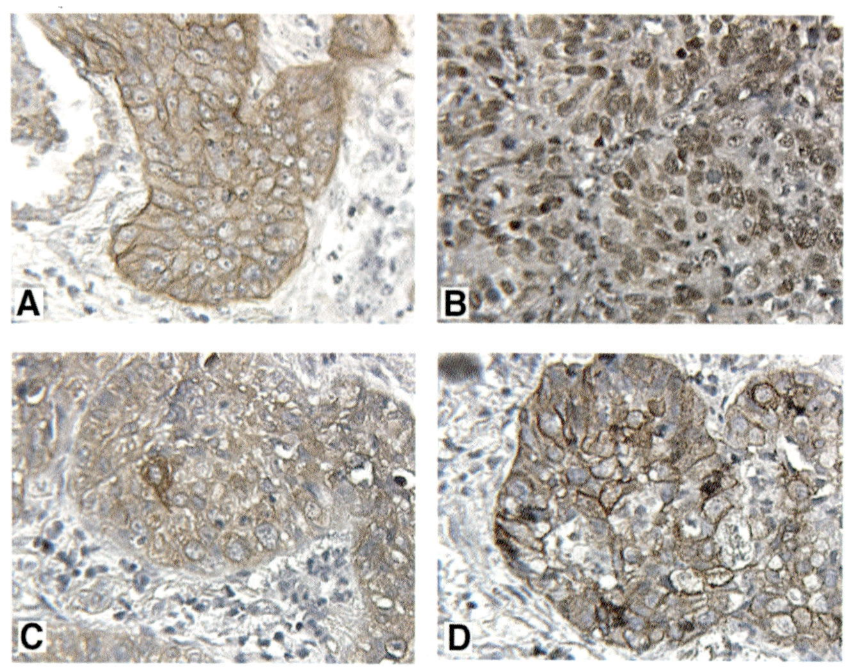

FIGURE 4.2

Targeting the Epidermal Growth Factor Receptor in the Clinic

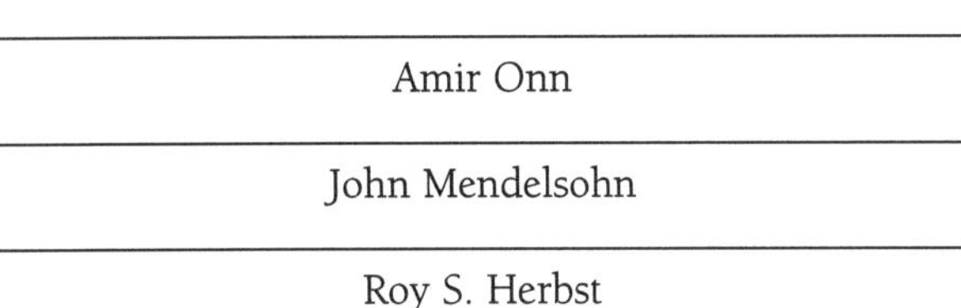
Amir Onn

John Mendelsohn

Roy S. Herbst

Advances in our understanding of cancer biology have led to the discovery of a number of potential molecular targets and the development of novel, biologically targeted agents that, unlike conventional cytotoxic agents, specifically target tumor cells.[1–3] Two such therapies include imatinib, a small molecule inhibitor of the intracellular tyrosine kinase BCR-ABL, which was approved by the Food and Drug Administration for the treatment of chronic myeloid leukemia in 2001, and the monoclonal antibody trastuzumab, which targets a membrane-bound growth factor receptor and was approved in 1998 for the treatment of metastatic breast cancer.

In parallel, agents have been developed to target the epidermal growth factor receptor (EGFR) signaling pathway, which is activated in many tumor cells but strictly controlled in normal cells.[3,4] The EGFR family comprises EGFR (HER1), HER2, HER3, and HER4, which are present in the cell as inactive monomers and, upon ligand binding, form homodimers or heterodimers. This results in autophosphorylation of the intracellular tyrosine kinase domains and activation of signaling pathways that induce tumorigenic processes such as proliferation, angiogenesis, metastatic spread, and decreased apoptosis (Figure 4.1).[2,5] Heterodimerization of EGFR with HER2, which share 80% homology, is the preferred option and, in comparison with other heterodimers, has a longer and greater proliferative signal.[2,6]

The EGFR is highly expressed in a number of common solid tumors and at all disease stages.[7] The proportion of tumors expressing EGFR varies within tumor type (Table 4.1),[3] and may be due to different detection methods or because no accepted standards define normal or elevated levels of expression.[8] High levels of expression have been associated with poor outcome in many solid tumors; however, this is controversial in lung cancer.[3,8,9] Between 25-30% of invasive breast cancers have increased expression of HER2, which has been correlated with poor disease-free survival, and resistance to chemotherapy and endocrine therapy.[10-14]

The EGFR was proposed as an anticancer target following preclinical studies with monoclonal antibodies raised against the EGFR of A431, a human epider-

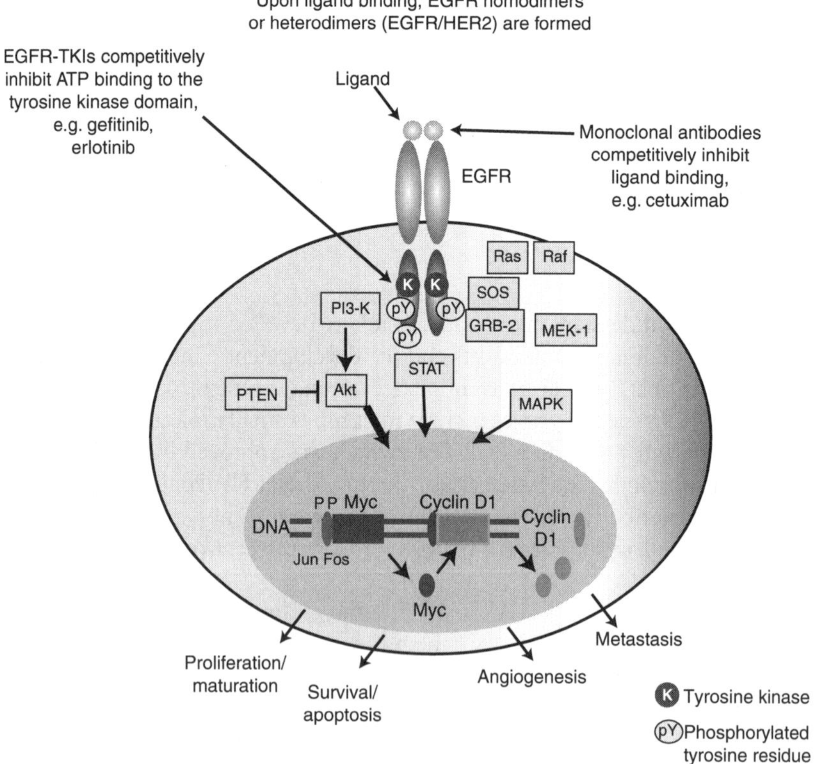

FIGURE 4.1 EGFR signaling pathway and inhibition by EGFR-targeted agents. Adapted with permission from AlphaMed Press ©.[29]

TABLE 4.1 List of Human Cancers That Express EGFR and the Percentage of Expression.[a]

Tumor Type	Expression	Prognostic significance
NSCLC	40–80	Potentially shorter overall survival, although this is controversial
Head and neck	80–100	Shorter disease-free and overall survival
Renal cell	50–90	Poor prognosis, shorter survival in positive tumors
Bladder	31–46	More prevalent in recurrent invasive tumors
Gastric	40	Shorter survival in tumors positive for TGF-α and EGFR
Pancreatic	30–50	Coexpression with ligands was associated with reduced survival
Colon	25–77	Higher proportion of tumor cells expressing EGFR was associated with poor patient outcome
Breast	14–91	Associated with worse overall survival and steroid-receptor-negative tumors
Ovary	35–70	Associated with reduced disease-free survival, overall survival, and drug resistance
Glioma	40–50	Most common tumor exhibiting the EGFR VIII mutation

NSCLC, non-small-cell lung cancer; TGF-α, transforming growth factor α; EGFR, epidermal growth factor receptor
[a]Reprinted with permission from Elsevier.[3]

moid carcinoma cell line.[15-17] Based on structure and function, two main approaches have developed inhibitors to block EGFR signaling. One approach was to develop orally active EGFR–TKIs (EGFR tyrosine kinase inhibitors). These competitively inhibit adenosine triphosphate binding to the TK domain of the receptor, directly inhibiting EGFR autophosphorylation. Examples include gefitinib (Iressa[a] ZDI839), erlotinib (Tarceva,[b] OSI-774), CI-1033, PKI-1066, GW2016, and EKB-569. Apart from CI-I033 and EKB-569, the EGFR-TKIs have a reversible mechanism of action.[2] Additionally, both CI–1033 and GW20/16 can inhibit the EGFR and HER2 kinases directly, with potential therapeutic advantages in HER2-dependent breast cancer tumors.[4,18,19]

Preclinical data showing antitumor activity in cancer cell lines and human tumor xenografts have provided a rationale for the clinical development of these

[a]Iressa is a trademark of AstraZeneca.
[b]Tarceva is a trademark of OSI Pharmaceuticals, Inc.

agents.[5,20–22] Currently, both gefitinib and erlotinib are in Phase III development, while the other EGFR-TKIs listed are in Phase I development. In 2002, based on promising results from Phase II trials involving patients with non-small-cell lung cancer (NSCLC), gefitinib became the first approved EGFR-targeted agent for use in patients with previously treated advanced NSCLC in Japan, followed by the USA and other countries in 2003.

An alternative approach developed monoclonal antibodies such as cetuximab (Erbitux,[c] IMC-C225) that are administered intravenously. Cetuximab recognizes the EGFR's extracellular domain, competes for ligand binding, and indirectly inhibits EGFR-TK.[23] In preclinical studies, cetuximab inhibits EGFR signaling in EGFR–dependent cells[24–26] and has antitumor activity against human tumor xenografts.[5,16,22,27,28] Cetuximab is in Phase III development, while other humanized monoclonal antibodies, EMD72000, ABX–EGF and h-R3, are in Phase I/II clinical development.[2,4]

Alternative strategies to target the EGFR include bispecific antibodies such as MDX-447 that also target epitopes on the surface of immune cells, cytotoxic single-chain fragment variable antibodies conjugated to toxins, EGF vaccines such as EGF-P64k, and antisense oligonucleotides that block translation of the EGFR or its ligands (Figure 4.1).[29]

CLINICAL TRIALS

Cytotoxic agents are relatively nonselective, therefore antitumor activity and toxic effects generally occur within a similar dose range, and in clinical trials the maximum tolerated dose (MTD) is the surrogate endpoint for potential antitumor activity. For biologically targeted agents, the optimum biologic dose (OBD; the dose at which the target molecule is maximally inhibited) often has greater clinical relevance and may be below the MTD. The three agents furthest on in clinical development, gefitinib, erlotinib, and cetuximab, have been investigated in patients with a range of tumor types (Tables 4.2 and 4.3). However, this chapter will concentrate on those tumors for which substantial clinical data are available: NSCLC; squamous-cell carcinoma of the head and neck (SCCHN); breast cancer. For completeness, Table 4.4 summarizes Phase I/II clinical trials involving other EGFR-TKIs and monoclonal antibodies.

Monotherapy

Gefitinib In four Phase I studies, gefitinib demonstrated favorable tolerability and encouraging antitumor activity, particularly in patients with NSCLC. On this basis, two large-scale, multicenter, dose-randomized, double-blind, parallel-group Phase II trials (Iressa Dose Evaluation in Advanced Lung cancer [IDEAL]

[c]Erbitux is a trademark of ImClone Systems, Inc.

TABLE 4.2 Ongoing Phase II/III Monotherapy Trials

Agent (Phase)	Tumor Type	No. of Patients	Dose (mg/day)	Regimen	Toxicities	Activity	Reference	Comments
Gefitinib (II)	SCCHN	30	250	Once daily	Skin, anorexia, nausea, diarrhea, dyspnea, increased transaminases, hypercalcemia	PR 1; SD 8	90	Patients must have recurrent of metastatic disease not amenable to curative therapy
Gefitinib (II)	Breast	33	500	Loading dose of 1000 mg on day 1, then 500 mg once daily	Rash, diarrhea, nausea, vomiting, alopecia, lethargy	ER-positive: PR 1, SD 5; ER-negative: PR 1, SD 1	40	
Gefitinib (II)	Breast	58	500	Once daily	Facial rash, nausea, vomiting, bowel disturbance, pruritus, peripheral edema, weakness. Grade 3: exanthema, diarrhea, noninfectious wound	PR 1	42	Patients must have received previous chemotherapy
Gefitinib (II)	Glioblastoma	57	500	Patients receive gefitinib once daily plus dexamethasone and/or CYP3A4 escalated to 1000 mg every 4 weeks	Rash, diarrhea	PR 1, SD 22	91	
Gefitinib (II)	Ovarian or primary peritoneal	27	500	Once daily	Grade 3/4: neutropenia, dermatological, diarrhea, nausea, vomiting, dyspepsia, hypokalemia, metabolic, pain, infection, constitutional stomatitis	PR/SD 4	92	Patients must have recurrent or persistent disease
Gefitinib (II)	Cervical	15	500	Once daily	Grade 3/4: diarrhea, dyspnea	SD 4	93	
Gefitinib (II)	Renal	28	500	Once daily	Skin rash, diarrhea. Grade 3/4 neutropenia, diarrhea (1 patient each)	SD 13	94	

(continued)

TABLE 4.2 ***Continued***

Agent (Phase)	Tumor Type	No. of Patients	Dose (mg/day)	Regimen	Toxicities	Activity	Reference	Comments
Gefitinib (II)	Renal	21	500	Once daily	Skin, diarrhea, fatigue, bleeding, pain, nausea, neurology, brain metastases, eyes, edema, cough, shortness of breath, constipation, anorexia, alopecia, reflux, vomiting, infection	SD 8	95	Stage IV or inoperable recurrent renal-cell carcinoma
Gefitinib (II)	Gastric	75	250 or 500	Once daily	Diarrhea, rash, anorexia	PR 1 (250 mg/day), SD 12 (4 250 mg/day; 8 500 mg/day)	96	
Gefitinib (II)	Prostate	51	500	Once daily	Rash, diarrhea	PSA 1 (PSA with a ≥50% decrease in serum PSA compared with trial entry)	97	
Gefitinib (II)	Malignant mesothelioma	43	500	Once daily	Grade 3/4 dehydration. Grade 3 diarrhea, nausea, vomiting, fatigue, skin rash, increased alanine aminotransferase	PR 2%, SD 46%	98	
Erlotinib (II)	Esophageal	13	150	Once daily over 4 week treatment cycles	Dermatological, fatigue, nausea, hepatic (grade 3)	SD 1	99	
Erlotinib (II)	Hepatocellular and biliary carcinomas	46	150	Once daily for 28 days	Grade 3/4: nausea, vomiting, fatigue, skin rash, bilirubin, dyspnea, hypokalemia, hypotension, sensory neuropathy, weight loss	NA	100	Patients must have unresectable disease

SCCHN, squamous-cell carcinoma of the head and neck; PR, partial response, SD, stable disease; ER, estrogen receptor; PSA, prostate-specific antigen; NA, not available

TABLE 4.3 Ongoing Phase II/III Combination Trials

Agent (Phase)	Tumor Type	No. of Patients	Dose	Regimen	Toxicities	Activity	Reference	Comments
Gefitinib (II)	NSCLC	Group A: 24; group B: 6	Gefitinib 250 mg/day; docetaxel 75 mg/m^2	Gefitinib administered once daily; docetaxel administered once every 3 weeks	Diarrhea, rash, dry skin, nausea, asthenia, alopecia, mucositis, erythema, dry eyes, increased transminases, neuropathy, pruritus, psoriasis, vomiting	Group A: PR 6, SD 8; group B: SD 4	56	Group A consists of patients who have progressed during or after platinum-based chemotherapy. Group B includes patients unsuitable for platinum-based chemotherapy
Gefitinib (II)	Breast	9	Gefitinib 250 mg/day; epidoxorubicin 20–40 mg/m^2	Gefitinib administered once daily. Epidoxorubicin is administered once weekly for 6 weeks, followed by a 2-week rest period	Vomiting, nausea, diarrhea, constipation, skin rash, dyspnea, asthenia, leukopenia, neutropenia, anemia	PR 1, SD 3	57	Part A is recruiting patients to determine the MTD of epidoxorubicin in combination with gefitinib. Part B will investigate response
Gefitinib (II)	Colorectal	Group A: 16; group B:16	Gefitinib 55 mg/day	Cycle 1 FOLFOX-4. Cycle 2 FOLFOX-4 with gefitinib. Each cycle consists of 14 days	Grade 3/4 diarrhea, nausea, neutropenia, vomiting	Group A: PR 9/12; group B: 3/13	101	Group A consists of patients who have not undergone prior therapy for metastatic disease. Group B consists of patients who have had prior therapy for metastatic disease
Erlotinib (II)	Ovarian	34	Erlotinib 150 mg/day; carboplatin AUC=5	Erlotinib administered once daily; carboplatin administered every 21 days	Acneiform rash, fatigue, diarrhea, nausea, dry skin	NA	102	Patients must have received ≤2 prior chemotherapy regimens, the first of which contained platinum
Cetuximab (I/II)	NSCLC	35	Cetuximab loading dose 400 mg/m^2, then weekly at 250 mg/m^2. Carboplatin (AUC=5 day one), gemcitabine 1000 mg/m^2	Cetuximab administered weekly. Carboplatin and gemcitabine administered every 3 weeks	Acneiform rash, dry skin, fatigue, anemia, thrombocytopenia, leukopenia, infection	PR 8, SD 14	62	Patients must have stage IV EGFR-positive NSCLC and have received no prior chemotherapy

((*continued*)

TABLE 4.3 Continued

Agent (Phase)	Tumor Type	No. of Patients	Dose	Regimen	Toxicities	Activity	Reference	Comments
Cetuximab (I/II)	NSCLC	31	Cetuximab loading dose 400 mg/m^2, then weekly at 250 mg/m^2. Paclitaxel 225 mg/m^2. Carboplatin (AUC=6)	Cetuximab administered weekly; chemotherapy administered every 3 weeks	Acneiform rash, hypersensitivity, fever/chills, nausea/vomiting, mucositis/stomatitis, diarrhea, fatigue/malaise, leukopenia/neutropenia, myalgia/arthraligia, neuropathy, pulmonary embolus	PR 9, SD 11	61	Chemonaive patients with stage IV NSCLC
Cetuximab (II)	Colorectal	Low-dose group 6; high-dose group 15	Cetuximab loading dose 400 mg/m^2, then weekly at 250 mg/m^2; irinotecan 80 mg/m^2, folinic acid 500 mg/m^2, 5-FU 1500 mg/m^2 in low-dose group and 2000 mg/m^2 in high-dose group	Both cetuximab and chemotherapy were administered weekly for 6 weeks	NA	PR 2, SD 12	103	
Cetuximab (II)	Nasopharyngeal carcinoma	56	Cetuximab loading dose of 400 mg/m^2 initially followed by 250 mg/m^2; carboplatin AUC=5	Cetuximab administered weekly; carboplatin administered every 3 weeks	Skin rash, nausea, vomiting, asthenia, anemia, thrombocytopenia	PR 9, PR 1 (not confirmed), SD 25	104	Patients with disease progression on or within 12 months after the end of platinum-based chemotherapy
Cetuximab (II)	Colorectal	18	Cetuximab loading dose of 400 mg/m^2 initially followed by 250 mg/m^2; irinotecan 180 mg/m^2; folinic acid 400 mg/m^2; 5-FU low-dose group 300 mg/m^2 (bolus) and infusional 2000 $mg/m^2/46$ h or 5-FU high-dose group 400 mg/m^2 (bolus) and infusional 2400 $mg/m^2/46$ h	Cetuximab administered weekly; FOLFIRI administered every 2 weeks	3 DLTs in high-dose group	PR 12, SD 4	105	

NSCLC, non-small-cell lung cancer; PR, partial respnose; SD, stable disease; MTD, maximum tolerated dose; EGFR, epidermal growth factor receptor; NA, not available

TABLE 4.4 Clinical Trials Involving Additional EGFR-TKIs and Monoclonal Antibodies.[a]

Agent (Phase)	Tumor Type	No. of Patients	Dose (mg/day)	Regimen	MTD	Toxicities	Activity	Reference	Comments
EGFR-TKIs									
CI-1033 (I)	Several	68	2–220	Days 1–14, then every 3 wks Days 1–21, then every 4 wks Days 1–28; then every 5 wks	NA	Stomatitis, skin rash	NA	106	
CI-1033 (I)	Several	34	100–560	Weekly for 3 wks, then every 4 wks	NA	Diarrhea, nausea, hypersensitivity	SD 2.9%	107	
PKI-166 (I)	Thyroid, renal, A-CUP, others	16 25	50–400 50–900	M-W-F Days 1–14, then every 2 wks	50 mg/day	Transaminase elevations, diarrhea, skin rash, nausea, vomiting	SD 18.7% SD 4.0%	108 109	DLT reached at 400 mg (M-W-F) and 900 mg (2 wks on, 2 wks off)
PKI-166 (I)	Colorectal, SCCHN, NSCLC	32	50–600	Continuous for at least 4 wks	NA	Transaminase elevations, diarrhea, skin rash, fatigue	PR 3%, SD 9%	110	
EKB-569 (I)	Colorectal, breast, SCCHN, NSCLC	30 11	25–125 24–50	Days 1–14, then every 4 wks continuous	75 mg/day	Diarrhea, skin rash, nausea, vomiting, stomatitis	NA	111	

((continued)

TABLE 4.4 Continued

Agent (Phase)	Tumor Type	No. of Patients	Dose (mg/day)	Regimen	MTD	Toxicities	Activity	Reference	Comments
Monoclonal antibodies									
EMD72000 (I)	SCCHN, colorectal, esophageal, cervical, others	22	400–2000 mg/wk	Weekly for 5 wks	1600 mg/wk	Headache, fever (dose limiting)	PR 23%, SD 17%	112	EGFR-expressing tumors
h-R3 (I)	SCCHN	12	Part A: 50–400 mg/wk	Weekly for 6 wks plus radiotherapy (60–66 Gy)	Not reached	Tremor, fever, chills, hypotension	CR 67%	113	Patients with advanced locoregional disease
		10	Part B: 200–400 mg/wk						
ABX-EGF (I)	Renal, prostate, NSCLC, pancreatic, esophageal, colorectal	33	0.01–2.5 mg/kg 1.0–2.5 mg/kg	Weekly for 4 wks, then every other wk	Not reached	Skin rash	MR 3%, SD 6%	114	EGFR-expressing tumors in part B
ABX-EGF (II)	Renal	88		Weekly	Not reached	Rigors, vomiting, diarrhea, skin rash	PR/MR 6%, SD 50%	115	20 patients per dose level planned in part 1 of the study; 40 additional patients will be treated with the two highest dose levels

NSCLC, non-small-cell lung cancer; SCCHN, squamous-cell carcinoma of the head and neck; OR, objective response; SD, stable disease; M-W-F, Monday, Wednesday, Friday; DLT, dose-limiting toxicity; NA not available; PR, partial response; EGFR, epidermal growth factor receptor; CR, complete response; MR, minor response

[a]Reprinted by permission of Oxford University Press.[2]

1 and 2) evaluated gefitinib 250 and 500 mg/day administered as monotherapy in patients with locally advanced or metastatic NSCLC.[30,31] Patients in IDEAL 1 (N = 209) had received one or two prior chemotherapy regimens, at least one of which contained platinum, while patients in IDEAL 2 (N = 216) had received at least two prior regimens, including platinum and docetaxel given either concurrently or separately. Both doses are much lower than the MTD of ≥700 mg/day; the 250 mg/day dose is higher than the lowest dose at which objective tumor regression was observed in Phase I studies, while 500 mg/day is the highest dose that was well tolerated over a long period. The two doses showed similar efficacy (Table 4.5) and treatment was generally well tolerated, with the majority of adverse events being National Cancer Institute Common Toxicity Criteria mild/moderate grade 1/2. The most common adverse events were an acneiform skin rash (47% and 43% in IDEAL 1 and 2, respectively) and diarrhea (40% and 48%, respectively). The 250 mg/day dose was associated with better tolerability and is therefore the recommended dose for patients with NSCLC.

By June 2003, over 37,000 NSCLC patients had received gefitinib monotherapy (250 mg/day) as part of the global Expanded Access Programme (EAP) allowing gefitinib to be given on a compassionate-use basis to cancer patients with no other treatment options. Data from this program have confirmed the antitumor activity and favorable tolerability of gefitinib monotherapy in this setting.[32–36]

An association was reported between EGFR expression and nonmucinous bronchioalveolar carcinoma (BAC) tumors, a histologic subtype of NSCLC that does not respond well to cytotoxic chemotherapy.[37] Preliminary data from a Phase II trial with gefitinib 500 mg/day show a response rate of 20% and 12%, and a median overall survival of 15 and 10 months for previously untreated and

TABLE 4.5 Efficacy Data from the IDEAL Trials

	IDEAL 1 1 or 2 Prior Regimens	IDEAL 2 ≥ 2 Prior Regimens
Response rate, %	18.4	11.8
Symptom improvement rate,[a] %	40.3	43.1
Disease control rate (partial response + stable disease), %	54.4	42.2
Median progression-free survival, months	2.7	1.9
Median overall survival, months	7.6	6.5

[a]Measured by the Lung Cancer Subscale of the Functional Assessment of Cancer Therapy-Lung questionnaire.[116]

treated patients, respectively. Both groups had a median progression-free survival of 4 months.[38]

Gefitinib (500 mg/day) showed antitumor activity in a Phase II study of patients with recurrent or metastatic SCCHN who had a poor prognosis and few treatment options. The response rate was 10.6% and the disease control rate (complete response + partial response + stable disease) was 53%, while median time to progression and survival were 3.4 and 8.1 months, respectively. Diarrhea was the only grade 3 toxicity, affecting 3 patients.[39] In patients with breast cancer, Phase II trials demonstrated that gefitinib monotherapy (500 mg/day) has antitumor activity and is well tolerated in both acquired tamoxifen-resistant estrogen-receptor (ER)-positive and ER-negative disease (Table 4.2).[40] In a second study, 10 of the 31 evaluable patients had disease stabilization for ≥ 3 months.[41] Gefitinib monotherapy was also generally well tolerated in patients with refractory breast cancer who had failed on previous chemotherapy. Although only 1 patient experienced a partial response, treatment was associated with an improved quality of life (35/52 evaluable patients) (Table 4.2).[42]

Erlotinib From Phase I studies involving 27 patients with advanced solid tumors, erlotinib 150 mg/day was the recommended dose for Phase II/III trials.[43,44] In Phase II studies, erlotinib showed promising antitumor activity in patients with advanced EGFR-expressing NSCLC that had progressed following platinum-based combination chemotherapy. Of the 57 patients enrolled into the study, 2 had a complete response, 5 had a partial response, and 22 had disease stabilization. The 1-year survival rate was 40%. The most common erlotinib-related adverse events were grade 1/2 maculopapular acneiform rash (67%), diarrhea (56%), dry skin (35%), and pruritus (35%).[45] Erlotinib 150 mg/day is also being investigated in patients with BAC. A partial response was observed in 9 of the 56 evaluable patients. Treatment was generally well tolerated, with common adverse events being rash and diarrhea.[46] In addition, erlotinib has promising activity in patients with recurrent SCCHN following previous induction therapy. Of the 78 patients evaluable for response, 13% had a partial response and 29% had disease stabilization. The most common adverse event was acneiform rash (72% of patients).[47] Preliminary results from a Phase II trial involving patients with metastatic colorectal cancer found that although 32% of patients had stable disease, treatment was associated with 24 grade 3 adverse events, including rash, diarrhea, nausea and vomiting, and 2 grade 4 adverse events of constipation.[48] This contrasts with the other trials, in which erlotinib treatment was generally well tolerated.

Cetuximab For cetuximab, a dosing schedule consisting of a loading dose of 400 mg/m^2 followed by a weekly maintenance dose of 250 mg/m^2 was selected for Phase II/III trials.[49] The most common adverse events are acneiform rash and allergic reactions[50]; the latter (grade 3/4) affect less than 4% of patients and typically occur during first infusion.[50]

Most Phase II clinical trials have involved cetuximab administered as combination therapy, but a number have assessed it as a single agent. A Phase II trial involving cetuximab administered as monotherapy is currently recruiting patients with NSCLC, and the results are awaited with interest. An additional Phase II trial has investigated the effect of cetuximab monotherapy in patients with EGFR-positive colorectal cancer that is refractory to both 5-fluorouracil and CPT-11. Treatment was well tolerated, with a partial response of 11% and a disease control rate of 33%.[51]

Safety of EGFR-targeted Agents

In clinical trials, these biologically targeted agents have been shown to be well tolerated. In particular, they are not generally associated with the severe hematologic toxicities that frequently occur with standard chemotherapy. The most common adverse events for EGFR-TKIs are skin and gastrointestinal toxicities, which resolve spontaneously in many cases. Gastrointestinal toxicities are dose limiting for these agents. However, if these adverse events do not spontaneously resolve, they can often be managed using suitable intentions (Table 4.6). Clinical trials with monoclonal antibodies first reported the acneiform rash associated with EGFR inhibitors, but the antibodies do not cause gastrointestinal toxicities. Recent reports from Japan have questioned the association of gefitinib with interstitial lung disease (ILD),[52] since a higher incidence has been observed in 39,600 Japanese patients treated with gefitinib (1.86%) compared with 53,150 patients treated worldwide (0.34%).[53] This may be due to increased awareness of ILD in Japan, differences in environmental exposures, or increased genetic susceptibility.

Combination Therapy with Conventional Chemotherapy

Preclinical studies combining EGFR-targeted therapies with either chemotherapy or radiotherapy demonstrated enhanced inhibition of cell growth, induction of apoptosis, and increased antitumor activity,[5,27,28] suggesting that combination therapy confers additional benefits over the agents alone. However, enhanced efficacy of these combinations has not always been observed in the clinic.

Gefitinib Two multinational, randomized, double-blind, placebo-controlled Phase III clinical trials evaluated gefitinib in combination with standard platinum-based chemotherapy in over 2100 chemonaive patients with advanced NSCLC, as part of the "Iressa" NSCLC Trial Assessing Combination Treatment (INTACT I gemcitabine/cisplatin; INTACT 2 carboplatin/paclitaxel.[54,55] Although there were no improvements in overall survival or other efficacy outcomes, the favorable safety profile of gefitinib was confirmed in a placebo-controlled setting. As predicted from Phase II trials, the only additional adverse events with combination therapy were dose-dependent diarrhea and skin rash. In INTACT 1 and 2, patients received combination therapy for 6 months, after which gefitinib was

TABLE 4.6 EGFR Inhibitors and Safety

Event	Treatment
Skin rash that does not resolve spontaneously	Emollients Topical or systemic antibiotics Steroid creams Topical or systemic antihistamines Retinoid creams
Diarrhea that does not resolve spontaneously[a]	Antidiarrheals (e.g. loperamide) Rehydration
Other adverse drug reactions	Dose reduction or interruption
Hypersensitivity (monoclonal antibodies)	Use corticosteroids, antihistamines and/or bronchodilators Prevent low-grade allergic reactions by increasing the infusion time

[a]Only with epidermal growth factor receptor tyrosine kinase inhibitors

continued as monotherapy. In the time-to-progression curve for INTACT 2, the placebo curve decline increases approximately 6 months after randomization, while the gefitinib curve continues to decline steadily. This suggests gefitinib may maintain the response after chemotherapy has been terminated and that optimal use of gefitinib could be in sequence with chemotherapy.

A Phase II trial is currently investigating the effect of gefitinib (250 mg/day) in combination with docetaxel in patients with NSCLC who have either progressed during or after platinum-based chemotherapy or who are unsuitable for platinum-based chemotherapy. Preliminary results indicate that combination therapy is associated with antitumor activity and good tolerability (Table 4.3).[56] A second Phase II trial is investigating the antitumor activity of gefitinib (250 mg/day) in combination with different doses of epidoxorubicin as second-line therapy in patients with advanced breast cancer. To date, no dose-limiting toxicities (DLTs) have been observed and therapy is well tolerated, with evidence of antitumor activity (Table 4.3).[57]

Erlotinib First-line treatment with erlotinib in combination with chemotherapy is being studied in two Phase III trials in patients with NSCLC.[58] The TRIBUTE trial is investigating whether or not addition of erlotinib to carboplatin and paclitaxel can improve the duration of patient survival, while the TALENT trial is examining the effect of erlotinib in combination with gemcitabine and cisplatin. Recent results reported that upon addition of erlotinib, patients with metastatic NSCLC did not have any improvement in overall survival. However, these combination therapies are being tested as second- and third-line treatments on patients with NSCLC, with the data expected at the beginning of 2004.

Cetuximab Cetuximab displayed synergistic effects in combination with both conventional chemotherapy agents and radiation in preclinical studies.[2,4,23] Patients with advanced NSCLC that is refractory to chemotherapy are currently involved in a Phase II trial to investigate cetuximab administered weekly in combination with docetaxel (75 mg/m^2) administered every 3 weeks. Of the 47 patients evaluable for response, 27.6% had a partial response and 17% had stable disease. Treatment was generally well tolerated, with the most common grade 3 toxicities being infection (21%), fatigue (21%), and acneiform rash (19%). However, 4 patients (8%) had an allergic reaction and withdrew from the trial.[59]

Three Phase II trials have investigated cetuximab administered in combination with chemotherapy in patients with advanced NSCLC. In the first trial, cetuximab administered in combination with cisplatin (80 mg/m^2) and vinorelbine (25 mg/m^2) was compared with chemotherapy alone. Preliminary data showed more patients receiving combination therapy (N = 18) responded to treatment than those receiving chemotherapy alone (N = 17); 50% vs. 29% respectively.[60] Cetuximab has also been investigated in combination with paclitaxel (225 mg/m^2) and carboplatin (AUC = 6) in chemonaive patients. Treatment was well tolerated, with a disease control rate of 64.5%.[61] A third study, involving 35 chemonaive patients, investigated cetuximab administered in combination with carboplatin (AUC = 5) and gemcitabine (1000 mg/m^2). Such treatment was associated with a disease control rate of 68.6%.[62]

Patients with SCCHN whose disease progressed after 2-4 cycles of platinum-based chemotherapy were treated with cetuximab plus cisplatin/carboplatin combination therapy in a Phase II trial. Of the 96 evaluable patients, 2.1% had a complete response, 12.5% had a partial response, and 39.6% had disease stabilization or a minor response for at least 6 weeks. Rash was the most common adverse event (45% of patients).[63] Phase III trials are comparing cetuximab and cisplatin combination therapy (N = 60) with cisplatin and a placebo (N = 63) in patients with untreated metastatic SCCHN. Preliminary data show that patients receiving combination therapy have a higher response rate (20%) than patients receiving chemotherapy alone (7.9%).[64]

In addition, cetuximab alone and in combination with irinotecan has been investigated in patients with EGFR-positive metastatic colorectal cancer whose disease has progressed on irinotecan therapy. The partial response rate with cetuximab alone (N = 111) was 10.8%, and with cetuximab and irinotecan (N = 218) was 22.8%. Patients receiving combination therapy had significantly higher rates of disease control (partial response + stable disease) and time to disease progression compared with patients receiving monotherapy (55.5% vs. 32.4% and 4.1 vs. 1.5 months, respectively) although combination therapy was associated with more grade 3/4 adverse events.[65]

Cocktails of Biologic Therapy

As there are myriad of ways that a cell may become cancerous and resistant to therapy, any of which might contribute to an individual tumor, combinations of biologically targeted agents may have to be used to maximize therapeutic benefit based on how these tumorigenic processes interact. An example of this approach is a Phase I/II trial investigating erlotinib in combination with bevacizumab in patients with recurrent NSCLC. Bevacizumab directly inhibits endothelial cells responding to vascular endothelial growth factor (VEGF), whereas erlotinib indirectly inhibits synthesis of VEGF, resulting in a two-pronged attack on the VEGF pathway. Three different dose regimens are under investigation involving 23 patients who have received at least 1 prior chemotherapy regimen. To date, treatment appears to be well tolerated, with 4 patients having a partial response and 5 having disease stabilization.[66]

In a similar study, gefitinib is administered in combination with rofecoxib, a cyclooxygenase (COX)-2 inhibitor, in patients with platinum-pretreated NSCLC. Almost all NSCLC tumors have COX-2 immunoreactivity, and activation of the EGFR may induce COX-2 in malignant cells. Both factors have a role in proliferation, cell survival, invasiveness, and angiogenesis. Preliminary results failed to reveal any pharmacokinetic interactions between the two agents, suggesting that this combination has a predictable safety profile with no unexpected toxicities. Of the 31 evaluable patients, 3 had a partial tumor response and 9 had stable disease, suggesting that this combination may be useful in the treatment of patients with pretreated NSCLC.[67]

LESSONS FROM RECENT TRIALS

Not all patients exhibit the same response to treatment with EGFR–TKIs, so research is focusing on identifying prognostic factors that may indicate which patients would benefit from treatment. This information could allow individual tailored therapies.

Molecular Predictors of Response

Potential biologic markers that may predict response to agents targeted to the EGFR include the EGFR itself and components of the EGFR signaling pathway. From preclinical work involving biologically targeted agents, the original hypothesis was that a relationship existed between receptor expression and susceptibility to receptor inhibition. Patients with tumors expressing high levels of EGFR were expected to benefit most from treatment. Expression is a strong prognostic indicator in head and neck, ovarian, cervical, bladder, and esophageal cancers and, in 70% of studies, increased EGFR expression was associated with reduced recurrence–free or overall survival rates. In gastric, breast, endometrial, and colorectal cancers, EGFR expression correlated with poor survival rates in 52% of studies. However, the initial study of cetuximab with irinotecan in colorectal cancer patients refractory to irinotecan first demonstrated that the level of EGFR expression did not predict response to treatment.[68] For NSCLC, only 30% of studies showed a relationship between EGFR expression and patient outcome.[8]

To clarify the potential prognostic value of EGFR expression for response to gefitinib in NSCLC, a retrospective exploratory analysis of baseline tumor biopsies from IDEAL 1 and 2 was undertaken. There was no evidence of a consistent relationship between EGFR expression levels and an objective response with gefitinib.[69,70] In patients with NSCLC, increased EGFR expression was more common among those with SCC and a correlation was found between increased EGFR expression and increased gene copy number per cell.[71]

A study involving 63 patients with pretreated advanced NSCLC investigated whether there was a correlation between HER2 expression and response to gefitinib. Of the 43 patients whose HER2/EGFR status was determined, there were no significant differences in the disease control rate (40.0 vs. 64.3%; P = 0.126), time to progression (3.5 vs. 3.7 months), or overall survival (5.7 vs. 6.8 months) between the 15 patients who expressed high levels of HER2 and the 28 patients who did not. This suggests HER2 expression may not influence efficacy, toxicity, or symptom outcome in patients with NSCLC treated with gefitinib.[72] Contrasting results have been found in a study that analyzed expression of EGFR, phosphorylated EGFR, TGF-α, and HER2 (Figure 4.2) as prognostic factors in patients with stage I NSCLC. There was an increased risk of recurrence in patients who had a synchronous increase in both EGFR and HER2 expression, and it has been suggested that this may predict decreased survival in patients with stage I NSCLC.[73]

Preclinical research is aiding identification of additional molecular factors that may be involved in resistance to EGFR-targeted therapies. A study investigating gefitinib and cetuximab in NSCLC cell lines found that persistent activity of either the extracellular signal-regulated kinase or Akt kinase pathways was involved in poor sensitivity to EGFR inhibitors,[74] suggesting a role for combining EGFR inhibitors with agents that target the extracellular signal-regulated kinase or Akt kinase pathways.

Disease Characteristics

Certain baseline factors appear to be predictive of improved clinical outcome in patients with advanced NSCLC receiving chemotherapy. In IDEAL 1, demographic prognostic factors showing a significant positive effect on response included performance status (PS) 0 or 1 (vs. 2), female gender, and adenocarcinoma histology (vs. other histologies).[30] In IDEAL 2, univariate analysis found an objective response was significantly more likely if the patient was

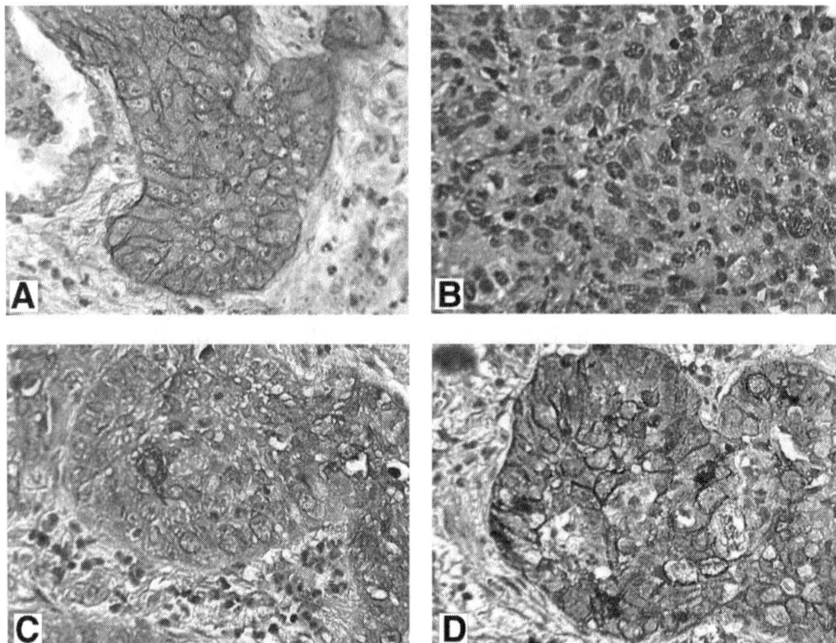

FIGURE 4.2 Representative findings on immunohistochemical staining for (A) EGFR, (B) phosphorylated EGFR, (C) TGF-α, and (D) HER2. Reprinted with permission from the American Association of Cancer Research, Inc.[73] (See p. 4 of color insert.)

female or had adenocarcinoma histology. For multivariate analysis, this held if the patient was female.[31] Prognostic factors indicating a significantly worse survival in INTACT 1 and 2 were a PS of 2, weight loss, bone and liver metastases, and squamous-cell, large-cell, or unspecified histology. In INTACT 2, male gender and brain metastases were also associated with poorer survival.[75]

For patients with advanced NSCLC following failure of platinum-based chemotherapy, treatment with erlotinib monotherapy was associated with higher objective response rates and 1-year survival rates in patients who had previously been treated with docetaxel compared with the entire group (26.7% vs. 12.3% and 47% vs. 40%, respectively). Time since last chemotherapy, time since diagnosis, and Eastern Cooperative Oncology Group PS also predicted for response or survival.[76]

Skin as a Surrogate Marker for Response

Most patients receiving EGFR-targeted agents who experience a response or stable disease also have a skin rash, suggesting that rash may predict response to these agents.[39,68,77,78] For example, treatment with erlotinib monotherapy in patients with advanced NSCLC after failure on platinum-based chemotherapy found cutaneous rash was associated with patients having an objective response or stable disease. Patients experiencing a rash had significantly longer survival, which increased with rash severity; 1.5, 8.5 or 19.6, months for patients experiencing no rash, grade 1 rash, or grade 213 rash, respectively.[76] However, responders are likely to remain on treatment for longer than those with progressive disease and have a greater chance of developing rash, meaning it may be more appropriate to investigate an association of early-onset skin toxicity with response. For gefitinib, analysis of data from IDEAL 1 demonstrated that both responders and nonresponders had the same incidence of rash, and patients from IDEAL 2 demonstrated no statistically significant difference in response rate between those with or without early-onset skin toxicity.[79,80]

Pharmacodynamic Data as a Surrogate Marker for Response

Phase I studies involving paired skin biopsies from patients receiving gefitinib (150-1000 mg/day) found that after gefitinib treatment there was a reduction in activated EGFR, although this was only significant in one study. In addition, there was a significant decrease in the proliferation markers mitogen-activated protein kinase (MAPK) and Ki-67, and a significant increase in the cyclin-dependent kinase inhibitor p27^{KIP-1}, as predicted from preclinical studies (Figure 4.3).[81] Such responses were not significantly associated with the development of skin reactions and there were no noteworthy dose- or plasma-concentration response effects.[82,83] In a Phase I study investigating the effects of erlotinib (25-200 mg/day), normal skin tissue was collected from patients at baseline and after the last dose of the drug during the first course of treatment. Although there was a significant decrease in activated EGFR, this was not related to the administered dose. In contrast to gefitinib, p27 was upregulated in a dose-related manner.[84]

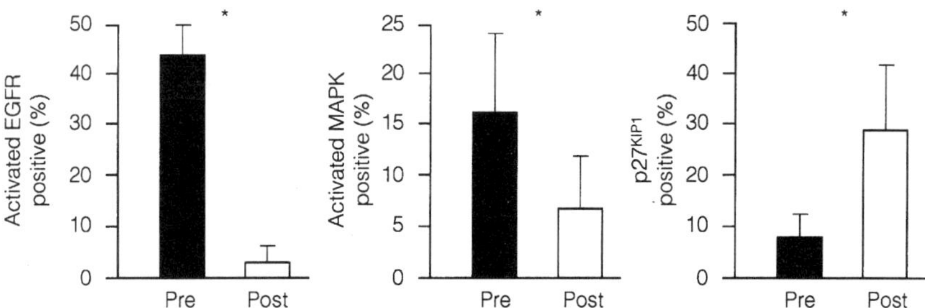

*p<0.001
EGFR, epidermal growth factor receptor; MAPK, mitogen-activated protein kinase

FIGURE 4.3 Activation of EGFR and MAPK and expression of p27^{KIP-1} before and after gefitinib treatment. Adapted with permission from the American Society of Clinical Oncology.[82]

From a study involving patients with SCCHN, activated ERKl/2 was suggested as a potential marker of inhibition of EGFR function. ERKl/2 has a vital role in the EGFR downstream signaling pathway, and the majority of SCCHN primary tumors have increased levels of this protein, which has been associated with advanced lymph node metastasis, higher proliferation, and an increased risk of relapse. Both gefitinib and cetuximab inhibited proliferation of EGFR-dependent cell lines at concentrations that inhibited ERKl/2 activation, and skin biopsies from patients treated with cetuximab had lower levels of activated ERKl/2 compared with untreated control samples.[85] An additional marker was identified by gene expression analysis and has been called the "gefitinib resistance gene I" (GRG1). This gene has been shown to be upregulated in gefitinib-resistant tumors.[86]

CONCLUSIONS AND FUTURE DIRECTIONS

Although much progress has been made in the development of these new biologic agents, further research is required to better understand the role of the EGFR in specific cancers. For example, in NSCLC the EGFR is present, but its significance in individual tumors has not yet been identified. Progress will require the development of standardized techniques to determine EGFR expression, levels of phosphorylated EGFR, and levels of EGF and TGF-α, which may also be relevant. As demonstrated in studies involving skin biopsies, it is possible that downstream molecules in the EGFR pathway have a more important influence than EGFR or ligand expression. Levels of these molecules should be measured in future trials to see which of these prognostic factors may identify patients likely to benefit from treatment. EGFR–TKIs and antibody inhibitors differ in a number of ways, including molecular size, pharmacology, and route of administration. Importantly, they also differ in gastrointestinal toxicity and clinical activity. For example, cetuximab alone produces 11% responses in advanced colorectal cancer.[65] Although no such responses were observed with gefitinib administered as monotherapy, 33% of patients had disease stabilization, including two patients who had been heavily pretreated.[87] Furthermore, preclinical studies show additive effects of cetuximab in combination with either gefitinib or erlotinib.[88,89] Such data suggest the need for clinical trials that investigate combination therapy involving agents that have different mechanisms of action for targeting the EGFR. For combination therapy, current preclinical models failed in many cases to correctly predict clinical outcome, therefore better animal models are required to predict the outcome of biologic and conventional therapies. In addition, new clinical trial designs need to be implemented to determine the settings in which these agents can best be used. One important consideration is that, in contrast to conventional agents, biologically targeted agents should be administered at their OBD rather than their MTD.

SUMMARY

In the clinic, agents that block EGFR activity offer beneficial alternative therapeutic strategies to patients with limited treatment options and are generally well tolerated, with a more favorable adverse event profile than conventional anticancer agents. Selecting patients most likely to benefit from therapy and the most appropriate schedule of administration, incorporating pharmacodynamic markers into clinical studies, and identifying surrogate markers of patient outcomes may achieve optimal use of biologically targeted agents. The response to combination therapies varies with the agents used and the target tumor, indicating that additional clinical trials are required. Ongoing research and innovative clinical trials should help to elucidate the clinical settings and patient populations in which these agents can best be used.

REFERENCES

1. Mendelsohn J, Baselga J. The EGF receptor family as targets for cancer therapy. Oncogene 2000;19:6550–6565.
2. Grünwald V, Hidalgo M. Developing inhibitors of the epidermal growth factor receptor for cancer treatment. J Natl Cancer Inst 2003;95:851–867.
3. Ritter CA, Arteaga CL. The epidennal growth factor receptor-tyrosine kinase: a promising therapeutic target in solid tumors. Semin Oncol 2003;30:3–11.
4. Mendelsohn J, Baselga J. Status of epidermal growth factor receptor antagonists in the biology and treatment of cancer. J Clin Oncol 2003;21:2787–2799.
5. Ciardiello F, Tortora G. A novel approach in the treatment of cancer: targeting the epidermal growth factor receptor. Clin Cancer Res 2001;7:2958–2970.
6. Graus-Porta D, Beerii RR, Daly JM, Hynes NE. ErbB-2, the preferred heterodimerization partner of all ErbB receptors, is a mediator of lateral signaling. EMBO J 1997;16:1647–1655.
7. Salomon DS, Brandt R, Ciardiello F, Normanno N. Epidermal growth factor-related peptides and their receptors in human malignancies. Crit Rev Oncol Hematol 1995;19:183–232.
8. Nicholson RI, Gee JMW, Harper ME. EGFR and cancer prognosis. Eur J Cancer 2001;37 (Suppl4):S9–15.
9. Brabender J, Danenberg KD, Metzger R, et al. Epidermal growth factor receptor and HER2-neu mRNA expression in non-small cell lung cancer is correlated with survival. Clin Cancer Res 2001;7:1850–1855.
10. Slamon DJ, Leyland-Jones B, Shak S, et al. Use of chemotherapy plus a monoclonal antibody against HER2 for metastatic breast cancer that overexpresses HER2. N Engl J Med 2001;344: 783–792.
11. Bianco AR, De Laurentiis M, Carlomagno C, et al. HER2 overexpression predicts adjuvant tamoxifen (TAM) failure for early breast cancer (EBC): complete data at 20 yr of the Naples GUN randomized trial. Proc Am Soc Clin Oncol 2000;19:75a, Abstr 289.
12. Paik S, Bryant J, Park C, Fisher B, et al. ErbB-2 and response to doxorubicin in patients with axillary lymph node–positive, hormone receptor–negative breast cancer. J Natl Cancer Inst 1998;90:1361–1370.
13. Slamon DJ, Clark GM, Wong SG, et al. Human breast cancer:correlation of relapse and survival with amplification of the HER–2/neu oncogene. Science 1987;235:177–182.

14. Thor AD, Berry DA, Budman DR, et al. ErbB-2, p53, and efficacy of adjuvant therapy in lymph node–positive breast cancer. J Natl Cancer Inst 1998;90:1346–1360.

15. Kawamoto T, Sato JD, Le A, et al. Growth stimulation of A431 cells by epidermal growth factor:identification of high–affinity receptors for epidermal growth factor by an anti-receptor monoclonal antibody. Proc Natl Acad Sci USA 1983;80:1337–1341.

16. Masui H, Kawamoto T, Sato JD, et al. Growth inhibition of human tumor cells in athymic mice by anti-epidermal growth factor receptor monoclonal antibodies. Cancer Res 1984;44:1002–1007.

17. Sato JD, Kawamoto T, Le AD, et al. Biological effects in vitro of monoclonal antibodies to human epidermal growth factor receptors. Mol Biol Med 1983;1:511–529.

18. Arteaga CL. The epidermal growth factor receptor: from mutant oncogene in nonhuman cancers to therapeutic target in human neoplasia. J Clin Oncol 2001;19:32s–40s.

19. Nelson JM, Fry DW. Akt, MAPK (Erkl/2), and p38 act in concert to promote apoptosis in response to ErbB receptor family inhibition. J Biol Chem 2001;276:14842–14847.

20. Moyer JD, Barbacci EG, Iwata KK, et al. Induction of apoptosis and cell cycle arrest by CP-358,774, an inhibitor of epidermal growth factor receptor tyrosine kinase. Cancer Res 1997;57:4838-4848.

21. Pollack VA, Savage DM, Baker DA, et al. Inhibition of epidermal growth factor receptor–associated tyrosine phosphorylation in human carcinomas with CP-358,774:dynamics of receptor inhibition in situ and antitumor effects in athymic mice. J Pharmacol Exp Ther 1999;291:739–748.

22. Ciardiello F, Caputo R, Bianco R, et al. Antitumor effect and potentiation of cytotoxic drugs activity in human cancer cells by ZD–1839 (Iressa), an epidermal growth factor receptor–selective tyrosine kinase inhibitor. Clin Cancer Res 2000;6:2053–2063.

23. Mendelsohn J. Targeting the epidermal growth factor receptor for cancer therapy. J Clin Oncol 2002;20:Is–13s.

24. Gill GN, Kawamoto T, Cochet C, et al. Monoclonal anti-epidermal growth factor receptor antibodies which are inhibitors of epidermal growth factor binding and antagonists of epidermal growth factor–stimulated tyrosine protein kinase activity. J Biol Chem 1984;259:7755–7760.

25. Goldstein NI, Prewett M, Zuklys K, et al. Biological efficacy of a chimeric antibody to the epidermal growth factor receptor in a human tumor xenograft model. Clin Cancer Res 1995;1:1311–1318.

26. Wu X, Fan Z, Masui H, et al. Apoptosis induced by an anti-epidermal growth factor receptor monoclonal antibody in a human colorectal carcinoma cell line and its delay by insulin. J Clin Invest 1995;95:1897–1905.

27. Baselga J, Norton L, Masui H, et al. Antitumor effects of doxorubicin in combination with anti-epidermal growth factor receptor monoclonal antibodies. J Natl Cancer Inst 1993;85 1327–1333.

28. Fan Z, Baselga J, Masui H, Mendelsohn J. Antitumor effect of anti-epidermal growth factor receptor monoclonal antibodies plus *cis*-diamminedichloroplatinum on well established A431 cell xenografts. Cancer Res 1993;53:4637–4642.

29. Baselga J. Why the epidermal growth factor receptor? The rationale for cancer therapy. Oncologist 2002;7 (Suppl 4):2–8.

30. Fukuoka M, Yano S, Giaccone G, et al. Multi-institutional randomized phase II trial of gefitinib for previously treated patients with advanced non-small cell lung cancer. J Clin Oncol 2003;21:2237–2246.

31. Kris MG, Natale RB, Herbst RS, et al. Efficacy of gefitinib, an inhibitor of the epidermal growth factor receptor tyrosine kinase, in symptomatic patients with non-small cell lung cancer. A randomized trial. JAMA 2003;290:2149–2158.

32. Argiris A, Mittal N, Masters G. Gefitinib (Iressa, ZD1839) is active as first-line, compassionate use therapy in patients with advanced non-small cell lung cancer (NSCLC). Lung Cancer 2003;41 (Suppl 2):S247, Abstr P-612.

33. Park J, Park B–B, Lee S-H, et al. Gefitinib ('Iressa', ZD1839) monotherapy as a salvage regimen for previously treated advanced non-small cell lung cancer. Poster presented at the WCLC, Vancouver, Canada, August 10–14, 2003. Lung Cancer 2003;41(suppl 2):S249, Abstr P-620.

34. Gips M, Heching Y, Levitt M, et al. The Israeli experience with gefitinib ('Iressa', ZD1839) as single agent treatment of advanced non-small cell lung cancer. Lung Cancer 2003;41 (Suppl 2):S247, Abstr P-613.

35. Haringhuizen A, Vaessen HFR, Baas P, van Zandwijk N. Gefinitib ('Iressa', ZD1839) as a last option for patients with recurrent non-small cell lung cancer (NSCLC). Poster P-617 presented at the WCLC, Vancouver, Canada, August 10–14, 2003. Lung Cancer 2003;41(suppl 2):S248, Abstr P-617.

36. Janne PA, Gurubhagavatula S, Lucca J, et al. Clinical benefits in patients with advanced non-small cell lung cancer treated with gefitinib ("Iressa", ZD1839) in the compassionate use program. Lung Cancer 2003;41 (Suppl2):S71, Abstr 0-243.

37. Franklin WA, Gumeriock PH, Crowley J, et al. EGFR, HER2 and ERB–B pathway activation in bronchioloalveolar carcinoma (BAC): analysis of SWOG 9417 and lung SPORE tissue samples. Proc Am Soc Clin Oncol 2003;22:620, Abstr 2493.

38. West HL, Franklin WA, Gumerlock P, et al. ZD1839 (Iressa) in advanced bronchioloalveolar carcinoma (BAC):a preliminary report of SWOG S0126. Lung Cancer 2003;41 (Suppl 2):S56, Abstr 0-187.

39. Cohen EEW, Rosen F, Stadler WM, et al. Phase II trial of ZD 1839 in recurrent or metastatic squamous cell carcinoma of the head and neck. J Clin Oncol 2003;21:1980–1987.

40. Robertson JFR, Gutteridge E, Cheung KL, et al. Gefitinib ('Iressa', ZD1839) is active in acquired tamoxifen–resistant oestrogen receptor (ER)–positive and ER–negative breast cancer:results from a phase II study. Poster 23 presented at the ASCO, Chicago, IL, May 31–June 3, 2003. Proc Am Soc Clin Oncol 2003;22:7, Abstr 23.

41. Baselga J, Albanell J, Ruiz A, et al. Phase II and tumor pharmacodynamic study of gefitinib (ZD1839) in patients with advanced breast cancer. Proc Am Soc Clin Oncol 2003;22:7, Abstr 24.

42. von Minckwitz G, Jonat W, Beckmann M, et al. A multicenter Phase II trial to evaluate gefitinib ('Iressa', ZD1839) 500 mg/day in patients with metastatic breast cancer after previous chemotherapy treatment. Poster 437 presented at the ECCO, Copenhagen, Denmark, September 21–25, 2003. Eur J Cancer 2003;l(Suppl 5):S133, Abstr 437.

43. Kim TE, Murren JR. Erlotinib OSI/Roche/Genentech. Curr Opin Investig Drugs 2002;3: 1385–1395.

44. Siu LL, Hidalgo M, Nemunaitis J, et al. Dose and schedule–duration escalation of the epidermal growth factor receptor (EGFR) tyrosine kinase (TK) inhibitor CP-358, 774:a phase I and pharmacokinetic (PK) study. Proc Am Soc Clin Oncol 1999;18:388a, Abstr 1498.

45. Perez–Soler R, Dai Q, Ling Y–H, et al. Molecular mechanisms of sensitivity and resistance to the HERl/EGFR–tyrosine kinase inhibitor erlotinib (Tarceva™). Lung Cancer 2003;41 (Suppl 2):S72, Abstr 0-247.

46. Patel JD, Miller VA, Kris MG, et al. Encouraging activity and durable responses demonstrated by the epithelial growth factor receptor–tyrosine kinase inhibitor, erlotinib (Tarceva TM, OSI774), in patients with advanced bronchioloalveolar (BAC) cell carcinoma. Lung Cancer 2003;41 (Suppl 2):S56, Abstr 0-188.

47. Soulieres D, Senzer NN, Vokes EE, et al. Multicenter phase II study of erlotinib, an oral epidermal growth factor receptor tyrosine kinase inhibitor, in patients with recurrent or metastatic squamous cell cancer of the head and neck. J Clin Oncol 2004; 22:77–85.

48. Oza AM, Townsley CA, Siu LL, et al. Phase II study of erlotinib (OSI-774) in patients with metastatic colorectal cancer. Proc Am Soc Clin Oncol 2003;22:196, Abstr 785.

49. Baselga J, Pfister D, Cooper MR, et al. Phase I studies of anti-epidermal growth factor receptor chimeric antibody C225 alone and in combination with cisplatin. J Clin Oncol 2000;18: 904–914.

50. Cohen RB. Epidermal growth factor receptor as a therapeutic target in colorectal cancer. Clin Colorectal Cancer 2003;2:246–251.

51. Saltz L, Meropol NJ, Loehrer PJ, et al. Single agent IMC-C225 (Erbitux™) has activity in CPT-11–refractory colorectal cancer (CRC) that expresses the epidermal growth factor receptor (EGFR). Proc Am Soc Clin Oncol 2002;21:127a, Abstr 504.

52. Inoue A, Saijo Y, Maemondo M, et al. Severe acute interstitial pneumonia and gefitinib. Lancet 2003;361:137–139.

53. Forsythe B, Faulkner K. Safety and tolerability of gefitinib ('Iressa', ZD1839) in advanced NSCLC:overview of clinical experience. Poster P327 presented at the ERS, Vienna, Austria, September 27–October 1,2003. Eur Respir J 2003;22(suppl 45):32s, Abstr P327.

54. Giaccone G, Herbst RS, Manegold C, et al. Gefitinib in combination with gemcitabine and cisplatin in advanced non-small cell lung cancer in phase III trial—INTACT 1. J Clin Oncol 2004; 22:777–784.

55. Herbst RS, Giaccone G, Schiller JH, et al. Gefitinib in combination with paclitaxel and carboplatin in advanced non-small cell lung cancer: a phase III trial—INTACT 2. J Clin Oncol 2004; 22:785–794.

56. Rixe O, LeMarie E, Chomy F, et al. Phase II combination of gefitinib (Tressa', ZD1839) and docetaxel for non-small cell lung cancer:clinical results and biological monitoring. Poster 2659 presented at the ASCO, Chicago, IL, USA, May 31–June 3, 2003. Proc Am Soc Clin Oncol 2003;22:661, Abstr 2659.

57. Magnani E, Sarmiento R, Fanelli M, et al. Gefitinib ('Iressa', ZD1839) combined with weekly epidoxorubicin as second-line therapy of advanced breast cancer:results of a dose finding study. Poster 177 presented at the ASCO, Chicago, IL, USA, May 31–June 3, 2003. Proc Am Soc Clin Oncol 2003;22:44, Abstr 177.

58. Adis International Ltd. Erlotinib. CP 358774, NSC 718781, OSI 774, R 1415. Drugs R D 2003;4:243–248.

59. Kim ES, Mauer AM, Tran HT, et al. A phase II study ofcetuximab, an epidermal growth factor receptor (EGFR) blocking antibody, in combination with docetaxel in chemotherapy refractory/resistant patients with advanced non-small cell lung cancer:Final report. Proc Am Soc Clin Oncol 2003;22:642, Abstr 2581.

60. Gatzemeier U, Rosell R, Ramlau R, et al. Cetuximab (C225) in combination with cisplatin/vinorelbine vs. cisplatin/vinorelbine alone in the first-line treatment of patients (pts) with epidermal growth factor receptor (EGFR) positive advanced non-small cell lung cancer (NSCLC). Proc Am Soc Clin Oncol 2003;22:642, Abstr 2582.

61. Kelly K, Hanna N, Rosenberg A, et al. A multicenter phase I/II study of cetuximab in combination with paclitaxel and carboplatin in untreated patients with stage IV non-small cell lung cancer. Poster 2592 presented at the ASCO, Chicago, IL, May 31–June 3, 2003. Proc Am Soc Clin Oncol 2003;22:644, Abstr 2592.

62. Robert F, Blumenschein G, Dicke K, et al. Phase Ib/IIa study of anti-epidermal growth factor receptor (EGFR) antibody, cetuximab, in combination with gemcitabine/carboplatin in patients with advanced non-small cell lung cancer (NSCLC). Proc Am Soc Clin Oncol 2003;22:643, Abstr 2587.

63. Baselga J, Trigo JM, Bourhis J, et al. Cetuximab (C225) plus cisplatin/carboplatin is active in patients (pts) with recurrent/metastatic squamous cell carcinoma of the head and neck

(SCCHN) progressing on a same dose and schedule platinum–based regimen. Proc Am Soc Clin Oncol 2002;21:226a, Abstr 900.

64. Burtness BA, Li Y, Flood W. Phase III trial comparing cisplatin and placebo to cisplatin and anti-epidermal growth factor antibody C225 in patients with metastatic or recurrent head & neck cancer. Poster 901 presented at the ASCO, Chicago, BL, May 31–June 3, 2002. Proc Am Soc Clin Oncol 2002;21:226a, Abstr 901.

65. Cunningham D, Humblet Y, Siena S, et al. Cetuximab (Erbitux™) or in combination with irinotecan or as a single agent in patients with EGFR–expressing, irinotecan–refractory metastatic colorectal cancer. Poster 1012 presented at the ASCO, Chicago, IL, May 31–June 3, 2003. Proc Am Soc Clin Oncol 2003;22:252, Abstr 1012.

66. Herbst RS, Mininberg E, Henderson T, et al. Phase I/II trial evaluating blockade of tumour blood supply and tumour cell proliferation with combined bevacizumab and erlotinib HC1 as targeted cancer therapy in patients with recurrent non-small cell lung cancer. Poster 977 presented at the ECCO 12, Copenhagen, Denmark, September 21–25,2003. Eur J Cancer 2003;l(Suppl5):S293, Abstr 977.

67. O'Byrne KJ, Clarke L, Dunlop D, et al. Clinical evaluation of gefitinib (Iressa, ZD1839) in combination with rofecoxib in cisplatin pre–treated relapsed non-small cell lung cancer. Lung Cancer 2003;41 (Suppl 2):S36, Abstr 0-113.

68. Saltz L, Rubin M, Hochster H, et al. Cetuximab (IMC–C225) plus irinotecan (CPT–11) is active in CPT–11–refractory colorectal cancer (CRC) that expresses epidermal growth factor receptor (EGFR). Proc Am Soc Clin Oncol 2001;20 (1 of2):3a, Abstr 7.

69. Bailey LR, Kris M, Wolf M, et al. Tumor EGFR membrane staining is not clinically relevant for predicting response in patients receiving gefitinib ('Iressa'JZD 1839) monotherapy for pretreated advanced non-small cell lung cancer:IDEAL 1 and 2. Poster LB–170 presented at the AACR, Washington, DC, USA, July 11–14, 2003. Proc Am Assoc Cancer Res 2003;44:1362, Abstr LB–170.

70. Janas M, Franklin WA, Schmidt K, Bailey LR. Interobserver reproducibility of visually interpreted EGFR immunohistochemical staining in non-small cell lung cancer. Poster LB–213 presented at the AACR, Washington, DC, USA, July 11–14, 2003. Proc Am Assoc Cancer Res 2003;44:Abstr LB–213.

71. Hirsch FR, Varella–Garcia M, Bunn PA, Jr., et al. Epidermal growth factor receptor in non-small cell lung carcinomas:correlation between gene copy number and protein expression and impact on prognosis. J Clin Oncol 2003;21:3798–3807.

72. Cappuzzo F, Gregorc V, Rossi E, et al. Gefitinib in pretreated non-small cell lung cancer (NSCLC):analysis of efficacy and correlation with HER2 and epidermal growth receptor expression in locally advanced or metastatic NSCLC. J Clin Oncol 2003;21:2658–2663.

73. Onn A, Correa AM, Gilcrease M, et al. Synchronous overexpression of epidermal growth factor receptor and HER2–neu protein is a predictor of poor outcome in patients with stage I non-small cell lung cancer. Clin Cancer Res 2004;10:136–143.

74. Janmaat ML, Kruyt FAE, Rodriguez JA, Giaccone G. Inhibition of the epidermal growth factor receptor induces apoptosis in A431 cells, but not in non-small-cell lung cancer cell lines. Proc Am Assoc Cancer Res 2002; 43:abstr 3901.

75. Giaccone G, Johnson D, Scagliotti GV, et al. Results of a multivariate analysis of prognostic factors of overall survival of patients with advanced non-small cell lung cancer (NSCLC) treated with gefitinib (ZD1839) in combination with platinum–based chemotherapy (CT) in two large phase in trials (INTACT 1 and 2). Proc Am Soc Clin Oncol 2003;22:627, Abstr 2522.

76. Perez–Soler R, Chachoua A, Huberman M, et al. Final results from a phase II study of erlotinib (Tarceva™) monotherapy in patients with advanced non-small cell lung cancer following failure of platinum–based chemotherapy. Poster P-611 presented at the WCLC, Vancouver, Canada, August 10–14, 2003. Lung Cancer 2003;41(suppl 2):S426, Abstr P-611.

77. Kies MS, Arquette MA, Nabell L, et al. Final report of the efficacy and safety of the anti-epidermal growth factor antibody Erbitux (IMC–C225), in combination with cisplatin in patients with recurrent squamous cell carcinoma of the head and neck (SCCHN) refractory to cisplatin containing chemotherapy. Proc Am Soc Clin Oncol 2002;21:232a, Abstr 925.

78. Perez–Soler R, Chachoua A, Huberman M, et al. A phase n trial of the epidermal growth factor receptor (EGFR) tyrosine kinase inhibitor OSI-774, following platinum-based chemotherapy, in patients (pts) with advanced, EGFR–expressing, non-small cell lung cancer (NSCLC). Proc Am Soc Clin Oncol 2001;20:310a, Abstr 1235.

79. Fukuoka M, Kris M, Giaccone G, et al. Phase II trials of gefitinib ('Iressa', ZD1839):rapid and durable objective responses in patients with advanced non-small cell lung cancer (IDEAL 1 and IDEAL 2). Lung Cancer 2003a;41 (Suppl 2):S247–S248, Abstr P-615.

80. Baselga J, Yano S, Giaccone G, et al. Initial results from a Phase II trial ofZD1839 ('Iressa') as second-and third-line monotherapy for patients with advanced non-small cell lung cancer (IDEAL 1). Poster 630A presented at the AACR–NCI–EORTC, Miami Beach, Florida, USA, October 29–November 2, 2001. Proc AACR–NCI–EORTC 2001;Abstr 630A.

81. Wu X, Rubin M, Fan Z, et al. Involvement of p27KJDPl in Gl arrest mediated by an anti-epidermal growth factor receptor monoclonal antibody. Oncogene 1996;12:1397–1403.

82. Albanell J, Rojo F, Averbuch S, et al. Pharmacodynamic studies of the epidermal growth factor receptor inhibitor ZD1839 in skin from cancer patients:histopathologic and molecular consequences of receptor inhibition. J Clin Oncol 2002;20:110–124.

83. Herbst RS, Maddox AM, Rothenberg ML, et al. Selective oral epidermal growth factor receptor tyrosine kinase inhibitor ZD1839 is generally well–tolerated and has activity in non-small cell lung cancer and other solid tumors:results of a phase I trial. J Clin Oncol 2002;20:3815–3825.

84. Malik SN, Siu LL, Rowinsky EK, et al. Pharmacodynamic evaluation of the epidermal growth factor receptor inhibitor OSI-774 in human epidermis of cancer patients. Clin Cancer Res 2003;9:2478–2486.

85. Albanell J, Codony–Servat J, Rojo F, et al. Activated extracellular signal-regulated kinases:association with epidermal growth factor receptor/transforming growth factor alpha expression in head and neck squamous carcinoma and inhibition by anti- epidermal growth factor receptor treatments. Cancer Res 2001;61:6500–6510.

86. Natale RB, Shak S, Aronson N, et al. Quantitative gene expression in non-small cell lung cancer from paraffin–embedded tissue specimens:predicting response to gefitinib, and EGFR kinase inhibitor. Proc Am Soc Clin Oncol 2003;22:190. Abstr 763.

87. Goss G, Stewart D, Hirte H, et al. Initial results of part 2 of a phase I/II pharmacokinetics (PK), phamiacodynamic (PD) and biological activity study of ZD1839 (Iressa):NCIC CTG IND.122. Poster 59 presented at the ASCO, Orlando, FL, May 18–21, 2002. Proc Am Soc Clin Oncol 2002;21:16a, Abstr 59.

88. Matar P, Rojo F, Guzman M, et al. Combined anti- epidermal growth factor receptor (EGFR) treatment with a tyrosine kinase inhibitor gefitinib (ZD1839, 'Iressa') and a monoclonal antibody (IMC–C225):evidence of synergy. Proc 2003;44:Abstr 4007.

89. Huang S–M, Armstrong E, Chinnaiyan P, Harari PM. Dual agent molecular targeting of the epidermal growth factor receptor:combining anti-HERl/EGFR monoclonal antibody with tyrosine kinase inhibitor. Proc Am Assoc Cancer Res 2003;44:Abstr 3777.

90. Cohen EEW, Stenson K, Gustin D, Lamont E, Mauer A, Blair E, Stadler W, Dekker A, Mallon W, Vokes EE. A phase II study of 250-mg gefitinib (ZD1839) monotherapy in recurrent and/or metastatic squamous cell carcinoma of the head and neck. Poster 2021 presented at the ASCO, Chicago, IL, May 31–June 3, 2003b. Proc Am Soc Clin Oncol 2003; 22: 502, abs 2021.

91. Peery TS, Reardon DA, Quinn J, Ochs J, Wikstrand CJ, Stenzel TT, Bigner DD, Friedman HS, Rich JN, Dancey J. Phase II trial of ZD1839 for patients with first relapse glioblastoma. Proc Am Soc Clin Oncol 2003; 22: 99, abs 396.

92. Schilder RJ, Kohn E., Sill MW, Lewandowski G, Lee RB, Decesare SL. Phase II trial of gefitinib (Iressa™) in patients with recurrent ovarian or primary peritoneal cancer: Gynecology Oncology Group 170C. Poster 1814 presented at the ASCO, Chicago, IL, May 31–June 3, 2003. Proc Am Soc Clin Oncol 2003; 22: 451, abs 1814.

93. Viens P, Lhommé C, Extra JM, Gladieff L, Kalla S, Fabbro M. A phase II trial to evaluate the efficacy and safety of gefitinib ('Iressa', ZD1839) in patients with locoregionally advanced or metastatic squamous-cell carcinoma of the cervix. Poster 1833 presented at the ASCO, Chicago, IL, May 31–June 3, 2003. Proc Am Soc Clin Oncol 2003; 22: 456, abs 1833.

94. Jermann M, Pless M, Salzberg M, Jörger M, Gillessen S, Morant R, Egli F, Rhyner K, Bauer JA, Stahel RA. An open-label phase II trial to evaluate the efficacy and safety of gefitnib ('Iressa', ZD1839) in patients with locally advanced, relapsed, or metastatic renal-cell carcinoma. Poster 1681 presented at the ASCO, Chicago, IL, May 31–June 3, 2003. Proc Am Soc Clin Oncol 2003; 22: 418, abs 1681.

95. Dawson NA, Guo C, Zak R, Dorsey B, Smoot J, Wong J, Hussain A. A phase II trial of ZD1839 in stage IV and recurrent renal cell carcinoma. Poster 1623 presented at the ASCO, Chicago, IL, May 31–June 3, 2003. Proc Am Soc Clin Oncol 2003; 22: 404, abs 1623.

96. Doi T, Koizumi W, Siena S, Cascinu S, Ohtsu A, Michael M, Takiuchi H, Swaisland H, Gallagher N, Van Cutsem E. Efficacy, tolerability, and pharmacokinetics of gefitinib ('Iressa', ZD 1839) in pretreated patients with metastatic gastric cancer. Poster 1036 presented at the ASCO, Chicago, IL, May 31–June 3, 2003. Proc Am Soc Clin Oncol 2003; 22: 258, abs 1036.

97. Rosenthal MA, Toner GC, Gurney H, Davis ID, Underhill C, Boyer MJ, Kotasek D. Inhibition of the epidermal growth factor receptor (EGFR) in hormone-refractory prostate cancer (HRPC): initial results of a phase II trial of gefitinib ('Iressa', ZD1839). Poster 1671 presented at the ASCO, Chicago, IL, May 31–June 3, 2003. Proc Am Soc Clin Oncol 2003; 22: 416, abs 1671.

98. Govindan R, Kratzke RA, Herndon JE, Niehans GA, Vollmer R, Watson D, Green M, Kindler HL. Gefitinib in patients with malignant mesothelioma (MM): A phase II study by the Cancer and Leukemia Group B (CALGB 30101). Proc Am Soc Clin Oncol 2003; 22; 630, abs 2535.

99. Radovich D, Kelsen D, Packer S, Klimstra D, Gonzales SG, Wilson KB, Ilson DH. Phase II trial of OSI-774 in advanced esophageal cancer. Proc Am Soc Clin Oncol 2003; 22: 337, abs 1352.

100. Philip PA, Geyer SM, Thomas JP, Pitot HC, Donehower R, Kim GP, Picus J, Fitch TR, Mahoney MR, Erlichman C. Tolerability of OSI-774 (Tarceva) in locally advanced or metastatic hepatocellular (HCC) and biliary (BILI) carcinomas: An interim report. Proc Am Soc Clin Oncol 2003; 22: 364, abs 1461.

101. Cho CD, Fisher GA, Halsey J, Jambalos CN, Advani RH, Wakelee H, Lum BL, Sikic BI. A phase II study of gefitinib in combination with FOLFOX-4 (IFOX) in patients with unresectable or metastatic colorectal cancer. Poster 1062 presented at the ASCO, Chicago, IL, May 31–June 3, 2003. Proc Am Soc Clin Oncol 2003; 22: 265, abs 1062.

102. Hirte H, Oza A, Hoskins P, Ellard S, Grimshaw R, Dubuc-Lissoir J, Kerr I, Fisher B, Seymour L. Phase II study of OSI-774 given in combination with carboplatin in patients (pts) with recurrent epithelial ovarian cancer (EOC): NCIC ctg ind. 149. Eur J Cancer Suppl 2003; 1: S51, abs 159.

103. Folprecht G, Lutz MP, Schoeffski P, Seufferlein T, Haag C, Beutel G, Nolting A, Mueser M, Pollert P, Koehne C-H. Pharmacokinetic (PK) evaluation of ctuximab in combination with weekly irinotecan (CPT-11) and 24h infusional 5-FU/folinic acid (FA) as first line treatment in patients (pts) with epidermal growth factor receptor (EGFR)-positive metastatic colorectal cancer (MCRC). Proc Am Soc Clin Oncol 2003; 22: 222, abs 890.

104. Chan ATC, Hsu MM, Goh BC, Hui EP, Liu TW, Millward M, Chang AY, Ma BB, Hong RL, Lin X, for the Cancer Therapeutics Research Group. A phase II study of cetuximab (C225) in combination with carboplatin in patients (pts) with recurrent or metastatic nasopharyngeal carcinoma (NPC) who failed to a platinum-based chemotherapy. Proc Am Soc Clin Oncol 2003; 22; 497, abs 2000.

105. Van Laethem J-L, Raoul J-L, Mitry E, Brezault C, Husseini F, Cals L, Vedovato J-C, Mueser MM, Rougier P. Cetuximab (C225) in combination with bi-weekly irinotecan (CPT-11), infusional 5-Fluorouracil (5-FU) and folinic acid (FA) in patients (pts) with metastatic colorectal cancer (CRC) expressing the epidermal growth factor receptor (EGFR). Preliminary safety and efficacy results. Proc Am Soc Clin Oncol 2003; 22; 264, abs 1058.

106. Rinehart JJ, Wilding G, Willson J, Krishnamurthi S, Natale R, Mani S, Burnett D, Olson S, Bycott P, Owens-Grillo JK, Hes M, Lenehan P. A phase I clinical and pharmacokinetic study of oral CI-1033, a pan-erB tyrosine kinase inhibitor, in patients with advanced solid tumors. Proc Am Soc Clin Oncol 2002; 21: 11a, abs 41.

107. Garrison MA, Tolcher A, McCreery H, Rowinsky EK, Schott A, Mace J, Drengler R, Patnaik A, Denis L, Lenehan P, Eiseman I, Bycott P, Olson S, Baker L. A phase I and pharmacokinetic study of CI-1033, a pan-ErbB tyrosine kinase inhibitor, given orally on days 1, 8, and 15 every 28 days to patients with solid tumors. Proc Am Soc Clin Oncol 2001; 20 (1 of 2): 72a, abs 283.

108. Dumez H, Hoekstra R, Eskens F, Sizer S, Vaidyanathan S, Ravera C, van Oosterom A, Verweij J, Gasthuisberg UZ. A phase I pharmacological study of PKI166, an epidermal growth factor receptor (EGFR) tyrosine kinase inhibitor, administered orally 3 times a week to patients with advanced cancer. Proc Am Soc Clin Oncol 2002; 21; 86a, abs 341.

109. Hoekstra R, Dumez H, van Oosterom AT, Sizer KC, Ravera C, Vaidyanathan S, Verweij J, Eskens FA. A phase I and pharmacological study of PK1166, an epidermal growth factor receptor (EGFR) tyrosine kinase inhibitor, administered orally in a two weeks on, two weeks off scheme to patients with advanced cancer. Proc Am Soc Clin Oncol 2002; 21: 86a, abs 340.

110. Murren JR, Papadimitrakopoulou VA, Sizer KC, Vaidyanathan S, Ravera C, Abbruzzese JL. A phase I dose-escalating study to evaluate the biological activity and pharmacokinetics of PKI166, a novel tyrosine kinase inhibitor, in patients with advanced cancers. Proc Am Soc Clin Oncol 2002; 21: 95a, abs 377.

111. Hidalgo M, Erlichman C. Rowinsky EK, Koepp-Norris J, Jensen K, Boni J, Korth-Bradley J, Quinn S, Zacharchuk C. Phase I trial of EKB-569, an irreversible inhibitor of the epidermal growth factor receptor (EGFR), in patients with advanced solid tumors. Proc Am Soc Clin Oncol 2002; 21: 17a, abs 65.

112. Tewes M, Schleucher N, Dirsch O, Schmid KW, Rosen O, Arens H-J, Kovar A, Seeber S, Harstrick A, Vanhoefer U. Results of a phase I trial of the humanized anti epidermal growth factor receptor (EGFR) monoclonal antibody EMD 72000 in patients with EGFR expressing solid tumors. Proc Am Soc Clin Oncol 2002; 21: 95a, abs 378.

113. Crombet T, Osorio M, Cruz T, Figueredo R, Koropatnick J, Reginfo E, Torres O, Pérez R, Lage A. Use of the anti-EGFR antibody h-R3 in combination with radiotherapy in the treatment of advanced head and neck cancer. Proc Am Soc Clin Oncol 2002; 21; 14a, abs 53.

114. Figlin RA, Belldegrun AS, Crawford J, Lohner M, Roskos L, Yang X-D, Foon KA, Schwab G, Weiner L. ABX-EGF, a fully human anti-epidermal growth factor receptor (EGFR) monoclonal antibody (mAb) in patients with advanced cancer: phase I clinical results. Proc Am Soc Clin Oncol 2002; 21: 10a, abs 35.

115. Schwartz G, Dutcher JP, Vogelzang NJ, Gollob J, Thompson J, Bukowski RM, Figlin RA, Lohner M, Roskos L, Hwang CC, Foon KA, Schwab G, Rowinsky EK. Phase 2 clinical trial evaluating the safety and effectiveness of ABX-EGF in renal cell cancer (RCC). Proc Am Soc Clin Oncol 2002; 21: 24a, abs 91.

116. Cella D, Eton DT, Fairclough DL, Bonomi P, Heyes AE, Silberman C, Wolf MK, Johnson DH. What is a clinically meaningful change on the Functional Assessment of Cancer Therapy-Lung (FACT-L) Questionnaire? Results from Eastern Cooperative Oncology Group (ECOG) Study 5592. J Clin Epidemiol 2002; 55: 285–295.

Chapter 5

Histone Acetyltransferases and Histone Deacetylases in Gene Regulation and as Drug Targets

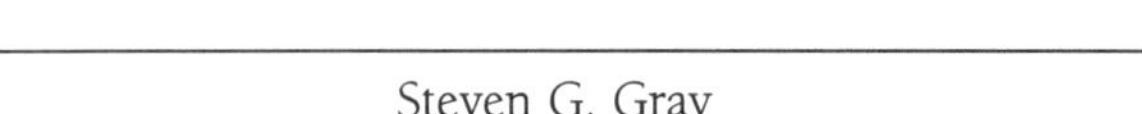

Steven G. Gray

Following the isolation and biochemical characterization of the histone deacetylases (HDACs) and histone acetyltransferases (HATs), new paradigms in the regulation of gene expression have emerged. These regulatory enzymes alter the acetylation status of histones and other proteins, and play critical roles in many cellular processes including transcription, cell cycle progression, differentiation and apoptosis.[1,2] Many of the processes to which these enzymes are linked are critical to carcinogenesis/tumorigenesis, and as such, these enzymes represent major targets for therapeutic intervention strategies and increasingly are being evaluated in clinical settings. Using breast cancer as an example, I will discuss how histone acetyltransferases and histone deacetylases are important in regulating gene expression in this cancer and how they are therefore appropriate drug targets for the treatment of cancer in general.

HISTONE ACETYLTRANSFERASES (HATS) AND HISTONE DEACETYLASES (HDACs)

On the basis of sequence similarity to yeast proteins, HATs can be grouped loosely into a single superfamily consisting of five subfamilies including the GNAT (GCN5-related N-acetyltransferase), and MYST families.[3] In a similar manner, HDACs can be grouped into a superfamily of proteins including bacterial members.[4–6] The mammalian HDACs also can be separated into three subfamilies based on their similarity to three yeast proteins.[1,2]

Currently, 18 members of the HDAC superfamily have been identified in humans. However, to complicate matters alternative splicing also has been observed for several HDAC family members including: HDAC3,[7] HDAC8,[8–10] HDAC9,[11,12] HDAC10,[13–15] and HDAC11.[17]

ADDITIONAL FUNCTIONS OF HATs/HDACs

The name histone acetyltransferase is in some ways a misnomer, as clearly they have been shown to acetylate proteins other than histones, which has led to them being described as FATs.[18] To my knowledge, at present up to 60 proteins are acetylated by histone acetyltransferases, and no doubt this number will increase in the future. The available evidence for histone deacetylases is less clear, but some studies have demonstrated that these enzymes have the ability to catalyze the removal of acetyl moities from proteins other than histones. Indeed, two histone deacetylases have additional roles where they act as tubulin deacetylases.[19–22]

Regulating the Activity of Histone Acetyltransferases and Histone Deacetylases

It is becoming increasingly clear that the timely regulation of histone acetyltransferase and histone deacetylase activity is important. An emerging picture indicates that several mechanisms are used by the cell to achieve such regulation, including specific interacting proteins, direct modifications of the enzymes themselves, and/or intracellular sequestration of HATs/HDACs, which are discussed in the following sections.

Protein Modifications

Acetylation One of the modifications identified to affect the activities of HATs/HDACs is that of acetylation itself. Autoacetylation of several histone acetyltransferases has been documented including CBP,[23] P/CAF,[24] and ESA1, which is a yeast histone acetyltransferase.[25]

In addition, acetylation of BCL6 has been shown to prevent its association with HDACs, and as such regulates its ability to repress gene transcription.[26]

Methylation At present only one HAT protein, CBP, is regulated by methylation. Two domains have been identified that are methylated. Of these, methylation of the KIX domain negates CBP binding ability.[27–29]

Phosphorylation Phosphorylation of various histone acetyltransferases and histone deacetylases has been shown to modulate their activities. PKCdelta phosphorylates CBP, resulting in the inhibition of its acetyltransferase activity.[30] Recruitment of p300 by C/EBP-β triggers the phosphorylation of p300, which appears to be functionally important, as mutation of the phosphorylation sites subtantially affects CBP activity.[18] Phosphorylation of Tip60 inhibits its histone acetyltransferase activity.[31] The mitogen-activated/extracellular response kinase kinase 1 (MEKK1) has been shown to enhance p300-mediated transcription. In their work, See et al show that MEKK1 has the ability to phosphorylate p300 in vitro and, therefore, it is possible that this may be a functional event and responsible for the enhanced transcription.[32] HDAC1 is phosphorylated in vitro by cAMP-dependent kinase and casein kinase II,[33] and mutation of identified sites of phosphorylation results in a reduction of its enzymatic activity, and ability to form complexes.[34] Finally, the kinase CK2 binds to and phosphorylates HDAC2,[35] which enhances its DNA binding capabilities. Similar to HDAC1, treatments that remove the phosphorylation result in decreased enzymatic activity.

Ubiquitination Ubiquitination is another posttranslational modification that occurs on HATs/HDACs. Ubiquitination of proteins normally targets them for degradation in the proteasome. Degradation of p300 occurs via the ubiquitin mediated pathway following retinoic acid differentiation of F9 cells.[36] Likewise, ubiquitination of SRC-1 also has been demonstrated. The function of this is unknown, but presumably it directs this HAT to the proteasome for degradation.[37]

Early evidence linking ubiquitin and deacetylase activity came from data published by Mezquita and colleagues, who found a heat-stable factor that stimulated histone deacetylase in vitro, which they identified as ubiquitin.[38] This is unusual, as more recently, the histone deacetylase inhibitor valproic acid was found to selectively cause the ubiquitination of HDAC2 and its subsequent degradation.[39] However, both HDAC5 and HDAC6 have been shown to be ubiquitinated in vivo. The ubiquitinated forms of these enzymes are not targeted for degradation and their functional significance at this time is unknown, but if the early evidence of Mezquita et al holds true, then the ubiquitination of these proteins may result in enhanced enzymatic activity.[40,41]

A Class III histone deacetylase is modified by ubiquitination also. CDC14B has been shown to provoke an exit from cellular mitosis, and it is suggested that part of the mechanism used in this process involves the ubiquitination and subsequent degradation of SIRT2.[42]

Sumoylation Sumoylation of HDACs 1, 4, 6 and 9 reduce their biological activity.[43–46] The adenovirus early protein GAM1 is crucial for virus replication and induces certain cellular genes by inactivating HDAC1. More recently it has been shown to interfere with the sumoylation of HDAC1, and does not seem to be absolutely required for HDAC1 biological activity.[47] HDAC3 also is associated with PIASxβ, a protein used in the sumoylation process.[48]

Sumoylation of p300 mediates repression of gene transcription,[49] while sumoylation of SRC-1 alters the kinetics of transfer between the nucleus and cytoplasm, overexpressing SUMO causes SRC-1 to be retained within the nucleus.[37]

Direct Interactions Inhibiting HATs/HDACs

Many viral proteins modulate histone acetyltransferase activity by interacting directly with HATs. The HIV protein Tat directly inhibits histone acetyltransferase activity.[50–52] The viral interferon regulatory factor (vIRF) binds to and inhibits p300 HAT activity,[53] whereas SV40 T antigen binds to CBP and enhances its HAT activity.[54] Adenovirus E1A binds to and inhibits HATs.[55–57] Latency-associated nuclear antigen (LANA) of Kaposi's sarcoma-associated herpesvirus (KSHV) binds to and inhibits the histone acetyltransferase activity of CBP.[58] Some viral proteins inhibit HDACs. In chicken, the CELO adenovirus protein GAM1 binds to HDAC1 and inactivates HDAC1.[59,60] It may be that the inactivation of HDAC1 by Gam1 may be caused in part by interference with the sumoylation of this protein.[61]

PU.1 is an Ets family transcription factor that is required for the development of myeloid and lymphoid cells. Recently, it was shown to bind both CBP and P/CAF, resulting in the inhibition of their histone acetyltransferase activity.[62] Two dominant-negative mutants of hepatocyte nuclear factor-1alpha (HNF-1alpha) that arise in maturity onset diabetes of the young (MODY3) patients recruit CBP and P/CAF, but have a greatly reduced HAT activity.[63] Early B cell factor (EBF) is a DNA binding protein required for early B-cell development. It also binds to the histone acetyltransferase domain of and inhibits its HAT activity both in vivo and in vitro.[64] Another protein that binds to p300/CBP is EID-1 (E1A-like inhibitor of differentiation 1). EID-1 binds to CBP/p300, inhibits its acetyltransferase activity and acts as a negative regulator of muscle differentiation.[65,66] The recently identified cell cycle regulator p34SEI-1 binds to CBP also, and suppresses transcription, but whether this is by directly inhibiting its acetyltransferase activity has yet to be determined.[67] The HOX Homeodomain Proteins are a family of transcription factors with fundamental importance for body patterning during embryonic development. Alterations to their expression also have been reported in cancer. They have been shown to bind with, and block, the histone acetyltransferase activity of CBP.[68] The bHLH Protein Twist is involved in craniofacial and limb development, binds both p300 and PCAF, and inhibits their HAT activity both in vitro and in vivo.[69] The general transcription factor, TFIID, consists of the TATA-binding protein (TBP) associated with a series of TBP-associated factors (TAFs) that together participate in the assembly of the transcription preinitiation complex. These include $TAF_{II}55$ and the HAT $TAF_{II}250$. $TAF_{II}55$ binds directly to $TAF_{II}250$ and inhibits its acetyltransferase activity, and therefore may play direct roles in regulating transcription initiation.[70]

A multiprotein histone acetyltransferase inhibitory complex (INHAT) has been isolated that functions by histone masking, preventing histone acetyltransferases from finding their targets.[71,72] Mitogen-regulated RSK2-CBP interaction controls their kinase and acetylase activities.[73]

HATs have been shown to activate p53 by acetylation.[74] MDM2 inhibits p300-mediated p53 acetylation and activation by forming a ternary complex with the two proteins.[75]

Intracellular Sequestration In recent years it has become apparent that one mechanism by which a cell can modulate histone deacetylase activity is through intracellular sequestration. For example, the class III HDAC SIRT3 is localized specifically to the mitochondria.[76] Ikappa-Balpha (Iκ-Bα) binds HDAC proteins through ankyrin-repeats, and in the case of HDAC3 this results in the partial redirection of this histone deacetylase to the cytoplasm.[77] In addition, IκBα was shown to associate with the nuclear factor-κB (NF-κB) member p65. This results in the translocation of the nuclear corepressors SMRT/N-CoR to the cytoplasm and consequent upregulation in transcription of Notch-dependent genes.[78] Several of the class II HDACs utilize nucleocytoplasmic shuttling to regulate gene expression in muscle and neuronal settings.[79–87] Expansion of polyglutamine repeats within the androgen receptor sequesters CBP in spinal and bulbar muscular atrophy (SBMA).[88]

Tubulin is a cellular microfilament that is posttranslationally modified by acetylation, and histone deacetylases recently were shown to mediate their deacetylation. Tubulin mediates the subcellular redistribution of the transcriptional coactivator p/CIP, and this is also known as ACTR, a protein with histone acetyltransferases activity.[89]

Intranuclear Bodies (Speckles) The importance of intracellular sequestration of HATs/HDACs in cellular events that can lead to pathogenesis is well documented for the autosomal dominant, late-onset neurodegenerative condition, Huntington's disease. The disease primarily is caused by an expansion of a polyglutamine repeat within the amino terminus of the predominantly cytosolic protein huntingtin.[90] Expansion of this repeat region results in nuclear translocation and aggregation of huntingtin, and has been implicated as the causative event in the pathogenesis of this disease.[91] Several studies have since shown that the repeat-containing huntingtin interacts directly with the HATs CBP and P/CAF.[92,93] One of the most important features of this association is that the nuclear localization of CBP is altered such that it aggregates into intranuclear inclusions in neuronal cells.[92,93] Thus, the major effects of this disease appear to be caused by a depletion of this HAT from its normal localization, resulting in aberrant transcriptional control. However, cell-free assays show that the mutant huntingtin protein has the ability to inhibit the activity of three HATs—CBP, p300 and P/CAF[93]—and, thus, a direct interference mechanism also may be involved. In addition, a cell line model of neuronal death caused by polyglutamine-expanded huntingtin found that this was associated with degradation of CBP, indicating that the mutant huntintin may function to actively eliminate CBP from the affected neurons.[94]

In addition to interacting with HATs, suggestive evidence indicates that huntingtin may functionally associate with HDACs. Two studies show that huntingtin associates with mSin3a and also to N-CoR, which indicates that a complex containing HDACs would be recruited.[93,95] Huntingtin has since been shown to directly associate with REST/NRSF (a histone deacetylase-containing complex) to modulate the transcription of NRSE-controlled neuronal genes.[96]

Another form of intracellular sequestration that involves HATs is that of the promyelocytic leukemia (PML) nuclear bodies (NBs). These are macromolecular nuclear domains present in virtually every mammalian cell, and have been functionally linked to several fundamental cellular processes, including transcriptional control, tumor suppression and apoptosis regulation.[97] A series of reports has demonstrated associations between histone acetyltransferases, histone deacetylases the PML protein, and the PML/PLZF RARαfusions.[74] It must be noted that PML NBs are not associated with sites of active transcription and do not localize with nascent DNA.[97] However, CBP has been shown to dynamically move into and out of the PML nuclear bodies in a cell type specific fashion.[98] As such, the idea that PML nuclear bodies can act as protein storage compartments[97] may be an important mechanism by which sequestration of HATs/HDACs and their subsequent appropriate release can be maintained and regulated.

IMPORTANCE OF HATS/HDACS IN THE PATHOGENESIS OF BREAST CANCER

It is becoming increasingly clear that histone acetyltransferases and histone deacetylases play important roles in the pathogenesis of breast cancer. The following sections will attempt to elaborate on some of the aspects to which these enzymes can impinge on breast cancer tumorigenesis.

BRCA1 and *BRCA2* are two critical breast cancer tumour suppressor genes. The BRCA2 protein itself has been shown to have intrinsic histone acetyltransferase activity,[99] but this is considered by some to be controversial, as it also has been shown to associate with the acetyltransferase P/CAF.[100] BRCA1 has been shown to associate with HDAC1 and HDAC2.[101]

Mutations of the histone acetyltransferase p300 have been identified, albeit with an extremely rare frequency, in primary breast cancers and cell lines.[102–104]

The nuclear hormone receptor superfamily has been shown to associate intimately with histone deacetylases and histone acetyltransferases. As a comprehensive overview of these complexes is beyond the scope of this review, I have chosen to focus on those with importance to breast cancer. For comprehensive overviews of this superfamily, readers are directed to the following reviews.[1,3,105–108]

Retinoic Acid Receptor

The best documented associations between retinoic acid receptors and histone deacetylases relate to the fusion translocations between the promyelocytic leukemia gene (*PML*), or the promyelolytic zinc finger gene (*PLZF*) to the retinoic acid receptor α gene (*RAR*-α).[1] Moreover, unliganded RAR complexes and or heterocomplexes of RAR/TR (thyroid hormone receptor) repress trancription by complexes containing HDACs,[1,109–116] predominantly through SMRT (of retinoic acid and thyroid hormone receptor).[1,2] Retinoic acid receptors play important roles in breast cancer[117,118] and epigenetic silencing of retinoic acid receptors is a frequent event in breast cancer.[119–121]

Histone acetyltransferases also are important to breast cancer tumorigenesis mediated via RAR. The cancer-amplified transcriptional coactivator (ASC-2) has altered expression in breast cancer and associates with RXR/RAR and CBP/p300 and SRC-1, and is essential for ligand-dependent transactivation by nuclear receptors in vivo.[122] ASC-2 is identical to the gene *AIB*-3 (amplified in breast cancer 3), which has been identified as either NRC, AIB3, ASC2, PRIP, TRBP, RAP250, or KIAA0181, leading to it being redefined as NCOA6.

Transforming Growth Factor

The transforming growth factors (TGFs) are an important superfamily of signalling molecules with important regulatory roles in several cellular processes including proliferation and differentiation.[123–125] It has become increasingly clear that the TGF-β signaling pathway is of great importance in carcinogenesis, including breast cancer.[126–129] Gene expression profiling of the TGF-β signaling network in a breast cancer cell line has defined that c-myc repression, a response that is key to the TGF-β program of cell cycle arrest, is selectively lost.[130] Additionally, a murine model of breast cancer TGF-β signaling impairs Neu-induced mammary tumorigenesis while promoting pulmonary metastasis.[131]

One mechanism by which TGF-β signaling regulates gene expression utilizes both HATs and HDACs. Following signaling by TGF-β at its receptors, Smads 1, 2, 3 and 4, AP-1, c-Jun and c-Fos were shown to interact with the histone acetyltransferase CBP/p300 to activate gene expression.[132–138] Down-regulation of Smad3 was shown to occur in high grade breast cancer, indicating that aberrant TGF-β signaling-mediated gene regulation may be occurring in these tumors.[139]

In addition to histone acetyltransferases, Smad 3, Smad6, and Smad7 were shown to functionally associate with class I histone deacetylases and direct repression.[140,141]. It is interesting to note that a recent study has indicated that Smad3 plays a pivitol role in TGF-β signaling via hierachical cascades.[142] As such, the importance of histone acetyltransferases and histone deacetylases takes on new significance with regard to aberrant transcriptional profiles in breast cancer tumorigenesis.

Two oncoproteins, Ski and Sno, have been demonstrated to be members of an SMRT/N-CoR/HDAC complex and act as transcriptional co-repressors in TGF-β signaling.[143–145] Moreover, the *sno* gene was shown to act as a tumor suppressor in mice indicating a potential role for HDACs in preventing tumor formation.[146] Other TGF-β related represson complexes have been isolated. In one of them, signaling by TGF-β1 recruits a p130/HDAC1 complex to repress gene expression.[147] Another smad transcriptional repressor, *TGIF*, has multiple modes by which it represses gene expression, and one of its modes of action is via an interaction with Smads 2 and 3 and recruitment of histone deacetylases to repress transcription.[148–150] An additional related gene, *TGIF2*, recruits HDACs to repress transcription.[151] One of the receptors for the TGF-β signaling pathway, the type two receptor (*TGFBR-II*) regulates at the level of expression via HDACs/HATs.[152]

Further evidence for important roles for the TGF signaling pathway in breast cancer has come from data demonstrating that TGF-β regulates the nuclear coreceptor amplified in breast cancer 1 (AIB1/NCOA3), and SMAD4, another member of the TGF signaling pathway, acts as a transcriptional corepressor for the estrogen receptor in breast cancer cells.[153] As the estrogen receptor plays important roles within the mammary gland (discussed below), this appears to be an important link in breast cancer.

Further evidence for the importance of histone deacetylases and the TGF signaling pathway comes from studies screening for TGF mimetics. The lead compound isolated from this screen was subsequently identified as a histone deacetylase inhibitor.[154]

Estrogen Receptors

The estrogen receptors play important roles in the pathogenesis of breast cancer.[117,155] The gene amplified in breast cancer, *AIB1*, is a nuclear coactivator intimately associated with estrogen receptors (ER).[156,157] AIB1 has many synonyms including: ACTR, AIB1, RAC3, SRC3, pCIP, CTG26, CAGH16, TNRC14, TNRC16, TRAM-1. It since has been renamed NCOA3 and is overexpressed in breast cancer.[156,158–167] One of the synonms previously used for NCOA3 is ACTR. This previously was shown to have intrinsic histone acetyltransferase activity.[116] Other histone acetyltransferases associate within the ER coactivator complex including p300 and P/CAF.[168–172] In addition, a TFTC-HAT complex is directed to ER-α.[3,173]

The major treatment of ER positive breast cancer cells is via tamoxifen, and NCOA3 has since been linked to tamoxifen resisistance in breast cancer; this would appear to be linked with histone acetyltransferases to cellular resistance to drug treatment.[143,144,161,162,174,175] Estradiol treatments in breast cancer cells altered the intranuclear distribution of ER and histone acetyltransferases, with both becoming tightly bound in the nucleus and associated with the nuclear matrix, while not affecting the intranuclear distribution of histone deacetylases, increasing histone acetylation levels and presumably up-regulating transcription of ER responsive genes.[176]

The estrogen receptor ? has been shown to be directly acetylated by p300, resulting in reduced hormone sensitivity and disrupted gene transcription.[177]

Histone deacetylases are involved also with ER regulation of gene transcription.[178,179] Fusions of the ER to N-CoR strongly inhibits estrogen-dependent responses in breast cancer cells,[180] while a direct association between ERbeta and NCoR/HDACs has been shown.[181]

Histone deacetylases have been implicated in tamoxifen-dependent interactions of N-CoR,[182,183] while microinjection of N-CoR into N-CoR$^{-/-}$ mouse embryo fibroblasts showed the presence of tamoxifen resulted in a decrease in transcriptional activation of ER.[184] A dominant-negative nuclear receptor corepressor was shown to relieve retinoic acid receptor-mediated transcriptional repression, but did not alter the agonist/antagonist activities of the tamoxifen-bound estrogen receptor.[185] Interestingly, insulin/IGF-I treatment of tamoxifen treated cells causes dissociation of N-CoR/SMRT from the ER, and results in the translocation of the ER back to the cytoplasm.[186] This opens new vistas in the potential treatment of tamoxifen-resistant breast cancer.

Regulation of ER gene expression involves histone deacetylases. BRCA1 mediates ligand independent repression of the estrogen receptor itself in a manner dependent upon histone deacetylase activity.[187] In breast cancer cells, pRb complexes containing HATs and HDACs have been shown to regulate the ER.[188].

Metastasis/MTA and the ER

Metastasis is a critical factor in cancer, and the metastasis-associated protein MTA1 is an important regulator of this process in cancer, including breast cancer.[189–191]

Recently, a variant of MTA1 was shown to sequester the ER in the cytoplasm.[192] The MTA1 protein was originally shown to associate with a chromatin remodeling complex (NURD) that contains histone deacetylases,[193] and further studies have found that both MTA1 and MTA2 associate with HDACs.[194,195]

HDAC directed repression by MTA1 occurs at estrogen receptor elements,[196] indicating that metastasis may be regulated in part through the ER. Further evidence shows that a novel MTA1 intercting protein MICoA also regulates estrogen receptor alpha transactivation functions,[197] while another interacting protein,

MTA1, associates with MTA1 to directly regulate the ER.[198] MTA3, another component of the NURD complex, also regulates an invasive growth pathway in breast cancer.[199] Finally, MTA1 regulates collagenase, a major component in the metastasis pathway in part through HDACs.[200] Clearly, targeting the ER/HAT/HDAC pathways appears to be a viable future therapeutic strategy in the treatment of breast cancer.

Androgen Receptor

Androgen receptors also utilize chromatin remodeling to regulate gene expression.[201] These receptors play important roles in breast cancer carcinogenesis.[202] Mutations of the androgen receptor have been found in breast cancers.[203] The TGF-β signaling pathway mediates androgen receptor regulation of gene expression,[204] further establishing the TGF-β pathway as a critical signaling pathway in breast cancer. In addition, direct associations between histone acetyltransferases and histone deacetylases and the androgen receptor have been identified.[205,206] As such, aberrant gene regulation by the androgen receptor through histone acetyltransferases and histone deacetylases may be a critical step in the pathogenesis of breast cancer. Mutations to BRCA1 have been linked to a loss of expression of the androgen receptor in 88% of the tumors studied.[207] Moreover, the *BRCA2* gene associates with histone acetyltransferases to regulate androgen receptor-mediated transcription.[207,208]

Progesterone Receptor

Another important hormone receptor in breast cancer is the progesterone receptor.[117,209–212] Loss of coordinate expression of progesterone receptors A and B is an early event in breast carcinogenesis.[213] Several studies have shown that the progesterone receptor associates with both histone acetyltransferases and histone deacetylases.[214–216] As such, the loss of progesterone receptor expression early in breast cancer development may lead to inappropriate gene regulation of critical genes by loss of histone acetyltransferase/histone deacetylase activity directed by the progesterone receptors.

Methylation-directed Gene Repression

It is well established that CpG methylation can direct methylbinding proteins such as MeCP2 to direct gene repression. It also is established that such methylbinding proteins can achieve gene repression through associations with histone deacetylases.[1] These proteins increasingly are being seen as important regulators in mammary gland development and tumorigenesis. Levels of MBD2 and MECP2 are up-regulated during the prenatal development of the human mammary gland, while MBD2 levels are significantly up-regulated and associated with breast cancer tumor size.[217] As such, aberrant transcription of specific genes by MBD2 via histone deacetylases may play an important role in breast cancer carcinogenesis. In support of this hypothesis, down-regulation of GISP-1 in breast cancer cells is directed by MBD2, although whether or not this is via histone deacetylases has yet to be elucidated.[218]

Summary

In conclusion, it is apparent that several proteins that utilize histone acetyltransferases and histone deacetylases to activate or repress transcription are also frequently affected in the pathogenesis of breast cancer. As such, targeting the histone acetyltransferases or histone deacetylases may be a viable therapeutic modality in the treatment of breast cancer. The following sections discuss the development and therapeutic potential of various inhibitors for these genes, and provide the available evidence demonstrating their potential efficacy in treating breast cancer.

SPECIFIC INHIBITORS FOR HDACs AND HATs

Generally, HDAC inhibitors can be separated into three categories: short chain fatty acids, naturally occurring compounds, and synthetic derivatives. Historically, sodium butyrate, a short chain fatty acid, was one of the first compounds shown to cause an increase in histone acetylation.[219,220] Sodium butyrate, however, has pleiotropic effects including the hypermethylation of DNA,[221] and does not represent a true histone deacetylase inhibitor *per se*. Several other butyrate or short chain fatty acid derivatives have since been shown to have histone deacetylase inhibitory activity.[222,223] In the second category, naturally occurring compounds, the first specific HDAC inhibitor described was trichostatin A (TSA), originally isolated as a fungistatic antibiotic from a streptomyces strain.[224]

Other naturally occurring compounds that have inhibitory effects include trapoxin,[225] apicidin,[226] HC toxin,[227] depudecin,[228] Psammaplins, 229 and FR901228.[230] Because of the interest in these inhibitors for their therapeutic potential, several synthetic compounds have been generated also, including hybrid polar compounds such as hydroxamic acids.[231–237] NVP-LAQ824,[238] valproic acid,[239,240] trifluoromethyl ketones,[241] cyclic tetrapeptides,[242,243] benzamides,[244,245] and others.[154,246,247]

Small molecule inhibitor screening increasingly is being used to identify and target for the most part histone deacetylases,[248–256] but some inhibitors for histone acetyltransferases have been identified also.[257–261]

One of the problems encountered with the current inhibitors of HATs has been the inability of these compounds to function efficently in mammalian cell culture models.[262] However, the successful use of various histone deacetylase inhibitors as an effective treatment in cell culture models of cancer has meant that several of these compounds, including sodium phenylbutyrate, SAHA and TSA, are currently undergoing clinical trials.[263–268]

HOW ARE HDAC INHIBITORS USEFUL IN THE TREATMENT OF BREAST CANCER?

Histone deacetylase inhibitors clearly have therapeutic potential in the treatment of cancer and currently are being evaluated in many clinical settings.[263,265–269] The following sections discuss the potential benefit of therapies targeted against histone deacetylases in the treatment of breast cancer.

Targeting Angiogenesis

Most solid tumors have reduced oxygen levels due to an imbalance in supply and consumption. A consequence of this is the stimulation of angiogenesis to increase tumor infiltration, which may increase the metastatic potential of the tumor by inducing certain genes.[270–272] Breast cancer is no exception, and angiogensis is an important factor in breast cancer carcinogens.[273]

Hypoxia-inducible transcription factor 1 (HIF-1) is an important angiogenesis transcription factor that binds to DNA at conserved hypoxia response elements to activate transcription of target genes.[270,272] A role for HATs in the HIF-1 signal transduction process has demonstrated that several histone acetyltransferases associate with hypoxia-inducible factor 1α (HIF-1α) and enhance its transactivation potential in a hypoxia-dependent manner.[274,275]

Histone deacetylases also directly regulate the angiogenesis process.[276] Both histone acetyltransferases and histone deacetylases appear to be extremely good targets for anti-angiogenic strategies in treating breast cancer. Several studies have shown that histone deacetylase inhibitors inhibit angiogeneis through inhibition of vascular endothelial growth factor (VEGF)[277–281] or prevent angiogensis by reducing endothelial nitric oxide synthase (eNOS) levels.[282] They also prevent angiogenesis by suppressing hypoxia inducible factor-α (HIFaβ).[278] More recently, HDAC inhibitors have been shown to inhibit angiogenesis through upregulation of RECK.[283]

Clearly, histone deacetylase inhibitors have the potential to inhibit angiogenesis and should be considered as a potential adjunct therapy in the treatment of breast cancer.

Targeting TGF-β Signaling

As described in the previous sections, the TGF-β signaling pathway plays important roles in breast cancer development and tumorigenesis. Histone deacetylase inhibitors have been shown to modulate many aspects of the TGF signaling process.

Transforming growth factor beta 1 and sodium butyrate differentially modulate urokinase plasminogen activator and plasminogen activator inhibitor-1 in human breast normal and cancer cells.[284] Up-regulation of TGF-β induces apoptosis in cell lines including breast cancer.[285] We have shown that TGF-β can be up-regulated by HDAC inhibitors in a hepatocellular cell culture model.[286] More importantly, we also demonstrated that the addition of exogenous insulin-like growth factor-II (IGF-II) amplified this response.[286]

The histone deacetylase inhibitor MS-275 selectively induces TGF-β type II receptor expression in human breast cancer cells and shows antiproliferative activity against all human breast cancer cell lines examined.[287]

Targeting Estrogen Receptor Signaling

Breast cancers can be classified into two types based on their expression of estrogen receptor (ER): ER positive and ER negative. A series of reports have shown that treating ER negative cells with histone deacetylase inhibitors reactivates expression of this gene, indicating that this may be a unique adjunt therapeutic option in the treatment of breast cancer.[288, 289] However, an early study also found that treating cells with sodium butyrate resulted in decreased expression of ER.[290]

Nevertheless, histone deacetylase inhibitors represent a strong therapeutic alternative in the treatment of breast cancer. Further studies have proven antineoplastic activity, increased apoptosis, and decreased cellular proliferation in mammary gland cells treated with histone deacetylase inhibitors, continuing to add weight to the argument for their inclusion into breast cancer treatment.[291–293]

Interestingly, insulin/IGF-I treatment of tamoxifen-treated cells causes dissociation of N-CoR/SMRT from the ER, and results in the translocation of the ER back to the cytoplasm,[186] indicating that this may be a further avenue for therapeutic intervention strategies.

Targeting Androgen Receptor

The influence of Smad3/Smad4 on the androgen receptor (AR) transactivation may involve histone acetylation, since treatment with trichostatin A or sodium butyrate can reverse Smad3/Smad4-repressed AR transactivation and the Smad3/Smad4 complex can decrease the acetylation level of AR.[294]

Targeting the Cell Cycle

One of the most common responses to treatment with histone deacetylase inhibitors is cell cycle arrest at the G_1/G_2M boundaries. The classical response of many cells to treatments with histone deacetylase inhibitors has been the induction or up-regulation of the cyclin-dependent kinase inhibitor (CKI) p21$^{WAF1/CIP1/Sdi1}$ (CDKN1A) induction.[295–302]

Up-regulation of the CKI p27^{Kip1} (CDKN1B) has been observed also in cell lines following inhibition of histone deacetylases.[303–307] In contrast, down-regulation of p57^{kip2} (CDKN1C) has been observed in a hepatocellular carcinoma-derived cell line.[308]

Inhibition of histone deacetylases also affects the expression of cyclins, including the down-regulation of cyclin A,[309,310] cyclin B1,[309–311] cyclin D1,[312] and cyclin E[296,313,314] However, the effects of histone deacetylase inhibitors also may be cell type specific, as elevated protein levels of cylin A and cyclin E have been observed in gastric and oral carcinoma cell lines following treatment with Trichostatin A.[315] Induction of cyclin D2[316] and cyclin D3[317] have been observed following treatment with histone deacetylase inhibitors.

Finally, treatments of hepatocytes with Trichostatin A have resulted in the loss of expresssion of CDC2 (CDK1).[318]

Overall, histone deacetylase inhibitors appear to be good candidates for disturbing appropriate cell cycle regulation. One caveat, however, is that these drugs also function to affect cell cycle regulation in normal breast epithelial cells.[319]

SUMMARY

Histone acetyltransferases and histone deacetylases appear to be critical regulators of many important cellular pathways. The availability of appropriate inhibitors for both of these enzymes has provided exciting new vistas in therapies for many human conditions including cancer. This chapter has focussed on the available data about breast cancer to explore the diverse areas by which histone acetylatransferases and histone deacetylases regulate gene expression, and has attempted to demonstrate how inhibitors of histone deacetylases may prove to be an exciting new therapeutic modality in the treatment of this cancer. The paucity of data currently available for the inhibitors of histone acetyltransferases of necessity precludes a discussion of their potential worth in the treatment of cancer. As new inhibitors for these enzymes become available, it will be of great interest to see if they too will prove to have therapeutic potential. Much more work is required within clinical settings to establish the value of these exciting drugs in the treatment of cancer, but the clinical studies that have been carried out are promising and warrant our further attention.

ACKNOWLEDGMENTS

I would like to apologize to all of the authors whose work I was unable to cite in this article due to space requirements.

REFERENCES

1. Gray SG, Teh BT. Histone acetylation/deacetylation and cancer: an "open" and "shut" case? Curr Mol Med 2001;1:401–429.
2. Gray SG, Ekström TJ. The human histone deacetylase family. Exp Cell Res 2001;262:75–83.
3. Carrozza MJ, Utley RT, Workman JL, Cote J. The diverse functions of histone acetyltransferase complexes. Trends Genet 2003;19:321–329.
4. Khochbin S, Wolffe AP. The origin and utility of histone deacetylases. FEBS Lett 1997;419157–419160.
5. Leipe DD, Landsman D. Histone deacetylases, acetoin utilization proteins and acetylpolyamine amidohydrolases are members of an ancient protein superfamily. Nucl Acids Res 1997;25: 3693–3697.
6. Trojer P, Brandtner EM, Brosch G et al. Histone deacetylases in fungi: novel members, new facts. Nucl Acids Res 2003;31:3971–3981.
7. Gray SG, Iglesias AH, Teh BT, Dangond F. Modulation of splicing events in histone deacetylase 3 by various extracellular and signal transduction pathways. Gene Expr 2003;11:13–21.
8. Buggy JJ, Sideris ML, Mak P et al. Cloning and characterization of a novel human histone deacetylase, HDAC8. Biochem J 2000;350:1199–1205.
9. Hu E, Chen Z, Fredrickson T et al. Cloning and characterization of a novel human class I histone deacetylase that functions as a transcription repressor. J Biol Chem 2000;275:15254–15264.
10. Van den Wyngaert I, de Vries W, Kremer A et al. Cloning and characterization of human histone deacetylase 8. FEBS Lett 2000;478:77–83.
11. Petrie K, Guidez F, Howell L et al. The histone deacetylase 9 gene encodes multiple protein isoforms. J Biol Chem 2003;278:16059–16072.
12. Zhou X, Marks PA, Rifkind RA, Richon VM. Cloning and characterization of a histone deacetylase, HDAC9. Proc Natl Acad Sci USA 2001;98:10572–10577.
13. Fischer DD, Cai R, Bhatia U et al. Isolation and characterization of a novel class II histone deacetylase, HDAC10. J Biol Chem 2002;277:6656–6666.
14. Guardiola AR, Yao TP. Molecular cloning and characterization of a novel histone deacetylase HDAC10. J Biol Chem 2002;277:3350–3356.
15. Kao HY, Lee CH, Komarov A, Han CC, Evans RM. Isolation and characterization of mammalian HDAC10, a novel histone deacetylase. J Biol Chem 2002;277:187–193.
16. Tong JJ, Liu J, Bertos NR, Yang XJ. Identification of HDAC10, a novel class II human histone deacetylase containing a leucine-rich domain. Nucl Acids Res 2002;30:1114–1123.
17. Gao L, Cueto MA, Asselbergs F, Atadja P. Cloning and functional characterization of HDAC11, a novel member of the human histone deacetylase family. J Biol Chem 2002;277:25748–25755.
18. Schwartz C, Beck K, Mink S et al. Recruitment of p300 by C/EBPbeta triggers phosphorylation of p300 and modulates coactivator activity. EMBO J 2003;22:882–892.
19. Hubbert C, Guardiola A, Shao R et al. HDAC6 is a microtubule-associated deacetylase. Nature 2002;417:455–458.
20. Matsuyama A, Shimazu T, Sumida Y et al. In vivo destabilization of dynamic microtubules by HDAC6-mediated deacetylation. EMBO J 2002;21:6820–6831.
21. North BJ, Marshall BL, Borra MT et al. The human Sir2 ortholog, SIRT2, is an NAD+-dependent tubulin deacetylase. Mol Cell 2003;11:437–444.

22. Zhang Y, Li N, Caron C et al. HDAC-6 interacts with and deacetylates tubulin and microtubules in vivo. EMBO J 2003;22:1168–1179.

23. Kalkhoven E, Teunissen H, Houweling A et al. The PHD type zinc finger is an integral part of the CBP acetyltransferase domain. Mol Cell Biol 2002;22:1961–1970.

24. Santos-Rosa H, Valls E, Kouzarides T, Martinez-Balbas M. Mechanisms of P/CAF auto-acetylation. Nucl Acids Res 2003;31:4285–4292.

25. Yan Y, Harper S, Speicher DW, Marmorstein R. The catalytic mechanism of the ESA1 histone acetyltransferase involves a self-acetylated intermediate. Nat Struct Biol 2002;9:862–869.

26. Bereshchenko OR, Gu W, Dalla-Favera R. Acetylation inactivates the transcriptional repressor BCL6. Nat Genet 2002;32:606–613.

27. Chevillard-Briet M, Trouche D, Vandel L. Control of CBP co-activating activity by arginine methylation. EMBO J 2002;21:5457–5466.

28. Wei Y, Horng JC, Vendel AC et al. Contribution to stability and folding of a buried polar residue at the CARM1 methylation site of the KIX domain of CBP. Biochemistry 2003;42:7044–7049.

29. Xu W, Chen H, Du K et al. A transcriptional switch mediated by cofactor methylation. Science 2001;294:2507–2511.

30. Yuan LW, Soh JW, Weinstein IB. Inhibition of histone acetyltransferase function of p300 by PKCdelta. Biochem Biophys Acta 2002;1592:205–211.

31. Lemercier C, Legube G, Caron C et al. Tip60 acetyltransferase activity is controlled by phosphorylation. J Biol Chem 2003;278:4713–4718.

32. See RH, Calvo D, Shi Y et al. Stimulation of p300-mediated transcription by the kinase MEKK1. J Biol Chem 2001;276:16310–16317.

33. Cai R, Kwon P, Yan-Neale Y et al. Mammalian histone deacetylase 1 protein is posttranslationally modified by phosphorylation. Biochem Biophys Res Commun 2001;283:445–453.

34. Pflum MK, Tong JK, Lane WS, Schreiber SL. Histone deacetylase 1 phosphorylation promotes enzymatic activity and complex formation. J Biol Chem 2001;276:47733–47741.

35. Sun JM, Chen HY, Moniwa M et al. The transcriptional repressor Sp3 is associated with CK2-phosphorylated histone deacetylase 2. J Biol Chem 2002;277:35783–35786.

36. Brouillard F, Cremisi CE. Concomitant increase of HAT activity and degradation of p300 during retinoic acid-induced differentiation of F9 cells. J Biol Chem 2003;278:39509–39516.

37. Chauchereau A, Amazit L, Quesne M et al. Sumoylation of the progesterone receptor and of the steroid receptor coactivator SRC-1. J Biol Chem 2003;278:12335–12343.

38. Mezquita J, Chiva M, Vidal S, Mezquita C. Effect of high mobility group nonhistone proteins HMG-20 (ubiquitin) and HMG-17 on histone deacetylase activity assayed in vitro. Nucl Acids Res 1982;10:1781–1797.

39. Kramer OH, Zhu P, Ostendorff HP et al. The histone deacetylase inhibitor valproic acid selectively induces proteasomal degradation of HDAC2. EMBO J 2003;22:3411–3420.

40. Hook SS, Orian A, Cowley SM, Eisenman RN. Histone deacetylase 6 binds polyubiquitin through its zinc finger (PAZ domain) and copurifies with deubiquitinating enzymes. PNAS 2002;99:13425–13430.

41. Seigneurin-Berny D, Verdel A, Curtet S et al. Identification of components of the murine histone deacetylase 6 complex: link between acetylation and ubiquitination signaling pathways. Mol Cell Biol 2001;21:8035–8044.

42. Dryden SC, Nahhas FA, Nowak JE et al. Role for human SIRT2 NAD-dependent deacetylase activity in control of mitotic exit in the cell cycle. Mol Cell Biol 2003;23:3173–3185.

43. Petrie K, Guidez F, Howell L et al. The histone deacetylase 9 gene encodes multiple protein isoforms. J Biol Chem 2003;278:16059–16072.

44. David G, Neptune MA, DePinho RA. SUMO-1 modification of histone deacetylase 1 (HDAC1) modulates its biological activities. J Biol Chem 2002;277:23658–23663.

45. Kirsh O, Seeler JS, Pichler A et al. The SUMO E3 ligase RanBP2 promotes modification of the HDAC4 deacetylase. EMBO J 2002;21:2682–2691.

46. Tatham MH, Jaffray E, Vaughan OA et al. Polymeric chains of SUMO-2 and SUMO-3 are conjugated to protein substrates by SAE1/SAE2 and Ubc9. J Biol Chem 2001;276:35368–35374.

47. Colombo R, Boggio R, Seiser C et al. The adenovirus protein Gam1 interferes with sumoylation of histone deacetylase 1. EMBO Rep 2002;3:1062–1068.

48. Tussie-Luna MI, Bayarsaihan D, Seto E et al. Physical and functional interactions of histone deacetylase 3 with TFII-I family proteins and PIASxbeta. PNAS 2002;99:12807–12812.

49. Girdwood D, Bumpass D, Vaughan OA et al. P300 transcriptional repression is mediated by SUMO modification. Mol Cell 2003;11:1043–1054.

50. Col E, Gilquin B, Caron C, Khochbin S. Tat-controlled protein acetylation. J Biol Chem 2002;277:37955–37960.

51. Weissman JD, Brown JA, Howcroft TK et al. HIV-1 Tat binds TAFII250 and represses TAFII250-dependent transcription of major histocompatibility class I genes. PNAS 1998;95: 11601–11606.

52. Harrod R, Nacsa J, van Lint C et al. Human immunodeficiency virus type-1 Tat/co-activator acetyltransferase interactions inhibit p53Lys-320 acetylation and p53-responsive transcription. J Biol Chem 2003;278:12310–12318.

53. Li M, Damania B, Alvarez X et al. Inhibition of p300 histone acetyltransferase by viral interferon regulatory factor. Mol Cell Biol 2000;20:8254–8263.

54. Valls E, de la Cruz X, Martinez-Balbas MA. The SV40 T antigen modulates CBP histone acetyltransferase activity. Nucl Acids Res 2003;31:3114–3122.

55. Perissi V, Dasen JS, Kurokawa R et al. Factor-specific modulation of CREB-binding protein acetyltransferase activity. Proc Natl Acad Sci USA 1999;96:3652–3657.

56. Chakravarti D, Ogryzko V, Kao HY et al. A viral mechanism for inhibition of p300 and PCAF acetyltransferase activity. Cell 1999;96:393–403.

57. Hamamori Y, Sartorelli V, Ogryzko V et al. Regulation of histone acetyltransferases p300 and PCAF by the bHLH protein twist and adenoviral oncoprotein E1A. Cell 1999;96:405–413.

58. Lim C, Gwack Y, Hwang S et al. The transcriptional activity of cAMP response element-binding protein-binding protein is modulated by the latency associated nuclear antigen of Kaposi's sarcoma-associated herpesvirus. J Biol Chem 2001;276:31016–31022.

59. Colombo R, Draetta GF, Chiocca S. Modulation of p120E4F transcriptional activity by the Gam1 adenoviral early protein. Oncogene 2003;22:2541–2547.

60. Chiocca S, Kurtev V, Colombo R et al. Histone deacetylase 1 inactivation by an adenovirus early gene product. Curr Biol 2002;12:594–598.

61. Colombo R, Boggio R, Seiser C et al. The adenovirus protein Gam1 interferes with sumoylation of histone deacetylase 1. EMBO Rep 2002;3:1062–1068.

62. Hong W, Kim AY, Ky S et al. Inhibition of CBP-mediated protein acetylation by the Ets family oncoprotein PU.1. Mol Cell Biol 2002;22:3729–3743.

63. Soutoglou E, Viollet B, Vaxillaire M et al. Transcription factor-dependent regulation of CBP and P/CAF histone acetyltransferase activity. EMBO J 2001;20:1984–1992.

64. Zhao F, McCarrick-Walmsley R, Akerblad P et al. Inhibition of p300/CBP by early B-cell factor. Mol Cell Biol 2003;23:3837–3846.

65. MacLellan WR, Xiao G, Abdellatif M, Schneider MD. A novel Rb- and p300-binding protein inhibits transactivation by MyoD. Mol Cell Biol 2000;20:8903–8915.

66. Miyake S, Sellers WR, Safran M et al. Cells degrade a novel inhibitor of differentiation with E1A-like properties upon exiting the cell cycle. Mol Cell Biol 2000;20:8889–8902.

67. Hirose T, Fujii R, Nakamura H et al. Regulation of CREB-mediated transcription by association of CDK4 binding protein p34SEI-1 with CBP. Int J Mol Med 2003;11:705–712.

68. Shen WF, Krishnan K, Lawrence HJ, Largman C. The HOX homeodomain proteins block CBP histone acetyltransferase activity. Mol Cell Biol 2001;21:7509–7522.

69. Hamamori Y, Sartorelli V, Ogryzko V et al. Regulation of histone acetyltransferases p300 and PCAF by the bHLH protein twist and adenoviral oncoprotein E1A. Cell 1999;96:405–413.

70. Gegonne A, Weissman JD, Singer DS. TAFII55 binding to TAFII250 inhibits its acetyltransferase activity. PNAS 2001;98:12432–12437.

71. Seo SB, Macfarlan T, McNamara P et al. Regulation of histone acetylation and transcription by nuclear protein pp32, a subunit of the INHAT complex. J Biol Chem 2002;277:14005–14010.

72. Seo SB, McNamara P, Heo S et al. Regulation of histone acetylation and transcription by INHAT, a human cellular complex containing the set oncoprotein. Cell 2001;104:119–130.

73. Merienne K, Pannetier S, Harel-Bellan A, Sassone-Corsi P. Mitogen-regulated RSK2-CBP interaction controls their kinase and acetylase activities. Mol Cell Biol 2001;21:7089–7096.

74. Gray SG, Teh BT. Histone acetylation/deacetylation and cancer: an "open" and "shut" case? Curr Mol Med 2001;1:401–429.

75. Kobet E, Zeng X, Zhu Y et al. MDM2 inhibits p300-mediated p53 acetylation and activation by forming a ternary complex with the two proteins. PNAS 2000;97:12547–12552.

76. Onyango P, Celic I, McCaffery JM et al. SIRT3, a human SIR2 homologue, is an NAD- dependent deacetylase localized to mitochondria. PNAS 2002;99:13653–13658.

77. Viatour P, Legrand-Poels S, van Lint C et al. Cytoplasmic Ikappa Balpha increases NF-kappa B-independent transcription through binding to HDAC1 and HDAC3. J Biol Chem 2003;278: 46541–46548.

78. Espinosa L, Ingles-Esteve J, Robert-Moreno A, Bigas A. Ikappa Balpha and p65 regulate the cytoplasmic shuttling of nuclear corepressors: cross-talk between notch and NFkappa B pathways . Mol Biol Cell 2003;14:491–502.

79. Chawla S, Vanhoutte P, Arnold FJ et al. Neuronal activity-dependent nucleocytoplasmic shuttling of HDAC4 and HDAC5. J Neurochem 2003;85:151–159.

80. McKinsey TA, Zhang CL, Olson EN. Identification of a signal-responsive nuclear export sequence in class II histone deacetylases. Mol Cell Biol 2001;21:6312–6321.

81. Zhang CL, McKinsey TA, Olson EN. The transcriptional corepressor MITR is a signal-responsive inhibitor of myogenesis. Proc Natl Acad Sci USA 2001;98:7354–7359.

82. Wu X, Li H, Park EJ, Chen JD. SMRTE inhibits MEF2C transcriptional activation by targeting HDAC4 and 5 to nuclear domains. J Biol Chem 2001;276:24177–24185.

83. Dressel U, Bailey PJ, Wang SC et al. A dynamic role for HDAC7 in MEF2-mediated muscle differentiation. J Biol Chem 2001;276:17007–17013.

84. McKinsey TA, Zhang CL, Olson EN. Activation of the myocyte enhancer factor-2 transcription factor by calcium/calmodulin-dependent protein kinase-stimulated binding of 14-3-3 to histone deacetylase 5. Proc Natl Acad Sci USA 2000;97:14400–14405.

85. McKinsey TA, Zhang CL, Lu J, Olson EN. Signal-dependent nuclear export of a histone deacetylase regulates muscle differentiation. Nature 2000;408:106–111.

86. Kao HY, Verdel A, Tsai CC et al. Mechanism for nucleocytoplasmic shuttling of histone deacetylase 7. J Biol Chem 2001;276:47496–47507.

87. Fischle W, Dequiedt F, Fillion M et al. Human HDAC7 histone deacetylase activity is associated with HDAC3 in vivo. J Biol Chem 2001;276:35826–35835.

88. McCampbell A, Taylor JP, Taye AA et al. CREB-binding protein sequestration by expanded polyglutamine. Hum Mol Genet 2000;9:2197–2202.

89. Qutob MS, Bhattacharjee RN, Pollari E et al. Microtubule-dependent subcellular redistribution of the transcriptional coactivator p/CIP. Mol Cell Biol 2002;22:6611–6626.

90. Group THDCR. A novel gene containing a trinucleotide repeat that is expanded and unstable on Huntington's disease chromosomes. Cell 1993;72:971–83.

91. Sieradzan KA, Mechan AO, Jones L et al. Huntington's disease intranuclear inclusions contain truncated, ubiquitinated huntingtin protein. Exp Neurol 1999;156:92–99.

92. Nucifora FC Jr, Sasaki M, Peters MF et al. Interference by huntingtin and atrophin-1 with cbp-mediated transcription leading to cellular toxicity. Science 2001;291:2423–2428.

93. Steffan JS, Kazantsev A, Spasic-Boskovic O et al. The Huntington's disease protein interacts with p53 and CREB-binding protein and represses transcription. Proc Natl Acad Sci USA 2000;97:6763–6768.

94. Jiang H, Nucifora FC Jr, Ross CA, DeFranco DB. Cell death triggered by polyglutamine-expanded huntingtin in a neuronal cell line is associated with degradation of CREB-binding protein. Hum Mol Genet 2003;12:1–12.

95. Boutell JM, Thomas P, Neal JW et al. Aberrant interactions of transcriptional repressor proteins with the Huntington's disease gene product, huntingtin. Hum Mol Genet 1999;8:1647–1655.

96. Zuccato C, Tartari M , Crotti A et al. Huntingtin interacts with REST/NRSF to modulate the transcription of NRSE-controlled neuronal genes. Nat Genet 2003;35:76–83.

97. Borden KLB. Pondering the promyelocytic leukemia protein (PML) puzzle: possible functions for PML nuclear bodies. Mol Cell Biol 2002;22:5259–5269.

98. Boisvert FM, Kruhlak MJ, Box AK et al. The transcription coactivator CBP is a dynamic component of the promyelocytic leukemia nuclear body. J Cell Biol 2001;152:1099–1106.

99. Siddique H, Zou JP, Rao VN, Reddy ES. The BRCA2 is a histone acetyltransferase. Oncogene 1998;16:2283–2285.

100. Fuks F, Milner J, Kouzarides T. BRCA2 associates with acetyltransferase activity when bound to P/CAF. Oncogene 1998;172531–172534.

101. Yarden RI, Brody LC. BRCA1 interacts with components of the histone deacetylase complex. Proc Natl Acad Sci USA 1999;96:4983–4988.

102. Bryan EJ, Jokubaitis VJ, Chamberlain NL et al. Mutation analysis of EP300 in colon, breast and ovarian carcinomas. Int J Cancer 2002;102:137–141.

103. Gayther SA, Batley SJ, Linger L et al. Mutations truncating the EP300 acetylase in human cancers. Nat Genet 2000;24:300–303.

104. Ozdag H, Batley SJ, Forsti A et al. Mutation analysis of CBP and PCAF reveals rare inactivating mutations in cancer cell lines but not in primary tumours. Br J Cancer 2002;87:1162–1165.

105. Belandia B, Parker MG. Nuclear receptors: a rendezvous for chromatin remodeling factors. Cell 2003;114:277–280.

106. Jones PL, Shi YB. N-CoR-HDAC corepressor complexes: roles in transcriptional regulation by nuclear hormone receptors. Curr Top Microbiol Immunol 2003;274:237–268.

107. Neely KE, Workman JL. The complexity of chromatin remodeling and its links to cancer. Biochim Biophys Acta 2002;1603:19–29.

108. Feng Q, Zhang Y. The NuRD complex: linking histone modification to nucleosome remodeling. Curr Top Microbiol Immunol 2003;274:269–290.

109. Minucci S, Horn V, Bhattacharyya N et al. A histone deacetylase inhibitor potentiates retinoid receptor action in embryonal carcinoma cells. Proc Natl Acad Sci USA 1997;94:11295–11300.

110. Soderstrom M, Vo A, Heinzel T et al. Differential effects of nuclear receptor corepressor (N-CoR) expression levels on retinoic acid receptor-mediated repression support the existence of dynamically regulated corepressor complexes. Mol Endocrinol 1997;11:682–692.

111. Laherty CD, Billin AN, Lavinsky RM et al. SAP30, a component of the mSin3 corepressor complex involved in N-CoR-mediated repression by specific transcription factors. Mol Cell 1998;2:33–42.

112. Wong J, Patterton D, Imhof A et al. Distinct requirements for chromatin assembly in transcriptional repression by thyroid hormone receptor and histone deacetylase. EMBO J 1998;17:520–534.

113. Wei LN, Farooqui M, Hu X. Ligand-dependent formation of retinoid receptors, receptor-interacting protein 140 (RIP140), and histone deacetylase complex is mediated by a novel receptor-interacting motif of RIP140. J Biol Chem 2001;276:16107–16112.

114. Li J, Wang J, Wang J et al. Both corepressor proteins SMRT and N-CoR exist in large protein complexes containing HDAC3. EMBO J 2000;19:4342–4350.

115. Cohen RN, Putney A, Wondisford FE, Hollenberg AN. The nuclear corepressors recognize distinct nuclear receptor complexes. Mol Endocrinol 2000;14:900–914.

116. Chen H, Lin RJ, Schiltz RL et al. Nuclear receptor coactivator ACTR is a novel histone acetyltransferase and forms a multimeric activation complex with P/CAF and CBP/p300. Cell 1997;90:569–580.

117. Keen JC, Davidson NE. The biology of breast carcinoma. Cancer 2003;97(suppl 3):825–833.

118. Yang Q, Sakurai T, Kakudo K. Retinoid, retinoic acid receptor beta and breast cancer. Breast Cancer Res Treat 2002;76:167–173.

119. Farias EF, Arapshian A, Bleiweiss IJ et al. Retinoic acid receptor alpha2 is a growth suppressor epigenetically silenced in MCF-7 human breast cancer cells. Cell Growth Differ 2002;13:335-341.

120. Sirchia SM, Ferguson AT, Sironi E et al. Evidence of epigenetic changes affecting the chromatin state of the retinoic acid receptor beta2 promoter in breast cancer cells. Oncogene 2000;19: 1556–1563.

121. Widschwendter M, Berger J, Muller HM et al. Epigenetic downregulation of the retinoic acid receptor-beta2 gene in breast cancer. J Mammary Gland Biol Neoplasia 2001;6:193–201.

122. Lee SK, Anzick SL, Choi JE et al. A nuclear factor, ASC-2, as a cancer-amplified transcriptional coactivator essential for ligand-dependent transactivation by nuclear receptors in vivo. J Biol Chem 1999;274:34283–34293.

123. Shi Y, Massague J. Mechanisms of TGF-beta signaling from cell membrane to the nucleus. Cell 2003;113:685–700.

124. Derynck R, Akhurst RJ, Balmain A. TGF-beta signaling in tumor suppression and cancer progression. Nat Genet 2001;29:117–129.

125. Wakefield LM, Yang YA, Dukhanina O. Transforming growth factor-beta and breast cancer: Lessons learned from genetically altered mouse models. Breast Cancer Res 2000;2:100–106.

126. Chang H, Brown CW, Matzuk MM. Genetic analysis of the mammalian transforming growth factor-{beta} superfamily. Endocr Rev 2002;23:787–823.

127. Dumont N, Arteaga CL. Transforming growth factor-beta and breast cancer: tumor promoting effects of transforming growth factor-beta. Breast Cancer Res 2000;2:125–132.

128. Koli KM, Arteaga CL. Complex role of tumor cell transforming growth factor (TGF)-beta s on breast carcinoma progression. J Mammary Gland Biol Neoplasia 1996;1:373–380.

129. Roberts AB, Wakefield LM. The two faces of transforming growth factor {beta} in carcinogenesis. PNAS 2003;100:8621–8623.

130. Chen CR, Kang Y, Massague J. Inaugural article: defective repression of c-myc in breast cancer cells: a loss at the core of the transforming growth factor beta growth arrest program. PNAS 2001;98:992–999.

131. Siegel PM, Shu W, Cardiff RD et al. Transforming growth factor {beta} signaling impairs Neu-induced mammary tumorigenesis while promoting pulmonary metastasis. PNAS 2003;100: 8430–8435.

132. Feng XH, Zhang Y, Wu RY, Derynck R. The tumor suppressor Smad4/DPC4 and transcriptional adaptor CBP/p300 are coactivators for smad3 in TGF-beta-induced transcriptional activation. Genes Dev 1998;12:2153–2163.

133. Zhang Y, Feng XH, Derynck R. Smad3 and Smad4 cooperate with c-Jun/c-Fos to mediate TFG-beta-induced transcription (1998;394:909). Nature 1998;396:491.

134. Topper JN, DiChiara MR, Brown JD et al. CREB binding protein is a required coactivator for Smad-dependent, transforming growth factor beta transcriptional responses in endothelial cells (1998;95:9506). Proc Natl Acad Sci USA 1998;95:12735.

135. Shen X, Hu PP, Liberati NT et al. TGF-beta-induced phosphorylation of Smad3 regulates its interaction with coactivator p300/CREB-binding protein. Mol Biol Cell 1998;9:3309–3319.

136. Wong C, Rougier-Chapman EM, Frederick JP et al. Smad3-Smad4 and AP-1 complexes synergize in transcriptional activation of the c-Jun promoter by transforming growth factor beta. Mol Cell Biol 1999;19:1821–1830.

137. Pearson KL, Hunter T, Janknecht R. Activation of Smad1-mediated transcription by p300/CBP. Biochim Biophys Acta 1999;1489:354–364.

138. Ghosh AK, Yuan W, Mori Y, Varga J. Smad-dependent stimulation of type I collagen gene expression in human skin fibroblasts by TGF-beta involves functional cooperation with p300/CBP transcriptional coactivators. Oncogene 2000;19:3546–3555.

139. Jeruss JS, Sturgis CD, Rademaker AW, Woodruff TK. Down-regulation of activin, activin receptors, and Smads in high-grade breast cancer. Cancer Res 2003;63:3783–3790.

140. Liberati NT, Moniwa M, Borton AJ et al. An essential role for Mad homology domain 1 in the association of Smad3 with histone deacetylase activity. J Biol Chem 2001;276:22595–22603.

141. Bai S, Cao X. A nuclear antagonistic mechanism of inhibitory Smads in transforming growth factor-beta signaling. J Biol Chem 2002;277:4176–4182.

142. Yang YC, Piek E, Zavadil J et al. Hierarchical model of gene regulation by transforming growth factor {beta}. PNAS 2003;100:10269–10274.

143. Akiyoshi S, Inoue H , Hanai J et al. c-Ski acts as a transcriptional co-repressor in transforming growth factor-beta signaling through interaction with Smads. J Biol Chem 1999;274:35269–35277.

144. Luo K, Stroschein SL, Wang W et al. The Ski oncoprotein interacts with the Smad proteins to repress TGFbeta signaling. Genes Dev 1999;13:2196–2206.

145. Nomura T, Khan MM, Kaul SC et al. Ski is a component of the histone deacetylase complex required for transcriptional repression by Mad and thyroid hormone receptor. Genes Dev 1999;13:412–423.

146. Shinagawa T, Dong HD, Xu M et al. The sno gene, which encodes a component of the histone deacetylase complex, acts as a tumor suppressor in mice. EMBO J 2000;19:2280–2291.

147. Bouzahzah B, Fu M, Iavarone A et al. Transforming growth factor-beta1 recruits histone deacetylase 1 to a p130 repressor complex in transgenic mice in vivo. Cancer Res 2000;60: 4531–4537.

148. Wotton D, Lo RS, Swaby LAC, Massague J. Multiple modes of repression by the Smad transcriptional corepressor TGIF. J Biol Chem 1999;274:37105–37110.

149. Wotton D, Lo RS, Lee S, Massague J. A Smad transcriptional corepressor. Cell 1999;97:29–39.

150. Wotton D, Knoepfler PS, Laherty CD et al. The Smad transcriptional corepressor TGIF recruits mSin3. Cell Growth Differ 2001;12:457–463.

151. Melhuish TA, Gallo CM, Wotton D. TGIF2 interacts with histone deacetylase 1 and represses transcription. J Biol Chem 2001;276:32109–32114.

152. Park SH, Lee SR, Kim BC et al. Transcriptional regulation of the transforming growth factor beta type II receptor gene by histone acetyltransferase and deacetylase is mediated by NF-Y in human breast cancer cells. J Biol Chem 2002;277:5168–5174.

153. Wu L, Wu Y, Gathings B et al. Smad4 as a transcription corepressor for estrogen receptor alpha. J Biol Chem 2003;278:15192–15200.

154. Glaser KB, Li J, Aakre ME et al. Transforming growth factor {beta} mimetics: discovery of 7-[4-(4-cyanophenyl)phenoxy]-heptanohydroxamic acid, a biaryl hydroxamate inhibitor of histone deacetylase. Mol Cancer Ther 2002;1:759–768.

155. Sommer S, Fuqua SAW. Estrogen receptor and breast cancer. Semin Cancer Biol 2001;11:339–352.

156. Bautista S, Valles H, Walker RL et al. In breast cancer, amplification of the steroid receptor coactivator gene AIB1 is correlated with estrogen and progesterone receptor positivity. Clin Cancer Res 1998;4:2925–2929.

157. Liao L, Kuang SQ, Yuan Y et al. Molecular structure and biological function of the cancer-amplified nuclear receptor coactivator SRC-3/AIB1. J Steroid Biochem Mol Biol 2002;83:3–14.

158. Zhao C, Yasui K, Lee CJ et al. Elevated expression levels of NCOA3, TOP1, and TFAP2C in breast tumors as predictors of poor prognosis. Cancer 2003;98:18–23.

159. Hudelist G, Czerwenka K, Kubista E et al. Expression of sex steroid receptors and their co-factors in normal and malignant breast tissue: AIB1 is a carcinoma-specific co-activator. Breast Cancer Res Treat 2003;78:193–204.

160. Girault I, Lerebours F, Amarir S et al. Expression analysis of estrogen receptor alpha coregulators in breast carcinoma: evidence that NCOR1 expression is predictive of the response to tamoxifen. Clin Cancer Res 2003;9:1259–1266.

161. Osborne CK, Bardou V, Hopp TA et al. Role of the estrogen receptor coactivator AIB1 (SRC-3) and HER-2/neu in tamoxifen resistance in breast cancer. J Natl Cancer Inst 2003;95:353–361.

162. Murphy LC, Leygue E, Niu Y et al. Relationship of coregulator and oestrogen receptor isoform expression to de novo tamoxifen resistance in human breast cancer. Br J Cancer 2002;87:1411–1416.

163. Reiter R, Wellstein A, Riegel AT. An isoform of the coactivator AIB1 that increases hormone and growth factor sensitivity is overexpressed in breast cancer. J Biol Chem 2001;276:39736–39741.

164. Shibata A, Hayashi Y, Imai T et al. Somatic gene alteration of AIB1 gene in patients with breast cancer. Endocr J 2001;48:199–204.

165. Murphy LC, Simon SL, Parkes A et al. Altered expression of estrogen receptor coregulators during human breast tumorigenesis. Cancer Res 2000;60:6266–6271.

166. Kurebayashi J, Otsuki T, Kunisue H et al. Expression levels of estrogen receptor-alpha, estrogen receptor-beta, coactivators, and corepressors in breast cancer. Clin Cancer Res 2000;6:512–518.

167. Anzick SL, Kononen J, Walker RL et al. AIB1, a steroid receptor coactivator amplified in breast and ovarian cancer. Science 1997;277:965–968.

168. Fan S, Ma YX, Wang C et al. p300 modulates the BRCA1 inhibition of estrogen receptor activity. Cancer Res 2002;62:141–151.

169. Hanstein B, Eckner R, DiRenzo J et al. p300 is a component of an estrogen receptor coactivator complex. Proc Natl Acad Sci USA 1996;93:11540–11545.

170. McMahon C, Suthiphongchai T, DiRenzo J, Ewen ME. P/CAF associates with cyclin D1 and potentiates its activation of the estrogen receptor. Proc Natl Acad Sci USA 1999;96:5382–5387.

171. Kraus WL, Kadonaga JT. p300 and estrogen receptor cooperatively activate transcription via differential enhancement of initiation and reinitiation. Gene Dev 1998;12:331–242.

172. Kraus WL, Manning ET, Kadonaga JT. Biochemical analysis of distinct activation functions in p300 that enhance transcription initiation with chromatin templates. Mol Cell Biol 1999;19:8123–8135.

173. Yanagisawa J, Kitagawa H, Yanagida M et al. Nuclear receptor function requires a TFTC-type histone acetyl transferase complex. Mol Cell 2002;9:553–562.

174. Schiff R, Massarweh S, Shou J, Osborne CK. Breast cancer endocrine resistance: how growth factor signaling and estrogen receptor coregulators modulate response. Clin Cancer Res 2003;9(1 Pt 2):447S–454S.

175. Sakamoto T, Eguchi H, Omoto Y et al. Estrogen receptor-mediated effects of tamoxifen on human endometrial cancer cells. Mol Cell Endocrinol 2002;192:93–104.

176. Sun JM, Chen HY, Davie JR. Effect of estradiol on histone acetylation dynamics in human breast cancer cells. J Biol Chem 2001;276:49435–49442.

177. Wang C, Fu M, Angeletti RH et al. Direct acetylation of the estrogen receptor alpha hinge region by p300 regulates transactivation and hormone sensitivity. J Biol Chem 2001;276:18375–18383.

178. Aranda A, Pascual A. Nuclear hormone receptors and gene expression. Physiol Rev 2001;81:1269–1304.

179. Tremblay GB, Giguere V. Coregulators of estrogen receptor action. Crit Rev Eukaryot Gene Expr 2002;12:1–22.

180. Chien PY, Ito M, Park Y et al. A fusion protein of the estrogen receptor (ER) and nuclear receptor corepressor (NCoR) strongly inhibits estrogen-dependent responses in breast cancer cells. Mol Endocrinol 1999;13:2122–2136.

181. Webb P, Valentine C , Nguyen P et al. ERbeta binds N-CoR in the presence of estrogens via an LXXLL-like motif in the N-CoR C-terminus. Nucl Recept 2003;1:4.

182. Shang Y, Brown M. Molecular determinants for the tissue specificity of SERMs. Science 2002;295:2465–2468.

183. Shang Y, Hu X, DiRenzo J et al. Cofactor dynamics and sufficiency in estrogen receptor-regulated transcription. Cell 2000;103:843–852.

184. Jepsen K, Hermanson O, Onami TM et al. Combinatorial roles of the nuclear receptor corepressor in transcription and development. Cell 2000;102:753–763.

185. Morrison AJ, Herrera RE, Heinsohn EC et al. Dominant-negative nuclear receptor corepressor relieves transcriptional inhibition of retinoic acid receptor but does not alter the agonist/antagonist activities of the tamoxifen-bound estrogen receptor. Mol Endocrinol 2003;17:1543–1554.

186. Carroll JS, Lynch DK, Swarbrick A et al. p27Kip1 induces quiescence and growth factor insensitivity in tamoxifen-treated breast cancer cells. Cancer Res 2003;63:4322–4326.

187. Zheng L, Annab LA, Afshari CA et al. BRCA1 mediates ligand-independent transcriptional repression of the estrogen receptor. Proc Natl Acad Sci USA 2001;98:9587–9592.

188. Macaluso M, Cinti C, Russo G et al. pRb2/p130-E2F4/5-HDAC1-SUV39H1-p300 and pRb2/p130-E2F4/5-HDAC1-SUV39H1-DNMT1 multimolecular complexes mediate the transcription of estrogen receptor-alpha in breast cancer. Oncogene 2003;22:3511–3517.

189. Nicolson GL, Nawa A, Toh Y et al. Tumor metastasis-associated human MTA1 gene and its MTA1 protein product: role in epithelial cancer cell invasion, proliferation and nuclear regulation. Clin Exp Metastasis 2003;20:19–24.

190. Nawa A, Nishimori K , Lin P et al. Tumor metastasis-associated human MTA1 gene: its deduced protein sequence, localization, and association with breast cancer cell proliferation using antisense phosphorothioate oligonucleotides. J Cell Biochem 2000;79:202–212.

191. Toh Y, Pencil SD, Nicolson GL. A novel candidate metastasis-associated gene, mta1, differentially expressed in highly metastatic mammary adenocarcinoma cell lines. cDNA cloning, expression, and protein analyses. J Biol Chem 1994;269:22958–22963.

192. Kumar R, Wang RA, Mazumdar A et al. A naturally occurring MTA1 variant sequesters oestrogen receptor-alpha in the cytoplasm. Nature 2002;418:654–657.

193. Xue Y, Wong J, Moreno GT et al. NURD, a novel complex with both ATP-dependent chromatin-remodeling and histone deacetylase activities. Mol Cell 1998;2:851–861.

194. Toh Y, Kuninaka S, Endo K et al. Molecular analysis of a candidate metastasis-associated gene, MTA1: possible interaction with histone deacetylase 1. J Exp Clin Cancer Res 2000;19:105–111.

195. Yao YL, Yang WM. The metastasis-associated proteins 1 and 2 form distinct protein complexes with histone deacetylase activity. J Biol Chem 2003;278:42560–42568.

196. Mazumdar A, Wang RA, Mishra SK et al. Transcriptional repression of oestrogen receptor by metastasis-associated protein 1 corepressor. Nat Cell Biol 2001;3:30–37.

197. Mishra SK, Mazumdar A, Vadlamudi RK et al. MICoA, a novel metastasis-associated protein 1 (MTA1) interacting protein coactivator, regulates estrogen receptor-{alpha} transactivation functions. J Biol Chem 2003;278:19209–19219.

198. Talukder AH, Mishra SK, Mandal M et al. MTA1 interacts with MAT1, a cyclin-dependent kinase-activating kinase complex ring finger factor, and regulates estrogen receptor transactivation functions. J Biol Chem 2003;278:11676–11685.

199. Fujita N, Jaye DL, Kajita M et al. MTA3, a Mi-2/NuRD complex subunit, regulates an invasive growth pathway in breast cancer. Cell 2003;113:207–219.

200. Yan C, Wang H, Toh Y, Boyd DD. Repression of 92-kDa type IV collagenase expression by MTA1 is mediated through direct interactions with the promoter via a mechanism, which is both dependent on and independent of histone deacetylation. J Biol Chem 2003;278:2309–2316.

201. Heinlein CA, Chang C. Androgen receptor (AR) coregulators: an overview. Endocr Rev 2002;23:175–200.

202. Lillie EO, Bernstein L, Ursin G. The role of androgens and polymorphisms in the androgen receptor in the epidemiology of breast cancer. Breast Cancer Res 2003;5:164–173.

203. Berns EM, Dirkzwager-Kiel MJ, Kuenen-Boumeester V et al. Androgen pathway dysregulation in BRCA1-mutated breast tumors. Breast Cancer Res Treat 2003;79:121–127.

204. Sharma M, Sun Z. 5'TG3" interacting factor interacts with Sin3A and represses AR-mediated transcription. Mol Endocrinol 2001;15:1918–1928.

205. Fu MF, Wang CG, Reutens AT et al. p300 and p300/cAMP-response element-binding protein-associated factor acetylate the androgen receptor at sites governing hormone-dependent transactivation. J Biol Chem 2000;275:20853–20860.

206. Sharma M, Zarnegar M, Li X et al. Androgen receptor interacts with a novel MYST protein, HBO1. J Biol Chem 2000;275:35200–35208.

207. Berns EM, Dirkzwager-Kiel MJ, Kuenen-Boumeester V et al. Androgen pathway dysregulation in BRCA1-mutated breast tumors. Breast Cancer Res Treat 2003;79:121–127.

208. Shin S, Verma IM. BRCA2 cooperates with histone acetyltransferases in androgen receptor-mediated transcription. Proc Natl Acad Sci USA 2003;100:7201–7206.

209. Lanari C, Molinolo AA. Progesterone receptors—animal models and cell signalling in breast cancer. Diverse activation pathways for the progesterone receptor: possible implications for breast biology and cancer. Breast Cancer Res 2002;4:240–243.

210. Anderson E. The role of oestrogen and progesterone receptors in human mammary development and tumorigenesis. Breast Cancer Res 2002;4:197–201.

211. Soyal S, Ismail PM, Li J et al. Progesterone's role in mammary gland development and tumorigenesis as disclosed by experimental mouse genetics. Breast Cancer Res 2002;4:191–196.

212. Gao X, Nawaz Z. Progesterone receptors-animal models and cell signaling in breast cancer: Role of steroid receptor coactivators and corepressors of progesterone receptors in breast cancer. Breast Cancer Res 2002;4:182–186.

213. Mote PA, Bartow S, Tran N, Clarke CL. Loss of co-ordinate expression of progesterone receptors A and B is an early event in breast carcinogenesis. Breast Cancer Res Treat 2002;72:163–172.

214. Liu Z, Wong J, Tsai SY, Tsai MJ, O'Malley BW. Steroid receptor coactivator-1 (SRC-1) enhances ligand-dependent and receptor-dependent cell-free transcription of chromatin. Proc Natl Acad Sci USA 1999;96:9485–9490.

215. Xu Y, Klein-Hitpass L, Bagchi MK. E1A-mediated repression of progesterone receptor-dependent transactivation involves inhibition of the assembly of a multisubunit coactivation complex. Mol Cell Biol 2000;20:2138–2146.

216. Li X, Wong J, Tsai SY et al. Progesterone and glucocorticoid receptors recruit distinct coactivator complexes and promote distinct patterns of local chromatin modification. Mol Cell Biol 2003;23:3763–3773.

217. Billard LM, Magdinier F, Lenoir GM et al. MeCP2 and MBD2 expression during normal and pathological growth of the human mammary gland. Oncogene 2002;21:2704–2712.

218. Lin X, Nelson WG. Methyl-CpG-binding domain protein-2 mediates transcriptional repression associated with hypermethylated GSTP1 CpG islands in MCF-7 breast cancer cells. Cancer Res 2003;63:498–504.

219. Boffa LC, Vidali G, Mann RS, Allfrey VG. Suppression of histone deacetylation in vivo and in vitro by sodium butyrate. J Biol Chem 1978;253:3364–3366.

220. Vidali G, Boffa LC, Bradbury EM, Allfrey VG. Butyrate suppression of histone deacetylation leads to accumulation of multiacetylated forms of histones H3 and H4 and increased DNase I sensitivity of the associated DNA sequences. Proc Natl Acad Sci USA 1978;75:2239–2243.

221. Boffa LC, Mariani MR, Parker MI. Selective hypermethylation of transcribed nucleosomal DNA by sodium butyrate. Exp Cell Res 1994;211:420–423.

222. Lea MA, Tulsyan N. Discordant effects of butyrate analogues on erythroleukemia cell proliferation, differentiation and histone deacetylase. Anticancer Res 1995;15:879–883.

223. Lea MA, Randolph VM. Induction of reporter gene expression by inhibitors of histone deacetylase. Anticancer Res 1998;18:2717–2122.

224. Yoshida M, Kijima M, Akita M, Beppu T. Potent and specific inhibition of mammalian histone deacetylase both in vivo and in vitro by trichostatin A. J Biol Chem 1990;265:17174–17179.

225. Kijima M, Yoshida M, Sugita K et al. Trapoxin, an antitumor cyclic tetrapeptide, is an irreversible inhibitor of mammalian histone deacetylase. J Biol Chem 1993;268:22429–22435.

226. Darkin-Rattray SJ, Gurnett AM, Myers RW et al. Apicidin: a novel antiprotozoal agent that inhibits parasite histone deacetylase. Proc Natl Acad Sci USA 1996;93:13143–13147.

227. Brosch G, Ransom R, Lechner T et al. Inhibition of maize histone deacetylases by HC toxin, the host-selective toxin of Cochliobolus carbonum. Plant Cell 1995;7:1941–1950.

228. Kwon HJ, Owa T, Hassig CA et al. Depudecin induces morphological reversion of transformed fibroblasts via the inhibition of histone deacetylase. Proc Natl Acad Sci USA 1998;95: 3356–3361.

229. Pina IC, Gautschi JT, Wang GY et al. Psammaplins from the sponge *Pseudoceratina purpurea*: inhibition of both histone deacetylase and DNA methyltransferase. J Org Chem 2003;68: 3866–3873.

230. Nakajima H, Kim YB, Terano H et al. FR901228, a potent antitumor antibiotic, is a novel histone deacetylase inhibitor. Exp Cell Res 1998;241:126–133.

231. Remiszewski SW, Sambucetti LC, Atadja P et al. Inhibitors of human histone deacetylase: synthesis and enzyme and cellular activity of straight chain hydroxamates. J Med Chem 2002;45:753–757.

232. Richon VM, Zhou X, Rifkind RA, Marks PA. Histone deacetylase inhibitors: development of suberoylanilide hydroxamic acid (SAHA) for the treatment of cancers. Blood Cells Mol Dis 2001;27:260–264.

233. Kapustin GV, Fejer G, Gronlund JL et al. Phosphorus-based SAHA analogues as histone deacetylase inhibitors. Org Lett 2003;5:3053–3056.

234. Wada CK, Frey RR, Ji Z et al. [alpha]-Keto amides as inhibitors of histone deacetylase. Bioorg Med Chem Lett 2003;13:3331–3335.

235. Dai Y, Guo Y, Guo J et al. Indole amide hydroxamic acids as potent inhibitors of histone deacetylases. Bioorg Med Chem Lett 2003;13:1897–1901.

236. Plumb JA, Finn PW, Williams RJ et al. Pharmacodynamic response and inhibition of growth of human tumor xenografts by the novel histone deacetylase inhibitor PXD101. Mol Cancer Ther 2003;2:721–728.

237. Kapustin GV, Fejer G, Gronlund JL et al. Phosphorus-based SAHA analogues as histone deacetylase inhibitors. Org Lett 2003;5:3053–3056.

238. Catley L, Weisberg E, Tai YT et al. NVP-LAQ824 is a potent novel histone deacetylase inhibitor with significant activity against multiple myeloma. Blood 2003;102:2615–2622.

239. Gottlicher M, Minucci S, Zhu P et al. Valproic acid defines a novel class of HDAC inhibitors inducing differentiation of transformed cells. EMBO J 2001;20:6969–6978.

240. Phiel CJ, Zhang F, Huang EY et al. Histone deacetylase is a direct target of valproic acid, a potent anticonvulsant, mood stabilizer, and teratogen. J Biol Chem 2001;276:36734–36741.

241. Frey RR, Wada CK, Garland RB et al. Trifluoromethyl ketones as inhibitors of histone deacetylase. Bioorg Med Chem Lett 2002;12:3443–3447.

242. Jung M, Hoffman K, Brosch G, Loidl P. Analogues of trichostain A and trapoxin B as histone deacetylase inhibitors. Bioorg Med Chem Lett 1997;7:1655–1658.

243. Taunton J, Collins JL, Schreiber SL. Synthesis of natural and modified trapoxins, useful reagents for exploring histone deacetylase function. J Am Chem Soc 1996;118:10412–10422.

244. Saito A, Yamashita T, Mariko Y et al. A synthetic inhibitor of histone deacetylase, MS-27-275, with marked in vivo antitumor activity against human tumors. Proc Natl Acad Sci USA 1999;96:4592–4597.

245. Kraker AJ, Mizzen CA, Hartl BG et al. Modulation of histone acetylation by [4-(acetylamino)-N-(2-amino-phenyl) benzamide] in HCT-8 colon carcinoma. Mol Cancer Ther 2003;2:401–408.

246. Kim YB, Lee KH, Sugita K et al. Oxamflatin is a novel antitumor compound that inhibits mammalian histone deacetylase. Oncogene 1999;18:2461–2470.

247. Van Ommeslaeghe K, Elaut G, Brecx V et al. Amide analogues of TSA: synthesis, binding mode analysis and HDAC inhibition. Bioorg Med Chem Lett 2003;13:1861–1864.

248. Bedalov A, Gatbonton T, Irvine WP et al. Identification of a small molecule inhibitor of Sir2p. Proc Natl Acad Sci USA 2001;98:15113–15118.

249. Grozinger CM, Chao ED, Blackwell HE et al. Identification of a class of small molecule inhibitors of the sirtuin family of NAD-dependent deacetylases by phenotypic screening. J Biol Chem 2001;276:38837–38843.

250. Grozinger CM, Schreiber SL. Deacetylase enzymes: biological functions and the use of small-molecule inhibitors. Chem Biol 2002;9:3–16.

251. Haggarty SJ, Koeller KM, Wong JC et al. Domain-selective small-molecule inhibitor of histone deacetylase 6 (HDAC6)-mediated tubulin deacetylation. Proc Natl Acad Sci USA 2003;100:4389–4394.

252. Haggarty SJ, Koeller KM, Wong JC et al. Multidimensional chemical genetic analysis of diversity-oriented synthesis-derived deacetylase inhibitors using cell-based assays. Chem Biol 2003;10:383–396.

253. Koeller KM, Haggarty SJ, Perkins BD et al. Chemical genetic modifier screens. Small molecule trichostatin suppressors as probes of intracellular histone and tubulin acetylation. Chem Biol 2003;10:397–410.

254. Sternson SM, Wong JC, Grozinger CM, Schreiber SL. Synthesis of 7200 small molecules based on a substructural analysis of the histone deacetylase inhibitors trichostatin and trapoxin. Org Lett 2001;3:4239–4242.

255. Wong JC, Hong R, Schreiber SL. Structural biasing elements for in-cell histone deacetylase paralog selectivity. J Am Chem Soc 2003;125:5586–5587.

256. Hu E, Dul E, Sung CM et al. Identification of novel isoform-selective inhibitors within class I histone deacetylases. J Pharmacol Exp Ther 2003;307:720–728.

257. Balasubramanyam K, Swaminathan V, Ranganathan A, Kundu TK. Small molecule modulators of histone acetyltransferase p300. J Biol Chem 2003;278:19134–19140.

258. Bandyopadhyay D, Okan NA, Bales E et al. Down-regulation of p300/CBP histone acetyltransferase activates a senescence checkpoint in human melanocytes. Cancer Res 2002;62:6231–6239.

259. Lau OD, Kundu TK, Soccio RE et al. HATs off: selective synthetic inhibitors of the histone acetyltransferases p300 and PCAF. Mol Cell 2000;5:589–595.

260. Thompson PR, Kurooka H, Nakatani Y, Cole PA. Transcriptional coactivator protein p300. Kinetic characterization of its histone acetyltransferase activity. J Biol Chem 2001;276:33721–33729.

261. Turlais F, Hardcastle A, Rowlands M et al. High-throughput screening for identification of small molecule inhibitors of histone acetyltransferases using scintillating microplates (FlashPlate). Anal Biochem 2001;298:62–68.

262. Cebrat M, Kim CM, Thompson PR et al. Synthesis and analysis of potential prodrugs of coenzyme A analogues for the inhibition of the histone acetyltransferase p300. Bioorg Med Chem 2003;11:3307–3313.

263. Johnstone RW. Histone-deacetylase inhibitors: novel drugs for the treatment of cancer. Nat Rev Drug Discov 2002;1:287–299.

264. Marks PA, Rifkind RA, Richon VM et al. Histone deacetylases and cancer: causes and therapies. Nat Rev Cancer 2001;1:194–202.

265. Remiszewski SW. Recent advances in the discovery of small molecule histone deacetylase inhibitors. Curr Opin Drug Discov Devel 2002;5:487–499.

266. Vigushin DM, Coombes RC. Histone deacetylase inhibitors in cancer treatment. Anticancer Drugs 2002;13:1–13.

267. Vigushin DM. FR-901228 Fujisawa/National Cancer Institute. Curr Opin Investig Drugs 2002;3:1396–1402.

268. Kelly WK, O'Connor OA, Marks PA. Histone deacetylase inhibitors: from target to clinical trials. Expert Opin Investig Drugs 2002;11:1695–1713.

269. Marks PA, Miller T, Richon VM. Histone deacetylases . Curr Opin Pharmacol 2003;3:344–351.

270. Choi KS, Bae MK, Jeong JW et al. Hypoxia-induced angiogenesis during carcinogenesis. J Biochem Mol Biol 2003;36:120–127.

271. Jain RK. Tumor angiogenesis and accessibility: role of vascular endothelial growth factor. Semin Oncol 2002;29(suppl 16):3–9.

272. Pugh CW, Ratcliffe PJ. Regulation of angiogenesis by hypoxia: role of the HIF system. Nat Med 2003;9:677–684.

273. Boudreau N, Myers C. Breast cancer-induced angiogenesis: multiple mechanisms and the role of the microenvironment. Breast Cancer Res 2003;5:140–146.

274. Carrero P, Okamoto K, Coumailleau P et al. Redox-regulated recruitment of the transcriptional coactivators CREB-binding protein and SRC-1 to hypoxia-inducible factor 1 alpha. Mol Cell Biol 2000;20:402–415.

275. Kallio PJ, Okamoto K, O'Brien S et al. Signal transduction in hypoxic cells: inducible nuclear translocation and recruitment of the CBP/p300 coactivator by the hypoxia-inducible factor-1alpha. EMBO J 1998;17:6573–6586.

276. Kim MS, Kwon HJ, Lee YM et al. Histone deacetylases induce angiogenesis by negative regulation of tumor suppressor genes. Nat Med 2001;7:437–443.

277. Sawa H, Murakami H, Ohshima Y et al. Histone deacetylase inhibitors such as sodium butyrate and trichostatin A inhibit vascular endothelial growth factor (VEGF) secretion from human glioblastoma cells. Brain Tumor Pathol 2002;19:77–81.

278. Mie LY, Kim SH, Kim HS et al. Inhibition of hypoxia-induced angiogenesis by FK228, a specific histone deacetylase inhibitor, via suppression of HIF-1alpha activity. Biochem Biophys Res Commun 2003;300:241–246.

279. Deroanne CF, Bonjean K, Servotte S et al. Histone deacetylases inhibitors as anti-angiogenic agents altering vascular endothelial growth factor signaling. Oncogene 2002;21:427–436.

280. Williams RJ. Trichostatin A, an inhibitor of histone deacetylase, inhibits hypoxia-induced angiogenesis. Expert Opin Investig Drugs 2001;10:1571–1573.

281. Kwon HJ, Kim MS, Kim MJ et al. Histone deacetylase inhibitor FK228 inhibits tumor angiogenesis. Int J Cancer 2002;97:290–296.

282. Rossig L, Li H, Fisslthaler B et al. Inhibitors of histone deacetylation downregulate the expression of endothelial nitric oxide synthase and compromise endothelial cell function in vasorelaxation and angiogenesis. Circ Res 2002;91:837–844.

283. Liu LT, Chang HC, Chiang LC, Hung WC. Histone deacetylase inhibitor up-regulates RECK to inhibit MMP-2 activation and cancer cell invasion. Cancer Res 2003;63:3069–3072.

284. Dong-Le Bourhis X, Lambrecht V, Boilly B. Transforming growth factor beta 1 and sodium butyrate differentially modulate urokinase plasminogen activator and plasminogen activator inhibitor-1 in human breast normal and cancer cells. Br J Cancer 1998;77:396–403.

285. Schuster N, Krieglstein K. Mechanisms of TGF-beta-mediated apoptosis. Cell Tissue Res 2002;307:1–14.

286. Gray SG, Yakovleva T, Hartmann W et al. IGF-II enhances trichostatin A-induced TGFbeta1 and p21(Waf1,Cip1, sdi1) expression in Hep3B cells. Exp Cell Res 1999;253:618–628.

287. Lee BI, Park SH, Kim JW et al. MS-275, a histone deacetylase inhibitor, selectively induces transforming growth factor {beta} type II receptor expression in human breast cancer cells. Cancer Res 2001;61:931–934.

288. Yang X, Ferguson AT , Nass SJ et al. Transcriptional activation of estrogen receptor alpha in human breast cancer cells by histone deacetylase inhibition. Cancer Res 2000;60:6890–6894.

289. Yang X, Phillips DL, Ferguson AT et al. Synergistic activation of functional estrogen receptor (ER)-alpha by DNA methyltransferase and histone deacetylase inhibition in human ER-alpha-negative breast cancer cells. Cancer Res 2001;61:7025–7029.

290. Stevens MS, Aliabadi Z, Moore MR. Associated effects of sodium butyrate on histone acetylation and estrogen receptor in the human breast cancer cell line MCF-7. Biochem Biophys Res Commun 1984;119:132–138.

291. Bovenzi V, Momparler RL. Antineoplastic action of 5-aza-2'-deoxycytidine and histone deacetylase inhibitor and their effect on the expression of retinoic acid receptor beta and estrogen receptor alpha genes in breast carcinoma cells. Cancer Chemother Pharmacol 2001;48:71–76.

292. Kennedy C, Byth K, Clarke CL, deFazio A. Cell proliferation in the normal mouse mammary gland and inhibition by phenylbutyrate. Mol Cancer Ther 2002;1:1025–1033.

293. Munster PN, Troso-Sandoval T, Rosen N et al. The histone deacetylase inhibitor suberoylanilide hydroxamic acid induces differentiation of human breast cancer cells. Cancer Res 2001;61: 8492–8497.

294. Kang HY, Huang KE, Chang SY et al. Differential modulation of androgen receptor-mediated transactivation by Smad3 and tumor suppressor Smad4. J Biol Chem 2002;277:43749–43756.

295. Gray SG, Yakovleva T, Hartmann W et al. IGF-II enhances trichostatin A-induced TGFbeta1 and p21(Waf1,Cip1, sdi1) expression in Hep3B cells. Exp Cell Res 1999;253:618–628.

296. Kim YB, Ki SW, Yoshida M, Horinouchi S. Mechanism of cell cycle arrest caused by histone deacetylase inhibitors in human carcinoma cells. J Antibiot (Tokyo) 2000;53:1191–1200.

297. Sowa Y, Orita T, Minamikawa-Hiranabe S et al. Sp3, but not Sp1, mediates the transcriptional activation of the p21/WAF1/Cip1 gene promoter by histone deacetylase inhibitor. Cancer Res 1999;59:4266–4270.

298. Xiao H, Hasegawa T, Isobe K. Both Sp1 and Sp3 are responsible for p21waf1 promoter activity induced by histone deacetylase inhibitor in NIH3T3 cells. J Cell Biochem 1999;73:291–302.

299. Archer SY, Meng S, Shei A, Hodin RA. p21(WAF1) is required for butyrate-mediated growth inhibition of human colon cancer cells. Proc Natl Acad Sci USA 1998;95:6791–6796.

300. Sowa Y, Orita T, Minamikawa S et al. Histone deacetylase inhibitor activates the WAF1/Cip1 gene promoter through the Sp1 sites. Biochem Biophys Res Commun 1997;241:142–150.

301. Sowa Y, Orita T, Hiranabe-Minamikawa S et al. Histone deacetylase inhibitor activates the p21/WAF1/Cip1 gene promoter through the Sp1 sites. Ann N Y Acad Sci 1999;886:195-199.

302. Xiao H, Hasegawa T, Isobe K. p300 collaborates with Sp1 and Sp3 in p21(waf1/cip1) promoter activation induced by histone deacetylase inhibitor. J Biol Chem 2000;275:1371–1376.

303. Klisovic DD, Katz SE, Effron D et al. Depsipeptide (FR901228) inhibits proliferation and induces apoptosis in primary and metastatic human uveal melanoma cell lines. Invest Ophthalmol Vis Sci 2003;44:2390–2398.

304. Park WH, Jung CW, Park JO et al. Trichostatin inhibits the growth of ACHN renal cell carcinoma cells via cell cycle arrest in association with p27, or apoptosis. Int J Oncol 2003;22: 1129–1134.

305. Wang ZM, Hu J, Zhou D et al. Trichostatin A inhibits proliferation and induces expression of $p21^{WAF}$ and p27 in human brain tumor cell lines. Ai Zheng 2002;21:1100–1105.

306. Strait KA, Dabbas B, Hammond EH et al. Cell cycle blockade and differentiation of ovarian cancer cells by the histone deacetylase inhibitor trichostatin A are associated with changes in p21, Rb, and Id proteins . Mol Cancer Ther 2002;1:1181–1190.

307. Finzer P, Kuntzen C , Soto U et al. Inhibitors of histone deacetylase arrest cell cycle and induce apoptosis in cervical carcinoma cells circumventing human papillomavirus oncogene expression. Oncogene 2001;20:4768–4776.

308. Gray SG, Ekström TJ. Effects of cell density and trichostatin A on the expression of HDAC1 and $p57^{Kip2}$ in Hep 3B cells. Biochem Biophys Res Commun 1998;245:423–427.

309. Nair AR, Boersma LJ, Schiltz L et al. Paradoxical effects of trichostatin A: inhibition of NF-Y-associated histone acetyltransferase activity, phosphorylation of hGCN5 and downregulation of cyclin A and B1 mRNA. Cancer Lett 2001;166:55–64.

310. Greenberg VL, Williams JM, Cogswell JP et al. Histone deacetylase inhibitors promote apoptosis and differential cell cycle arrest in anaplastic thyroid cancer cells. Thyroid 2001;11:315–325.

311. Katula KS, Fields A, Apple P, Rotruck T. Cell cycle specific changes in the human cyclin B1 gene regulatory region as revealed by response to trichostatin A. Arch Biochem Biophys 2002;401:271–276.

312. Lallemand F, Courilleau D, Sabbah M et al. Direct inhibition of the expression of cyclin D1 gene by sodium butyrate. Biochem Biophys Res Commun 1996;229:163–169.

313. Polanowska J, Fabbrizio E, Le Cam L et al. The periodic down regulation of Cyclin E gene expression from exit of mitosis to end of G(1) is controlled by a deacetylase- and E2F-associated bipartite repressor element. Oncogene 2001;20:4115–4127.

314. Bandyopadhyay D, Okan NA, Bales E et al. Down-regulation of p300/CBP histone acetyltransferase activates a senescence checkpoint in human melanocytes. Cancer Res 2002;62:6231–6239.

315. Suzuki T, Yokozaki H, Kuniyasu H et al. Effect of trichostatin A on cell growth and expression of cell cycle- and apoptosis-related molecules in human gastric and oral carcinoma cell lines. Int J Cancer 2000;88:992–997.

316. Bouchard C, Thieke K, Maier A et al. Direct induction of cyclin D2 by Myc contributes to cell cycle progression and sequestration of p27. EMBO J 1999;18:5321-5333.

317. Siavoshian S, Segain JP, Kornprobst M et al. Butyrate and trichostatin A effects on the proliferation/differentiation of human intestinal epithelial cells: induction of cyclin D3 and p21 expression. Gut 2000;46:507–514.

318. Papeleu P, Loyer P, Vanhaecke T et al. Trichostatin A induces differential cell cycle arrests but does not induce apoptosis in primary cultures of mitogen-stimulated rat hepatocytes. J Hepatol 2003;39:374–382.

319. Davis T, Kennedy C, Chiew YE et al. Histone deacetylase inhibitors decrease proliferation and modulate cell cycle gene expression in normal mammary epithelial cells. Clin Cancer Res 2000;6:4334–4342.

Chapter 6

Role of DNA Hypomethylating Agents in Cancer Treatment

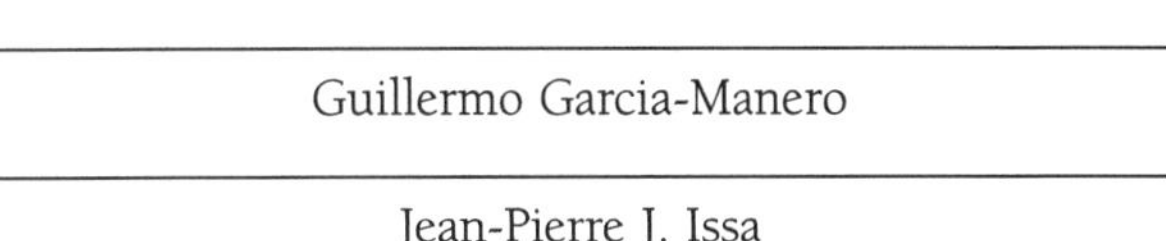

Guillermo Garcia-Manero

Jean-Pierre J. Issa

DNA methylation is a natural biochemical modification of the nucleic acid cytosine that is very prevalent in the human genome. DNA methylation has attracted significant attention since it was discovered that its presence at high density around gene promoters is associated with absent transcription and hence absent function of the affected gene. This epigenetic change is stable and thought to physiologically irreversible, as illustrated by the inactive X-chromosome in women where DNA methylation is required to maintain the inactive state. Cancer cells have been found to have profound alterations in DNA methylation, and this epigenetic change is now thought to be as powerful as genetic changes in altering the function of critical pathways through silencing of tumor-suppressor genes. The biochemistry of DNA methylation-associated gene inactivation has been clarified recently, which has led to intense efforts aimed at targeting this change for cancer treatment. Pharmacologic hypomethylation has been demonstrated following irreversible inhibition of the DNA-methyltransferase enzymes by the cytosine analogues 5-aza-2′-deoxycytidine (decitabine) and 5-azacytidine (azacytidine). Other approaches to inducing demethylation include antisense molecules to DNMT1, the major DNA methyltransferase enzyme, as well as drugs such as Procainamide and Zebularine, which have a less well defined mechanism of action. In clinical trials, azacytidine has shown clinical activity in the myelodysplastic syndrome (MDS) and decitabine has shown clinical activity in MDS as well as in chronic myelogenous leukemia (CML) and acute myelogenous leukemia (AML). These two drugs induce responses that are characteristically slow to emerge, suggesting a non-cytotoxic mechanism of action. Decitabine has been shown to induce hypomethylation in vivo and, consistent with its in vitro action on DNA methylation, appears to be more active at low doses than at high doses (where cytotoxicity is observed). Hypomethylating agents are the first of a new class of cancer therapy aimed at reactivating abnormally silenced genes. Other epigenetic acting agents such as histone deacetylase inhibitors also have shown promise in clinical trials, and it appears likely that this new form of cancer therapy will be incorporated in the routine management of cancer over the next decade.

EPIGENETIC MECHANISMS IN CANCER

Epigenetics

Epigenetics refers to the study of clonally inherited changes in gene expression without accompanying genetic changes.[1,2] In most cases, these changes in gene expression are not directly related to dosage of transcription factors. Thus, epigenetic silencing, which refers to near complete loss of gene expression, is achieved in the face of persistent levels of transcription factors for the silenced genes.[3] A compelling example of this process is X-inactivation in women where the active and silenced chromosomes coexist in the same cells with constant levels of transcription factors. There are three described mechanisms of epigenetic changes (typically silencing) in mammalian cells; DNA methylation, histone code changes and RNA interference.

Epigenetic changes were among the first identified characteristic features of neoplasia.[4] However, the absence of a defined mechanism for explaining such clonal inheritance has hampered research in the field. Over the past 20 years, DNA methylation has emerged as a mechanism of perpetuating epigenetic changes in gene expression through mitosis.[5] In particular, CpG island methylation has been shown to be a robust mechanism of gene silencing in normal cells, and evidence is accumulating that neoplastic cells use this mechanism to silence undesirable genes.[6–8] Recently, there is interest in histone modifications as mediators of epigenetic changes,[9] and there is considerable cross-talk between DNA methylation and these histone modifications.[10] Histone changes, either primary or associated with DNA methylation are also emerging as constant molecular characteristics of neoplastic cells.

CpG Island Methylation as a Mechanism of Epigenetic Silencing

The natural occurrence of 5-methyl-cytosine in mammalian DNA was discovered over 50 years ago, and its potential role in the regulation of gene expression began to be studied over 20 years ago.[11] Despite these decades of research, the physiological role of DNA methylation in human cells remains unclear. The most convincing evidence of the normal function of DNA methylation comes from studies where the process is inhibited either genetically or pharmacologically. These studies demonstrated an essential role for DNA methylation in mammalian development[12] and in allele-specific silencing of selected genes, such as genes on the inactive X-chromosome[13] and parentally imprinted genes.[14] It has been suggested also that methylation is involved as a mechanism of genome defense against the expression of inserted retroviruses and other recombinogenic repeats.[15] Evidence in support of this hypothesis is accumulating.[16]

In mammals, DNA methylation only affects cytosine when it is part of the cytosine–phospho-guanosine (CpG) dinucleotide. Methylated cytosines are hypermutable through spontaneous deamination to form the uracil base and possibly through slower repair.[17] Over evolution, this is thought to have resulted in a relative paucity of CpG sites in the human genome, where CpGs are found at only 20% of their statistically expected frequency. This CpG suppression is evident throughout the genome, except in small areas that are 0.5 to 2 kb in length where its frequency is at or substantially higher than expected.[18] These areas are referred to as CpG islands, and are thought to have escaped CpG depletion through evolution by being unmethylated in normal tissues. About half of all human genes contain a CpG island in their 5′ area, often encompassing the promoters and transcription start sites of the associated genes.

Much evidence has now accumulated linking promoter CpG island methylation with transcriptional silencing in human cells.[1,2,5] A role for methylation in the normal regulation of gene expression was suggested early on, but CpG islands were found to be generally free of methylation regardless of the expression status of the associated gene.[19] While not part of normal regulation of gene expression, CpG island methylation nevertheless was shown to be associated with absent transcription from the involved promoter, and this silencing appeared to be stably transmitted through mitosis, thus insuring clonal inheritance. This association between CpG island methylation and absent transcription is most striking when one considers the two physiological conditions where this process was described: X-inactivation[20] and imprinting.[21] In both cases, one of the two copies of the involved genes is transcriptionally silent, in association with promoter methylation, despite continued normal expression of the unmethylated allele. Evidence for a direct role of methylation in maintaining the silenced state came from studies where methylation was relieved via pharmacologic[22] or genetic[14] reduction in DNA methyltransferase activity. In most such studies, bi-allelic expression could be restored, in association with decreased methylation of the affected promoters.

DNA METHYLATION CHANGES IN CANCER

There are complex changes in DNA methylation in cancer.[7] For the most part, these changes involve simultaneous global demethylation, increased expression of DNA-methyltransferases (Mtases) and de novo methylation at previously unmethylated CpG islands. Demethylation was first discovered by studying overall 5-methyl-cytosine (5mC) content in tumors, and appears to involve primarily satellite DNA, repetitive sequences and CpG sites located in introns.[23,24] The cause of this demethylation remains unclear, although it could be related to alterations in proliferation or cell-cycle control.[25] The functional consequences of hypomethylation are equally unclear. Initial suggestions that gene-specific hypomethylation can cause increased oncogene expression, for the most part, have not been confirmed experimentally. An increased mutation rate was demonstrated in cells in which severe hypomethylation (>75%) was achieved by homozygous deletion of *DNMT1*, a major DNA-methyltransferase enzyme,[26] but it is not clear whether this degree of hypomethylation is ever achieved in neoplasms.[27] Increased enzymatic Mtase activity is a property of nearly all transformed cells.[28] Increased mRNA levels for *DNMT1*, *DNMT3a* and *DNMT3b* have been described also in some neoplasms including leukemias,[29–31] and these three Mtase genes probably account for the observed increase in activity. The causes and functional significance of these increases remain unclear.[32,33] In primary tumors and cell lines, no correlation was found between Mtase activity and gene silencing.[34,35] Nevertheless, simultaneous inhibition of multiple Mtases does inhibit cancer cell growth,[36] making them potential therapeutic targets.

In parallel to global hypomethylation and increased Mtase activity, there are distinct and frequent localized increases in methylation, often involving CpG islands.[6,7] Because CpG island methylation is associated with repressed transcription that is stably inherited through mitosis, this de novo methylation in transformed cells has been proposed as an alternate mechanism for inactivating tumor-suppressor genes. Indeed, several genes now have been shown to be transcriptionally silent in neoplasia, in association with CpG island methylation. The most convincing evidence for CpG island methylation as a true alternative to mutations in neoplasia came from studies of *RB1*,[37] *p16*,[38] *VHL*,[39] and *MLH1*.[40] For each of these genes, the tumor-spectrum of methylation events is virtually the same as that for mutations, and there are described cases where one allele of the gene is inactivated by methylation while the other is mutated, suggesting an equivalent growth advantage for each event in neoplasia. For example, in colorectal cancer, the HCT116 cell line carries one mutated unmethylated *p16* allele, while the second allele in this cell line is unmutated but densely hypermethylated and transcriptionally silent.[38]

Histone Modifications

Histones are small proteins that form a core around which DNA is wrapped, forming nucleosomes. Nucleosomes are the basic in vivo structural unit of DNA, and consist of eight histone molecules (2 each of histones H1, H2, H3 and H4) around which a loop of DNA is wrapped.[41] While H1 and H2 are thought to play primarily a structural role, it has become apparent that histones H3 and H4 and key integrators of a variety of signals that regulate gene transcription.[9,42,43] In particular, these two histone proteins have histone "tails" or strings of amino acids that protrude outside of the basic nucleosomal structure and make contact with DNA. Specific post-translational modifications of the amino acids in these histone tails (e.g., methylation, acetylation, ubiquination, sumoylation) interact with other proteins to create nucleosomes that are relaxed and promote transcription, or nucleosomes that are closed, exclude transcription factors and result in gene silencing. These histone modifications occur relatively dynamically and are mediated by specific histone modifying proteins. Targeting of these histone modifiers to specific gene promoters in turn is achieved by transcriptional activator/co-activator complexes in response to physiologic stimuli. Thus, histone modifications form a "code" that integrates gene activation/inactivation/silencing signals, such that the transcriptional activity of a given promoter can be predicted by looking at the specific histone modifications.

CpG Island Methylation and Histone Modifications

The mechanism whereby CpG island methylation suppresses gene transcription has been partially elucidated, at least in vitro.[44] Methylated CpG islands form excellent binding sites for methylated-DNA binding proteins (often with transcriptional repression properties), such MeCP2. MeCP2 binding is followed by the recruitment of a protein complex that includes histone deacetylases, and eventually leads to a closed chromatin configuration. This closed chromatin configuration results in exclusion of transcription factors, thus insuring allele-specific inactivation. Methylation-related epigenetic silencing is also associated with histone lysine 9 methylation.[9] Evidence from several laboratories[45–47] suggests that histone H3 lysine 9 methylation is the critical modification that is associated with closed chromatin. Histone H3 lysine 9 methylation itself appears to set-up a silencing loop by attracting more DNA methylation,[48] and may precede DNA hypermethylation in some cases.[49] These and other experiments suggest that gene silencing associated with DNA methylation in cancer results from a cascade of events that ultimately form a self-reinforcing loop. As described in Figure 6.1, the proposed model is that DNA methylation leads to binding by methyl-binding proteins, which attract histone deacetylases and histone methylases, which allow the sequential deacetylation and methylation of H3 lysine 9, which allows binding by HP1, which attracts a silencing complex that results in closed chromatin. In turn, H3 lysine 9 methylation and HP1-mediated silencing itself triggers DNA

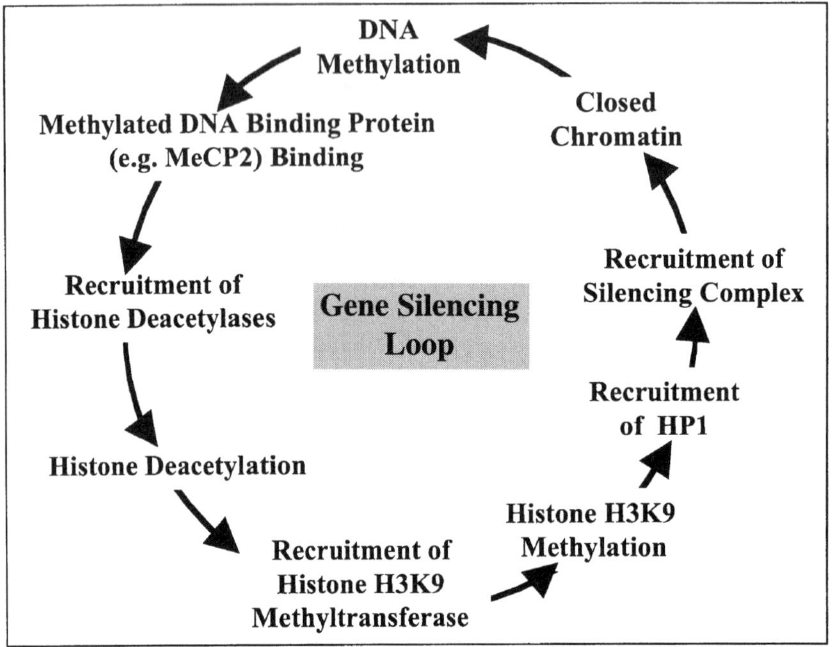

FIGURE 6.1 Model of DNA methylation associated gene silencing loop in cancer.

methylation. This loop accounts for the remarkable stability of the silencing process in cancer cells, and suggests that interventions aimed at breaking the silence could take advantage of any step, although the (presumed) first step (DNA methylation) and the last steps (HP1 binding) may be most critical.

Reversal of Gene Silencing in Cancer

Unlike mutations, epigenetic changes are potentially reversible via pharmacologic modulation. There is convincing evidence that reversing methylation results in functional reactivation of gene expression. For example, the MLH1 mismatch repair gene is unmutated but densely methylated in the mismatch repair deficient cell line RKO, and nearly normal levels of mismatch repair can be restored in this cell line by inhibiting Mtase activity using the DNA methylation inhibitor decitabine.[50] Also, signaling by the estrogen receptor ER-α[51] or the retinoid acid receptor RAR-β2[52] is inhibited by DNA methylation in the promoters of these genes. Reversing methylation restores ER-α signaling[53] or retinoic acid responsiveness in cancer cells.[54] These experiments have stimulated interest in inhibiting DNA methylation as a therapeutic strategy in the treatment of cancer.

HYPOMETHYLATING CYTOSINE ANALOGUES

Several cytidine analogues, of which cytosine arabinoside (ara-C) is the prototype, have been developed as chemotherapeutic agents for both solid tumors and hematological malignancies. Ara-C remains the most important component of combination therapy for patients with acute myelogenous leukemia (AML),[55] and other leukemias.[56] The activity of ara-C has triggered interest in the development of more active cytidine analogues with a better toxicity profile. Two of these cytidine analogues, 5-azacytidine (azacytidine) and 5-aza-2′-deoxycytidine (decitabine) were developed in the 1960s as potential new chemotherapeutic agents.[57] Azacytidine differs from cytosine only in that, at the 5 position, a nitrogen replaces a carbon. Because it is a ribose derivative, azacytidine incorporates into RNA but not DNA. Decitabine is the deoxyribose form of azacytidine, and incorporates efficiently into DNA.

Taylor and Jones first observed the biological importance of these agents.[58,59] In their classical experiments, these investigators reported that azacytidine could induce the differentiation of cultured cells into three distinct mesenchymal phenotypes: contractile striated muscle cells, and biochemically active adipocytes and chondrocytes. This phenotypic transformation required several days to weeks to occur, and was associated with the inhibition of methylation of newly synthesized DNA.[59] The dose-response curve for differentiation was remarkable; Initially, the agents induced dose-dependent efficient differentiation associated with hypomethylation. As the doses were increased, hypomethylation showed a plateau, and the differentiation effect was actually lost. An explanation for this phenomenon resides in the mechanism of DNA methylation inhibition by the drugs. Following incorporation into DNA, the cytosine analogues form irreversible covalent bonds with Mtases.[57] The complexes are then excised and degraded in the proteosome, resulting in depletion of active Mtases.[60] Cellular replication in the absence of DNA methylases results in passive demethylation and reactivation of gene expression. At high doses, the analogue/methylases complexes overwhelm the repair mechanisms of the cells and result in cell death rather than in hypomethylation.[61]

DECITABINE

Decitabine was first synthesized in the early sixties and it was first shown to have activity in a leukemia mouse model by Sorm and Vesely.[62] Decitabine is phosphorylated by deoxycytidine kinase, and the triphosphate form incorporates into DNA, traps Mtases and depletes them from the cell. Levels of Mtase activity have been inversely associated with the hypomethylating activity of decitabine,[28,61] suggesting that Mtase function is fundamental for the activity of decitabine. Jones et al. were the first to demonstrate that decitabine could induce reactivation of the X chromosome gene *HPRT*.[63] This effect on gene specific methylation has been observed in most of the methylated genes studied so far, and has become a paradigm in the field of DNA methylation.

In vitro, decitabine has been shown to induce differentiation of malignant cells and to have significant antineoplastic activity. At concentrations of 0.1 to 1 μg/mL, decitabine induced morphological differentiation of the leukemic cell line HL-60 into a more mature monocytoid phenotype.[64] This phenomenon also has been observed in human leukemic cells in suspension treated ex vivo with decitabine.[65] In these experiments, decitabine induced a reduction in 5-methylcytosine content and decreased cell colony formation.

Decitabine also has potent in vitro antileukemic activity in the L1210 leukemia cell line model. In clonogenic assays, decitabine showed a dose-dependent effect, and cellular survival decreased as exposure time increased up to 24 hours. Incubation of L1210 cells with decitabine at concentrations greater than 0.5 μg/mL for greater than or equal to 24 hours resulted in total inhibition of measurable cell growth for 72 to 96 hours. This effect was reversed by drug removal.[66] Mice inoculated with L1210 leukemia cells received decitabine at a total dose ranging from 0.5 mg/kg to 22 mg/kg. The DNA of L1210 leukemia cells was isolated from treated mice and studied for its ability to accept methyl groups. The methyl-accepting ability of leukemia cell DNA was found to be dependent on the dose of decitabine, thus indicating that decitabine produced a dose-dependent reduction in the 5-methylcytosine content of DNA.[67] In plasma and cerebrospinal fluid (CSF) pharmacokinetic assays, decitabine half-life was between 39 and 144 minutes depending on the animal model, and decitabine concentrations in the CSF were 27% to 58% of the plateau plasma concentration.[68]

Initial Phase I/II Studies of Decitabine

The original phase I study of decitabine was performed in Quebec by Rivard et al.[69] In this study 30 pediatric patients were treated with increasing doses and duration of decitabine. The starting dose was 0.75 mg/kg infused intravenously over 12 hours. Most patients had acute leukemias and the protocol required that they had received at least two to three prior chemotherapy regimens. Although the extent of toxicity was not clearly reported, significant toxicities only included diarrhea and alopecia at doses of 36 to 80 mg/kg infused over 36 to 44 hours. No maximally tolerated dose (MTD) was reported. Three patients with solid tumors and no bone marrow involvement were entered in the study in an attempt to evaluate marrow toxicity of decitabine. Significant myelotoxicity was observed in these patients with absolute neutrophils counts less than $0.1 \times 10^9\ L^{-1}$ and platelets less than $10 \times 10^9 L^{-1}$. Nadir was observed 9 to 12 days after initiation of therapy. The time to recovery was 24 to 42 days at doses of 36 to 80 mg/kg infused over 40 hours. Responses in leukemic patients were dose dependent. At low doses (range 0.75 to 30 mg/kg), decreased bone marrow leukemic blasts in excess of 50% was observed in 10 of 11 (90%) patients. No complete remission (CR) was observed. Symptomatic improvement was observed in seven patients. Duration of blast response was short lived, ranging from 5 to 34 days. At higher doses (36 to 80 mg), marrow remissions (blast less than 5%) were observed in three of nine (33%) patients. Duration of response ranged from 5 days to 50+ days. Of interest, one patient with acute lymphocytic leukemia (ALL) with central nervous system (CNS) involvement achieved a complete response in the CSF. Pharmacokinetic analysis was performed using an in vitro bioassay that measured growth inhibition of the L1210 leukemic cell line. The half-life was calculated to be 12 minutes, and the steady state plasma concentration at the end of a 24 to 40 hour infusion was estimated to have a mean value of 0.5 (μg/mL. CSF levels ranged between 0.06 and 0.2 μg/mL in two patients.

This study was subsequently expanded in a different cohort of pediatric and adult patients with acute leukemias using higher doses than in the original study.[70] In this second phase of the original phase I study, 27 patients, 21 with ALL and 6 with acute myelogenous leukemia (AML), were treated using a classic dose escalation model. The starting dose was 45 mg/kg (an equivalent of 1350 mg/m^2) infused over 40 hours. The highest dose level was 100 mg/kg (equivalent to 3000 mg/m^2) over 90 hours. Six patients (14%) achieved CR: four (19%) with ALL, and two (33%) with AML. Non-hematologic toxicity was rare, and no MTD was reported. The authors detected a 70% inhibition of DNA methylation but no evidence of blast differentiation.

Another phase I study was performed in the Netherlands.[71] In this study, 21 adult patients (age range 37 to 75 years) were treated using a modified Fibonacci scheme. Starting dose was 50 mg/m^2 IV in three divided doses given seven hours apart over one hour, except for the first three patients, who received it in two divided doses. Decitabine was escalated up to 300 mg/m^2. Treatments were repeated every three to six weeks. Most patients (33%) had colorectal cancer. Four patients died of progression of disease, but no drug-related deaths were observed. The dose limiting toxicity (DLT) was neutropenia. This was only severe in patients receiving 225 mg/m^2 of decitabine or more. Neutropenia was delayed (range 22 to 33 days), and peripheral counts did not recover until day 36 to 43. Mild thrombocytopenia was observed also, but platelet counts were never below $40 \times 10^9 L^{-1}$. Platelet nadir occurred earlier (days 14 to 22) and recovery was also faster (day 21 to 22) than that of neutrophils. Two patients had transient elevation of creatinine, and one patient developed acute interstitial nephritis that resolved several months after cessation of therapy. One patient with an undifferentiated carcinoma achieved a partial response that lasted in excess of 15 months. Pharmacokinetic studies were only informative at the 100 mg/m^2 dose.

The recommended phase II dose for solid tumors was 75 mg/m^2. The subsequent experience in solid tumors using this schedule in phase II studies in patients with solid tumors was disappointing. In an EORTC study in patients with different solid tumors receiving decitabine at a dose of 75 mg/m^2 in three divided doses every five weeks, only one partial response was observed in 101 treated patients.[72]

Another phase I clinical trial of decitabine administered by continuous infusion was recently reported.[73] The drug was given for 72 hours at dose levels of 20, 30 and 40 mg/m^2. Dose-limiting neutropenia was seen at 40 mg/m^2, a dose substantially lower than what can be given by bolus infusion, a finding that mirrors the experience with ara-C. At the higher doses, decitabine levels of 0.1 to 0.2 μM were achieved and these are at the lower range of effective demethylation in vitro. No responses were seen in 19 patients with solid tumors (mostly melanomas).

Early Experience with Decitabine in Human Leukemias

Decitabine has been widely studied in phase I to III trials in patients with acute and chronic leukemias, both as a single agent and in combination with other drugs. Decitabine was used in elderly patients with AML and MDS as single agent at doses of 15 to 90 mg/m^2 over four hours, three times a day for three days.[74] Using this schedule, 3 out of 20 patients (15%) achieved CR. Some degree of cell differentiation was observed in 12 (60%) patients. Non-hematological grade 3 toxicities complicated 13 treatment courses, including two cases of severe pulmonary toxicity. In a pilot study in newly diagnosed patients with poor prognosis AML, Petti et al. treated 12 patients with decitabine at doses of 90 to 120 mg/m^2 three times daily for three days.[75] The CR rate was 25%, and significant non-hematologic toxicity was minimal. A similar study was conducted in patients with advanced MDS.[76] In this study, 10 patients with refractory anemia with excess blasts or in transformation were treated with decitabine 45 mg/m^2 in three divided doses daily for three days or as a continuous infusion of 50 mg/m^2 daily for three days. Hematologic improvement and trilineage differentiation were observed in over 50% of the patients with mild non-hematologic toxicity. Decitabine has also been used as a continuous infusion at low doses in elderly patients with MDS. Using a 72 hour infusion, 54% of 19 patients achieved a hematological response, including eight (27%) CRs. The program was associated with significant myelosuppression, and five (17%) patients died during therapy.[77] Finally, decitabine was studied at high doses. Decitabine as a single agent at doses of 750 mg/m^2 had minimal activity in relapsed or refractory AML, resulting in a CR rate of 6% in 17 patients.[78]

Decitabine was then studied in combination. In a study of decitabine combined with m-amsacrine, 8 of 11 patients (72%) with relapsed disease and an initial CR duration of six months or more achieved a second CR with decitabine.

The dose of decitabine was 125 to 500 mg/m^2 twice daily for three to six days.[79] In a subsequent study, decitabine was combined with m-amsacrine or idarubicin in 22 patients with relapsed/refractory leukemia. The CR rate with this combination was 59%, but the treatment was associated with significant toxicities comparable to those observed with ara-C.[80] These studies encouraged the development of a phase II randomized study combining decitabine (125 mg/m^2 as a 6 hour infusion every 12 hours for 6 days) with m-amsacrine (120 mg/m^2 on days 6 and 7) or with idarubicin (12 mg/m^2 on days 5 to 7).[81] In this EORTC multicenter study, 68 adult patients with relapsed acute leukemia were enrolled. CR was achieved in 23 (36.5%) patients. As expected, patients with duration of first CR of more than one year had a better response rate (51% vs. 15%), as did patients with normal cytogenetics (61% vs. 15%). The CR rate was 27% for the m-amsacrine arm and 45% for the idarubicin arm. Non-hematologic toxicity was more frequently observed with idarubicin, in particular cardiac toxicity. Median disease-free survival was eight months, and only 20% of the patients remained in remission for more than one year. Decitabine also has been combined with daunorubicin, another anthracycline, in untreated patients with AML. The schedule consisted of decitabine as a four-hour IV infusion at a dose of 90 mg/m^2 daily × 5, with daunorubicin 50 mg/m^2 on days one to three. All six evaluable patients achieved CR after one or two courses of induction therapy.[82]

Several studies have analyzed the activity of decitabine in patients with chronic myelogenous leukemia (CML).[83,84] In two consecutive studies at the University of Texas M. D. Anderson Cancer Center, 130 patients with CML were treated with decitabine at doses of 75 mg/m^2 to 100 mg/m^2 infused over six hours every 12 hours for five days. Sixty-four patients had blastic phase disease, 51 were in accelerated phase, and 8 were in chronic phase. Four patients (3%) died during the first course of therapy and one of progressive disease. Six patients (9%) in blastic phase achieved complete hematologic response (CHR), and two patients (3%) achieved partial cytogenetic response. In accelerated phase, 12 (24%) patients achieved CHR, and 3 (6%) patients achieved a complete cytogenetic response. The major side effect was prolonged myelosuppression. This was dose related, especially for platelet count recovery. Non-hematologic toxicity was acceptable and consisted of diarrhea (5%), nausea and vomiting (4%), fatigue, cardiac events and alopecia (2% each). Of interest is the fact that, of the 55 patients that achieved a response, 31 (56%) patients required 3 or more courses of therapy.

Recent Experience Using Decitabine at Low Doses in Hematologic Malignancies

The results summarized above suggest that decitabine is active in myeloid malignancies, but this activity is difficult to distinguish from that of ara-C. At high doses of decitabine, it may well be that its main effect is cytotoxicity, and that as such, it is not superior to other cytotoxic agents including ara-C. However, as discussed earlier, the in vitro experience with decitabine suggests that relatively low doses are required to induce cell differentiation and gene re-expression, and that the effect may be lost at higher doses.[59] This has prompted renewed interest in examining lower dose schedules of this agent.

Wijermans et al first studied decitabine at low doses in patients with high risk MDS, primarily because they were interested in developing a less toxic regimen for use in elderly patients.[85] In this phase II multicenter study, 66 patients were treated. The dose of decitabine was 15 mg/m^2 infused over four hours every eight hours (45 mg/m^2 per day) for three consecutive days. Courses were repeated every six weeks for a maximum of six courses, depending on the response. Ten patients received only one course of therapy, with five patients experiencing toxic death. Thirteen patients (20%) achieved CR, and 28% either hematological improvement or partial response. Complete responses were more frequently observed in patients with refractory anemia with excess blasts or in transformation (26% and 22%, respectively) compared to those with refractory anemia (9%). Using the International Prognostic Scoring System (IPSS) score,[86] response rate were 64% for high risk patients, 48% for those with intermediate-II risk, and 25% for those with intermediate-I risk. These differences were statistically significant ($P = 0.01$). The mean number of cycles to achieve the best response was three. Of interest, increased platelet count was observed in 66% of patients. The median duration of response was 31 weeks. Median survival was 15 months for the whole group, and 19 months for those achieving a CR. The most frequent toxicity was fever that complicated 14% of the courses or 27% of patients, infection in 10% and 20%, sepsis in 4% and 10%, neutropenia 7% and 12%, and anemia 6% and 11%, respectively.

More recently, the same group updated the results of three consecutive trials[87] using decitabine 45 to 50 mg/m^2/d for three days in 169 patients. The median age was 70 years, 48 patients had intermediate-I disease, 50 intermediate-II, and 71 high-risk disease. Overall response rate was 49%, and the induction death rate was 7% (11 patients). As in previous experience, increments in platelet counts were observed in 63% of patients. The median duration of response was nine months, and the median survival 15 months. The response rate for patients with high-risk disease was 51% compared to 46% for those with intermediate-I disease. Decitabine therapy resulted in cytogenetic responses in a subset of these patients.[86] Karyotyping was available in 115 patients. Fifty-three percent had abnormal cytogenetics prior to therapy. Nineteen patients (31% with known karyotype) achieved a major cytogenetic response. Duration of these responses was 7.5 months. Survival was better for patients achieving a cytogenetic response compared to those that did not ($P = 0.02$). A phase III randomized study comparing decitabine at this dose schedule versus supportive care has been completed in the US, and results from this study are expected over the next year.

Decitabine was used at a low dose, outpatient regimen in patients with sickle cell anemia.[88,89] These studies demonstrated biological activity at these low doses. Encouraged by this experience, our group conducted a study of low dose decitabine in patients with relapsed or refractory leukemias.[78] In this study, 50 patients were treated with increasing doses of decitabine (5, 10, 15 and 20 mg/m^2 infused over 1 hour daily for 10 days). Two cohorts of patients received 15 mg/m^2 for 15 or 20 days. Median age was 60 years (range 2–84), 73% of patients had AML, most of whom had relapsed disease with duration of first CR of less than 12 months. Overall, nine patients (18%) achieved CR. The most striking feature of this study was the dose-response relationship. Patients who received cumulative doses of 150 mg/m^2 or less had significantly more responses than patients who received higher cumulative doses (14/31 or 45% vs. 2/19 or 11%). This low response rate at high doses was consistent with earlier studies discussed above.

Table 6.1 summarizes clinical trials of decitibine in myeloid malignancies.

Mechanisms of Response to Decitabine

Several lines of evidence suggest that responses to decitabine are via a non-cytotoxic effect and clearly distinguish this drug from ara-C. First, responses to this drug are typically slow to develop.[78] Studies in both MDS and CML suggested that the median number of courses to optimal response was around three.[84,85] Second, as discussed above, the drug was found to be consistently more effective at lower doses. Given that, in vitro, low doses favor hypomethylation while high doses favor cytotoxicity, the clinical observations are most consistent with a mechanism of action that involves loss of methylation in the cancer cell and downstream events rather than direct cell death. Third, responses have been observed in patients clearly refractory to ara-C.[78]

Evidence for in vivo hypomethylation following decitabine administration is accumulating. In the European MDS trials, twenty three patients were analyzed for gene specific methylation of the p15 and p16 genes prior and during therapy.[90] P15 methylation was observed in 15 (63%) patients whereas p16 was not methylated in any case. Among nine patients with p15 methylation, all (75%) achieved p15 demethylation, a phenomenon associated with clinical response. Induction of p15 expression was observed in four out of eight patients with pretreatment p15 methylation. In that study, methylation was measured at greater than one month interval following therapy, raising the possibility that the results were related to clonal selection rather than hypomethylation. However, in our own study, p15 methylation was measured 5 and 10 days after decitabine administration, and hypomethylation was observed also in this setting.[78] However, an association between p15 demethylation and clinical response was not observed in this study.

Methylation following decitabine exposure was determined using a novel assay that measures methylation of repetitive elements in the human genome. In

TABLE 6.1 Selected Decitabine Clinical Trials in Myeloid Malignancies

Author-Year	Therapy	Number	Response	Non-hematological Toxicity
Rivard[69] 1981	Decitabine 0.75–80 mg/kg for 8–44 h infusion	30 (pediatric)	10% marrow response	Mild diarrhea, alopecia
Momparler[70] 1985	Decitabine 45–100 mg/kg for 40–90 h	27	22% CR	Mild nausea, vomiting, mucositis
Pinto[74] 1989	Decitabine 45–270 mg/m^2 × 3 days	27	15% CR	Grade III hepatic, GI, renal, pulmonary
Richel[79] 1991	Decitabine 500–1000 mg/m^2 × 3–6 days or decitabine 250–500 mg/m^2 × 6 days with amsacrine 120 mg/m^2 days 6 and 7	16	72% CR	Sterile peritonitis, hepatotoxicity, GI bleed, hemiparesis, somnolence
Willemze[80] 1993	Decitabine 250 mg/m^2 × 6 days with amsacrine 120 mg/m^2 days 6–7 or idarubicin 12 mg/m^2 days 5–7	22	59% CR	Nausea/vomiting, diarrhea, peritonitis, CNS toxicity, weight loss, GI bleed
Petti[75] 1993	Decitabine 270–360 mg/m^2 × 3 days	12	25% CR	No grade III-IV
Zagonel[76] 1993	Decitabine 45–50 mg/m^2 × 3 days	10	50% HI	Nausea/vomiting, peritonitis
Willemze[81] 1997	Decitabine mg/m^2 × 6 randomized to amsacrine 120 mg/m^2 days 6–7 or idarubicin 12 mg/m^2 days 5–7	68	36% CR (27% amsa 45% ida)	Grade IV nausea, vomiting, diarrhea, cardiac
Kantarjian[78] 1993	Decitabine 750 mg/m^2	17	6%	NA
Wijermans[85] 2000	Decitabine 45 mg/m^2 × 3	66	20% CR	GI, pain, seizures, renal, cardiac
Wijermans[87] 2002	Decitabine 45–50 mg/m^2 × 3 days	169	49% CR+PR	NA
Issa[78] 2004	Decitabine 5–20 mg/m^2 × 10–20 days	50	18% CR, 14% PR	Hepatotoxicity

these studies, decitabine induced 10% to 40% hypomethylation within 5 to 10 days[27] (and Yang et al., manuscript submitted for publication). Induction of hypomethylation correlated with dose and with response in the low dose trial.

An unresolved question is what follows induction of hypomethylation, and what mediates responses in that setting. The broad range of genes hypermethylated in cancer[91] suggests multiple potential mechanisms (which could be operating in parallel), including induction of differentiation, apoptosis, senescence, or inhibited angiogenesis. However, it is unlikely that these mechanisms are the only ones operative here. First, it is unclear whether all the cells exposed to decitabine actually hypomethylate genes.[92] Second, this mechanism of action does not explain the peculiar dose-response observed in vivo. Thus, at higher doses, one should observe at least equal activity. An attractive possibility is that, at low doses, decitabine induces a pattern of gene expression that favors a bystander effect that would be lost at higher doses. Particularly intriguing is the possibility that decitabine exposure induces tumor antigens[93,94] (or possibly differentiation of malignant cells to dendritic cells), which would trigger a bystander effect via an immune response. At high doses, the cytotoxicity could abolish this immune response. Indirect evidence for this comes from the fact that, in animal studies, immune modulation potentiates the effect of decitabine.[95]

Decitabine: The Future

It is obvious from the above data that although decitabine, especially at lower doses, has significant effects in leukemia and MDS, its potential as an epigenetic drug has just begun to be investigated. Its future use likely will be in combination with other agents. Conceptually, we consider two types of combinations: combinations that augment its epigenetic effect, and combinations that take advantage of its epigenetic effects.

One of the most interesting combinations to augment epigenetic activation is that of decitabine and a histone deacetylase inhibitor (HDACI). Several HDACI are in clinical development (see below). Pharmacologic modulation of epigenetically repressed genes has provided important information regarding the role of DNA methylation and histone changes on gene expression. In several models, the HDACI trichostatin A alone could not increase gene expression despite increasing histone acetylation. In contrast, decitabine could induce it alone; however, the effect was significantly increased in combination with a HDACI.[47,96–98] This suggests that drugs that inhibit DNA methylation and those that inhibit histone deacetylation can reactivate silenced genes synergistically; thus, there is significant interest in these combinations in clinical practice. Other approaches to potentiate the epigenetic effects of decitabine are described later.

Taking advantage of decitabine-induced gene reactivation is a very promising approach that is currently in clinical trials. Indeed, the potential use of this drug as a modulator of gene expression renders its single agent activity relatively less important than its potential in combination. For example, resistance to platinum compounds in ovarian cancer has been linked to silencing of the *MLH1* gene and decitabine reverses drug resistance to cisplatin in vitro.[99] A clinical trial of this combination is underway. Another promising activity of decitabine is reactivation of several pro-apoptotic molecules.[100–102] Thus, decitabine may well augment the activity of cytotoxic agents that work through apoptosis induction. Moreover, decitabine reactivates or augments the expression of several genes involved in the activity of biological response modifiers. As discussed above, decitabine reactivates estrogen receptor and retinoic acid receptor function, possibly augmenting the effects of interventions targeted to these pathways. In vitro, decitabine also activates several interferon response genes,[103] raising the possibility of combining it with interferon-alpha (IFN-α).

Other potential combinations of interest include decitabine and a DNA topoisomerase inhibitor. These agents have the capacity to introduce double or single DNA strand breaks and have significant activity, especially DNA topoisomerase II inhibitors, in leukemia and MDS. Decitabine has in vitro synergy with a topoisomerase inhibitor.[104] A possible biologic explanation for the synergy of this combination resides in the fact that the boundaries of nucleosomes are enriched in DNA topoisomerase I and II consensus sequences.[105,106] The combination of these two agents in the right sequence may lead to significant disruption of the nucleosome architecture and anticancer activity. The combination of ara-C and a topoisomerase II inhibitor constitutes the standard induction therapy for patients with AML and is an important part of the therapy for ALL,[55,56] and, therefore, decitabine could be tested as a substitute to ara-C in this combination.

AZACYTIDINE

Azacytidine is a ribose analogue of cytosine and incorporates primarily into RNA. Azacytidine also can be converted intracellularly into decitabine, and is thus a prodrug for that agent. The low efficiency of this conversion makes azacytidine 5- to 30-fold less effective as a hypomethylating agent than decitabine at equimolar concentrations.[59] Nevertheless, azacytidine induces differentiation and gene reactivation in vitro as discussed earlier.

Azacytidine has been in clinical trials in the US for over two decades. These have been extensively summarized.[107–110] At various doses, azacytidine has shown disappointing results in solid tumors, but promising results in MDS. The Cancer and Leukemia Group B (CALGB) conducted a series of clinical trials with azacytidine in MDS. Initially, they tested a continuous infusion schedule of azacytidine at 75 mg/m^2/day for seven days, and showed complete or partial remission in 16 of 49 patients (33%). The mean number of courses to achieve the best response was 3.8. Side effects included mostly nausea/vomiting and diarrhea.[111] A second CALGB trial evaluated a subcutaneous formulation of azacytidine at the same total dose of 525 mg/m^2 per course. Complete and partial remissions were seen in 18 of 70 patients enrolled (26%).[112] This led to a pivotal phase III trial randomizing patients with MDS to either supportive care or azacytidine at 75 mg/m²/day subcutaneously for seven days every 28 days.[113] In that trial, patients who progressed while on supportive care were allowed to cross over to the azacytidine arm. This study of 191 patients revealed significantly higher responses in the azacytidine group, along with a lower probability of AML transformation (Table 6.2). Survival was not prolonged in this study, perhaps because of the cross over design. A confirmatory phase III study was recently announced.

The experience with azacytidine parallels some of the findings with decitabine described above. The drug is active at relatively low doses, responses are slow to develop, and MDS is the most responsive disease to this agent thus far. Further development of azacytidine mirrors what was described above for decitabine. Thus, ongoing trials are examining the combination of azacytidine with HDACI, and with other chemotherapeutic agents.

There has been no direct clinical comparison of azacytidine and decitabine. As mentioned earlier, these two drugs are actually different in that azacytidine incorporates primarily into RNA while decitabine incorporates into DNA. The in-vivo hypomethylating effects of azacytidine have not been described and will likely be less pronounced than decitabine, given that the latter agent is active at lower concentrations in vivo. Decitabine has shown more activity in CML than azacytidine, but these differences may reflect patient selection, etc. Neither drug is currently approved in the US, and the issue of the superiority of one over the other may become academic if one is approved but the other is not.

POTENTIAL DRAWBACKS TO HYPOMETHYLATING AGENTS

The two most important conceptual problems with the chronic use of hypomethylating agents in humans include their potential capacity to induce ma-

TABLE 6.2 Azacytidine in MDS: Results of a Phase III CALGB Study Comparing Azacytidine to Supportive Care[113]

	Supportive care	Azacytidine	*P* value
Patients evaluated, *N*	92	99	
Complete response, *N* (%)	0 (0)	7 (7)	
Partial response, *N* (%)	0 (0)	16 (16)	
Improved, *N* (%)	5 (5)	37 (37)	
Total response, *N* (%)	5 (5)	60 (60)	<0.001
Probability of transformation (%)	11	31	.003
Median time to transformation (months)	12	22	.003
Survival	14	18	.1

lignant transformation and their lack of specificity in gene reactivation. In vitro experience suggests that DNA methylation inhibitors may be carcinogenic. Azacytidine and/or decitabine are potential mutagens[114] and teratogens,[115,116] and have been shown to induce the transformation of non-tumorigenic NIH3T3 fibroblasts transfected with deregulated oncogenes.[117] Transient exposure to decitabine induced neoplastic transformation in a significant fraction of these cells.

In addition to direct mutagenesis, hypomethylation itself may be deleterious. DNA methylation is physiologically observed in non-malignant cells.[1] This methylation tends to occur in intergenic non-coding areas rich in repetitive DNA elements. In contrast, methylation of promoter associated CpG islands is probably only functionally relevant for imprinted genes or for genes located in the X chromosome in females, where DNA methylation is important to control gene dosage. A major concern of hypomethylating therapy is therefore activation of physiologically-silenced gene expression with potentially deleterious effects such as inducing malignant transformation. These could be mediated via different mechanisms including the induction of retroviral elements, of normally silenced oncogenes, or by causing chromosomal instability.

Different animal models have provided conflicting data regarding these observations. Rats exposed to methylation-poor diets that induce global hypomethylation developed liver tumors.[118] Abrogation of DNMT1 function in the MIN mouse model of adenomatous polyposis resulted in a reduced number of colon polyps.[119] This inhibitory effect could be tissue dependent. Lack of DNMT1 function in animals devoid of MLH1, which usually develop colon cancer, resulted in a decreased frequency of colon tumors but in an increased frequency of lymphomas.[120] More recently, Jaenisch et al. have develop a mouse model carrying only a hypomorphic allele of DNMT1,[121] as DNMT1 $^{-/-}$ animals die during gestation. Mice carrying the hypomorphic DNMT1 allele had reduced levels of global DNA methylation. These mice were runted and their weight was significantly decreased compared to wildtype animals. Of importance, these animals developed aggressive T cell lymphomas. Some of these data therefore suggest that the induction of hypomethylation with hypomethylating agents in vivo may induce second malignancies.

These data suggest that caution is indicated in hypomethylating therapies, but they also need to be considered in the context of human studies. Mouse modeling induces severe hypomethylation that may not be representative of the extent of hypomethylation observed in human malignancies or after hypomethylating therapy.[27] Indeed, no study has reported a second malignancy in patients treated with hypomethylating drugs. Although it is obvious that DNA methylation is not specific for the cancer cell, it is also possible that neoplastic cells are more sensitive to the effects of hypomethylating therapies either via selective uptake of the drug, or simply because cancer cells are more dependent on gene silencing than normal cells. Indeed, decitabine has been shown to affect cancer cells in-vitro more effectively than normal cells,[122] and we have observed no significant demethylation of the imprinted *H19* gene in patients treated with decitabine (Yang et al., manuscript submitted for publication).

It is clear that long-term use of hypomethylating agents is a risky proposition at present, and those patients exposed to this approach will have to be closely monitored for ill effects (including unexpected effects) before this approach is declared safe.

OTHER HYPOMETHYLATING AGENTS

MG98

This drug is an antisense molecule directed at DNMT1, the DNA methyltransferase enzymes showing the highest level of expression in adult cells.[123] As a therapeutic target, DNMT1 has been questioned because genetic ablation of this gene in a colon cancer cell line had little effect on gene expression.[12] However, somewhat surprisingly in light of the genetic experiment, MG98 shows effective inhibition of DNA methylation in vitro that is associated with gene-specific hypomethylation, reactivated expression of tumor-suppressor genes such as P16, and inhibited growth.[123,125] A phase I clinical trial of MG98, given as a two-hour IV infusion twice weekly for three weeks out of every four to patients with solid tumors, has been completed.[126] Toxicity was relatively minimal. No significant inhibition of DNMT1 was documented in this trial, and minimal clinical activity was observed. A 21-day continuous infusion schedule also was reported for this drug.[127] It was more toxic than the previous schedule and no modulation of methylation biomarkers or clinical responses were seen.

Genetic ablation experiments have shown that simultaneous inhibition of two DNA-methyltransferases, DNMT1 and DNMT3b, is likely to be the most effective way of reactivating gene expression[36] and RNA interference assays have confirmed this observation.[128] An antisense molecule directed at DNMT3b is in development,[129] and would be reasonable to test in combination with MG98.

Zebularine

This molecule was originally designed as an inhibitor of cytidine deaminase.[130] In an in vitro screen for hypomethylating agents, it was discovered that Zebularine was effective at reactivating gene expression, as well as at inducing hypomethylation and differentiation in vitro.[131] Zebularine is potentially orally bioavailable. It has been suggested that it is less toxic than hypomethylating cytosine analogues, and that it would be useful to maintain hypomethylation for prolonged periods of time.[132] However, the mechanism by which Zebularine inhibits Mtase activity and induces hypomethylation has not been unequivocally established, and high doses of the agent are required to achieve hypomethylation in vitro. Clinical trials of this agent have not yet been initiated.

Others

The anti-arrythmic Procainamide and the diuretic hydralazine are both associated with the development of autoimmune phenomena, which have been attributed to their ability to induce demethylation.[133] Procainamide is probably an allosteric inhibitor of DNMT1,[133] and gene-specific hypomethylation has been reported after treatment with the agent.[134] However, compared to decitabine, the hypomethylating activity of Procainamide is minimal, and it is unclear whether it is potent enough at bioavailable doses to achieve much in vivo demethylation. Clinical trials of Procainamide as a hypomethylating agent have not been reported.

Recently, the green tea polyphenol (-)-epigallocatechin-3-gallate (EGCG) has been reported to inhibit DNMT1 through interference with S-adenosyl-methionine binding.[135] In vitro hypomethylation and gene reactivation have been observed following treatment of cancer cell lines. The doses required for this effect are difficult to achieve systemically, but may be achieved locally in the oral mucosa for the treatment or prevention of oro-pharyngeal malignancies. Because EGCG is not efficiently absorbed, and is excreted in the bile, significant concentrations of EGCG can be found also in the large intestine, and could be tested for the treatment or prevention of colorectal tumors. However, the effects of EGCG on DNA methylation have not been confirmed, and clinical trials with this agent as a hypomethylating agent are years away.

OTHER EPIGENETIC ACTING AGENTS

Figure 6.1 describes the proposed silencing loop of biochemical modifications that are involved in gene silencing. Thus far, reversal of silencing has been discussed for the critical step of DNA methylation, but some degree of activity for drugs that target other steps in the pathway could be expected. Table 6.3 describes current therapeutic approaches now being testing or in development that are aimed at epigenetic processes. There are currently no known inhibitors of methyl-binding proteins, histone methyltransferases, or HP1 in clinical trials. However, inhibitors of histone deacetylases have been in clinical trials for several years.[136] The two early members of this class, butyrate and phenylbutyrate, show some activity in vitro but have been disappointing in clinical trials in vivo.[136] Two more recent members of this class of agents, depsipetide and SAHA, are currently in phase II studies, and complete responses to the agents have been reported in some cases.[137] Three other histone deacetylase inhibitors, MS275,[138] AN-9,[139] and LAQ824[140] are currently in phase I/II stud-

TABLE 6.3 Epigenetic Acting Molecules in Clinical Trials or in Development

Target	Molecules in Clinical Trials	Molecules in Development
DNA methylation	Azacytidine Decitabine MG98 (DNMT1 antisense)	Zebularine EGCG
Histone deacteylation	Butyrate Phenylbutyreate Valproate Depsipeptide SAHA LAQ824 MS275 AN9	
Histone lysine 9 methylation	None	In development
Methyl-binding proteins	None	In development
Heterochromatin protein 1 (HP1)	None	In development

Details are in the text.

ies. Finally, the approved antiseizure agent valproic acid is also a histone deacetylase inhibitor,[141] and clinical trials of this agent in cancer are ongoing. While these agents may end up having significant activity on their own, it is more likely that their eventual development and usage will be in biologically-guided combinations. As discussed earlier, hypomethylating agents show synergy with histone deacetylase inhibitors,[96] and clinical trials of this combination are eagerly awaited. Other potential ways of using histone deacetylase inhibitors are in combination with biologic response modifiers such as retinoic acid,[142] or in combination with chemotherapy.[143]

CONCLUSIONS

Hypomethylating agents reverse gene silencing, which appears critical to the neoplastic phenotype in some cases. These agents show significant promise in clinical trials, and their use will likely become widespread, at least for myeloid malignancies. Their promise, however, lies in the fact that they are prototypes for an emerging class of agents that potentially treat cancer via affecting epigenetic processes that regulate gene expression. We are only beginning to learn how best to use these drugs and their most impressive benefits will likely come from combination therapy approaches. In the long run, these agents promise to achieve a kinder and gentler approach to curing human malignancies.

ACKNOWLEDGMENTS

GGM is supported by an American Society of Clinical Oncology Career Development Award and the Physician-Scientist Program Award from the M.D. Anderson Cancer Center. Work in JPJI's laboratory is supported by grants from the National Institutes of Health, the Department of Defense and the George and Barbara Bush foundation for Cancer Research. JPJI and GGM have served as consultants to and have received research support from SuperGen (Dublin, CA).

REFERENCES

1. Jones PA, Takai D. The role of DNA methylation in mammalian epigenetics. Science 2001;293:1068–1070.
2. Bird A. DNA methylation patterns and epigenetic memory. Genes Dev 2002;16:6–21.
3. Wolffe AP, Matzke MA. Epigenetics: regulation through repression. Science 1999;286:481–486.
4. Pitot HC, Jost JP. Control of biochemical expression in morphologically related cells in vivo and in vitro. Natl Cancer Inst Monogr 1967;26:145–166.
5. Cedar H. DNA methylation and gene activity. Cell 1988;53:3–4.
6. Jones PA, Laird PW. Cancer epigenetics comes of age. Nat Genet 1999;21(163-167.
7. Baylin SB, Herman JG, Graff JR et al. Alterations in DNA methylation—A fundamental aspect of neoplasia. Adv Cancer Res 1998;72:141–196.
8. Herman JG, Baylin SB. Gene silencing in cancer in association with promoter hypermethylation. N Engl J Med 2003;349:2042–2054.
9. Jenuwein T, Allis CD. Translating the histone code. Science 2001;293:1074–1080.
10. Rountree MR, Bachman KE, Baylin SB. DNMT1 binds HDAC2 and a new co-repressor, DMAP1, to form a complex at replication foci. Nat Genet 2000;25:269–277.
11. Weissbach A. A chronicle of DNA methylation (1948-1975). EXS 1993;64:1–10.
12. Li E, Bestor TH, Jaenisch R. Targeted mutation of the DNA methyltransferase gene results in embryonic lethality. Cell 1992;69:915–926.
13. Panning B, Jaenisch R. DNA hypomethylation can activate Xist expression and silence X-linked genes. Genes Dev 1996;10:1991–2002.
14. Li E, Beard C, Jaenisch R. Role for DNA methylation in genomic imprinting. Nature 1993;366: 362–365.
15. Walsh CP, Chaillet JR, Bestor TH. Transcription of IAP endogenous retroviruses is constrained by cytosine methylation. Nat Genet 1998;20:116–117.
16. Miura A, Yonebayashi S, Watanabe K et al. Mobilization of transposons by a mutation abolishing full DNA methylation in Arabidopsis. Nature 2001;411:212–214.
17. Zingg JM, Jones PA. Genetic and epigenetic aspects of DNA methylation on genome expression, evolution, mutation and carcinogenesis. Carcinogenesis 1997;18:869–882.
18. Bird AP. CpG-rich islands and the function of DNA methylation. Nature 1986;321:209–213.
19. Bird A. The essentials of DNA methylation. Cell 1992;70:5–8.
20. Heard E, Clerc P, Avner P. X-chromosome inactivation in mammals. Annu Rev Genet 1997;31:571–610.
21. Barlow DP. Gametic imprinting in mammals. Science 1995;270:1610–1613.
22. Jones PA. Altering gene expression with 5-azacytidine. Cell 1985;40:485–486.

23. Ji W, Hernandez R, Zhang XY et al. DNA demethylation and pericentromeric rearrangements of chromosome 1. Mutat Res 1997;379:33–41.

24. Feinberg AP, Vogelstein B. Hypomethylation distinguishes genes of some human cancers from their normal counterparts. Nature 1983;301:89–92.

25. Goodman JI, Counts JL. Hypomethylation of dna: a possible nongenotoxic mechanism underlying the role of cell proliferation in carcinogenesis. Environ Health Perspect 1993;101(Suppl 5):169–172.

26. Chen RZ, Pettersson U, Beard C et al. DNA hypomethylation leads to elevated mutation rates. Nature 1998;395:89–93.

27. Yang AS, Estecio MR, Garcia-Manero G et al. Comment on "Chromosomal instability and tumors promoted by DNA hypomethylation" and "Induction of tumors in nice by genomic hypomethylation." Science 2003;302:1153.

28. Kautiainen TL, Jones PA. DNA methyltransferase levels in tumorigenic and nontumorigenic cells in culture. J Biol Chem 1986;261:1594–1598.

29. Issa JP, Vertino PM, Wu J et al. Increased cytosine DNA-methyltransferase activity during colon cancer progression. J Natl Cancer Inst 1993;85:1235–1240.

30. Eads CA, Danenberg KD, Kawakami K et al. CpG island hypermethylation in human colorectal tumors is not associated with DNA methyltransferase overexpression. Cancer Res 1999;59:2302–2306.

31. Robertson KD, Uzvolgyi E, Liang G et al. The human DNA methyltransferases (DNMTs) 1, 3a and 3b: coordinate mRNA expression in normal tissues and overexpression in tumors. Nucleic Acids Res 1999;27:2291–2298.

32. Szyf M, Kaplan F, Mann V et al. Cell cycle-dependent regulation of eukaryotic DNA methylase level. J Biol Chem 1985;260:8653–8656.

33. Lee PJ, Washer LL, Law DJ et al. Limited up-regulation of DNA methyltransferase in human colon cancer reflecting increased cell proliferation. Proc Natl Acad Sci USA 1996;93:10366–10370.

34. Toyota M, Ahuja N, Ohe-Toyota M et al. CpG island methylator phenotype in colorectal cancer. Proc Natl Acad Sci USA 1999;96:8681–8686.

35. Liang G, Salem CE, Yu MC et al. DNA methylation differences associated with tumor tissues identified by genome scanning analysis. Genomics 1998;53:260–268.

36. Rhee I, Bachman KE, Park BH et al. DNMT1 and DNMT3b cooperate to silence genes in human cancer cells. Nature 2002;416:552–556.

37. Sakai T, Toguchida J, Ohtani N et al. Allele-specific hypermethylation of the retinoblastoma tumor- suppressor gene. Am J Hum Genet 1991;48:880–888.

38. Myohanen SK, Baylin SB, Herman JG. Hypermethylation can selectively silence individual p16ink4A alleles in neoplasia. Cancer Res 1998;58:591–593.

39. Herman JG, Latif F, Weng Y et al. Silencing of the VHL tumor-suppressor gene by DNA methylation in renal carcinoma. Proc Natl Acad Sci USA 1994;91:9700–9704.

40. Kane MF, Loda M, Gaida GM et al. Methylation of the hMLH1 promoter correlates with lack of expression of hMLH1 in sporadic colon tumors and mismatch repair-defective human tumor cell lines. Cancer Res 1997;57:808–811.

41. Khorasanizadeh S. The nucleosome. From genomic organization to genomic regulation. Cell 2004;116:259–272.

42. Lachner M, Jenuwein T. The many faces of histone lysine methylation. Curr Opin Cell Biol 2002;14:286–298.

43. Rice JC, Allis CD. Histone methylation versus histone acetylation: new insights into epigenetic regulation. Curr Opin Cell Biol 2001;13:263–273.

44. Jones PL, Wolffe AP. Relationships between chromatin organization and DNA methylation in determining gene expression. Semin Cancer Biol 1999;9:339–347.

45. Nguyen CT, Weisenberger DJ, Velicescu M et al. Histone H3-lysine 9 methylation is associated with aberrant gene silencing in cancer cells and is rapidly reversed by 5-aza-2'-deoxycytidine. Cancer Res 2002;62:6456–6461.

46. Fahrner JA, Eguchi S, Herman JG, Baylin SB. Dependence of histone modifications and gene expression on DNA hypermethylation in cancer. Cancer Res 2002;62:7213–7218.

47. Kondo Y, Shen L, Issa JP. Critical role of histone methylation in tumor suppressor gene silencing in colorectal cancer. Mol Cell Biol 2003;23:206–215.

48. Tamaru H, Selker EU. A histone H3 methyltransferase controls DNA methylation in Neurospora crassa. Nature 2001;414:277–283.

49. Bachman KE, Park BH, Rhee I et al. Histone modifications and silencing prior to DNA methylation of a tumor suppressor gene. Cancer Cell 2003;3:89–95.

50. Herman JG, Umar A, Polyak K et al. Incidence and functional consequences of hMLH1 promoter hypermethylation in colorectal carcinoma. Proc Natl Acad Sci USA 1998;95:6870–6875.

51. Ottaviano YL, Issa JP, Parl FF et al. Methylation of the estrogen receptor gene CpG island marks loss of estrogen receptor expression in human breast cancer cells. Cancer Res 1994;54:2552–2555.

52. Cote S, Momparler RL. Activation of the retinoic acid receptor beta gene by 5-aza-2′-deoxycytidine in human DLD-1 colon carcinoma cells. Anticancer Drugs 1997;8:56–61.

53. Ferguson AT, Lapidus RG, Baylin SB, Davidson NE. Demethylation of the estrogen receptor gene in estrogen receptor- negative breast cancer cells can reactivate estrogen receptor gene expression. Cancer Res 1995;55:2279–2283.

54. Bovenzi V, Momparler RL. Antineoplastic action of 5-aza-2′-deoxycytidine and histone deacetylase inhibitor and their effect on the expression of retinoic acid receptor beta and estrogen receptor alpha genes in breast carcinoma cells. Cancer Chemother Pharmacol 2001;48:71–76.

55. Estey EH. Therapeutic options for acute myelogenous leukemia. Cancer 2001;92:1059–1073.

56. Garcia-Manero G, Thomas DA. Salvage therapy for refractory or relapsed acute lymphocytic leukemia. Hematol Oncol Clin North Am 2001;15:163–205.

57. Santini V, Kantarjian HM, Issa JP. Changes in DNA methylation in neoplasia: pathophysiology and therapeutic implications. Ann Intern Med 2001;134:573–586.

58. Taylor SM, Jones PA. Multiple new phenotypes induced in 10T1/2 and 3T3 cells treated with 5-azacytidine. Cell 1979;17:771–779.

59. Jones PA, Taylor SM. Cellular differentiation, cytidine analogs and DNA methylation. Cell 1980;20:85–93.

60. Ferguson AT, Vertino PM, Spitzner JR et al. Role of estrogen receptor gene demethylation and DNA methyltransferase.DNA adduct formation in 5-aza-2′deoxycytidine-induced cytotoxicity in human breast cancer cells. J Biol Chem 1997;272:32260–32266.

61. Juttermann R, Li E, Jaenisch R. Toxicity of 5-aza-2′-deoxycytidine to mammalian cells is mediated primarily by covalent trapping of DNA methyltransferase rather than DNA demethylation. Proc Natl Acad Sci USA 1994;91:11797–11801.

62. Sorm F, Vesely J. Effect of 5-aza-2′-deoxycytidine against leukemic and hemopoietic tissues in AKR mice. Neoplasma 1968;15:339–343.

63. Jones PA, Taylor SM, Mohandas T, Shapiro LJ. Cell cycle-specific reactivation of an inactive X-chromosome locus by 5-azadeoxycytidine. Proc Natl Acad Sci USA 1982;79:1215–1219.

64. Momparler RL, Bouchard J, Samson J. Induction of differentiation and inhibition of DNA methylation in HL-60 myeloid leukemic cells by 5-AZA-2'-deoxycytidine. Leuk Res 1985;9:1361–1366.

65. Pinto A, Attadia V, Fusco A et al. 5-Aza-2′-deoxycytidine induces terminal differentiation of leukemic blasts from patients with acute myeloid leukemias. Blood 1984;64:922–929.

66. Covey JM, Zaharko DS. Effects of dose and duration of exposure on 5-aza-2′-deoxycytidine cytotoxicity for L1210 leukemia in vitro. Cancer Treat Rep 1984;68:1475–1481.

67. Wilson VL, Jones PA, Momparler RL. Inhibition of DNA methylation in L1210 leukemic cells by 5-aza-2′-deoxycytidine as a possible mechanism of chemotherapeutic action. Cancer Res 1983;43:3493–3496.

68. Chabot GG, Rivard GE, Momparler RL. Plasma and cerebrospinal fluid pharmacokinetics of 5-Aza-2′-deoxycytidine in rabbits and dogs. Cancer Res 1983;43:592–597.

69. Rivard GE, Momparler RL, Demers J et al. Phase I study on 5-aza-2′-deoxycytidine in children with acute leukemia. Leuk Res 1981;5:453–462.

70. Momparler RL, Rivard GE, Gyger M. Clinical trial on 5-aza-2′–deoxycytidine in patients with acute leukemia. Pharmacol Ther 1985;30:277–286.

71. van Groeningen CJ, Leyva A, O'Brien AM et al. Phase I and pharmacokinetic study of 5-aza-2′-deoxycytidine (NSC 127716) in cancer patients. Cancer Res 1986;46:4831–4836.

72. Abele R, Clavel M, Dodion P et al. The EORTC Early Clinical Trials Cooperative Group experience with 5-aza-2′-deoxycytidine (NSC 127716) in patients with colo-rectal, head and neck, renal carcinomas and malignant melanomas. Eur J Cancer Clin Oncol 1987;23:1921–1924.

73. Aparicio A, Eads CA, Leong LA et al. Phase I trial of continuous infusion 5-aza-2′-deoxycytidine. Cancer Chemother Pharmacol 2003;51:231–239.

74. Pinto A, Zagonel V, Attadia V et al. 5-Aza-2'-deoxycytidine as a differentiation inducer in acute myeloid leukaemias and myelodysplastic syndromes of the elderly. Bone Marrow Transplant 1989;4(Suppl 3):28–32.

75. Petti MC, Mandelli F, Zagonel V et al. Pilot study of 5-aza-2′-deoxycytidine (Decitabine) in the treatment of poor prognosis acute myelogenous leukemia patients: preliminary results. Leukemia 1993;7(Suppl 1):36–41.

76. Zagonel V, Lo RG, Marotta G et al. 5-Aza-2'-deoxycytidine (Decitabine) induces trilineage response in unfavourable myelodysplastic syndromes. Leukemia 1993;7(Suppl 1):30–35.

77. Wijermans PW, Krulder JW, Huijgens PC, Neve P. Continuous infusion of low-dose 5-Aza-2′-deoxycytidine in elderly patients with high-risk myelodysplastic syndrome. Leukemia 1997;11(Suppl 1):S19–S23.

78. Issa JP, Garcia-Manero G, Giles FJ et al. Phase I study of low-dose prolonged exposure schedules of the hypomethylating agent 5-aza-2′-deoxycytidine (Decitabine) in hematopoietic malignancies. Blood 2004;103:1635–1640.

79. Richel DJ, Colly LP, Kluin-Nelemans JC, Willemze R. The antileukaemic activity of 5-Aza-2 deoxycytidine (Aza-dC) in patients with relapsed and resistant leukaemia. Br J Cancer 1991;64:144–148.

80. Willemze R, Archimbaud E, Muus P. Preliminary results with 5-aza-2′-deoxycytidine (DAC)-containing chemotherapy in patients with relapsed or refractory acute leukemia. The EORTC Leukemia Cooperative Group. Leukemia 1993;7(Suppl 1):49–50.

81. Willemze R, Suciu S, Archimbaud E et al. A randomized phase II study on the effects of 5-Aza-2'-deoxycytidine combined with either amsacrine or idarubicin in patients with relapsed acute leukemia: an EORTC Leukemia Cooperative Group phase II study (06893). Leukemia 1997;11(Suppl 1):S24–S27.

82. Schwartsmann G, Fernandes MS, Schaan MD et al. Decitabine (5-Aza-2′-deoxycytidine; DAC) plus daunorubicin as a first line treatment in patients with acute myeloid leukemia: preliminary observations. Leukemia 1997;11(Suppl 1):S28–S31.

83. Kantarjian HM, O'Brien SM, Keating M et al. Results of decitabine therapy in the accelerated and blastic phases of chronic myelogenous leukemia. Leukemia 1997;11:1617–1620.

84. Kantarjian HM, O'Brien S, Cortes J et al. Results of decitabine (5-aza-2'deoxycytidine) therapy in 130 patients with chronic myelogenous leukemia. Cancer 2003;98:522–528.

85. Wijermans P, Lubbert M, Verhoef G et al. Low-dose 5-aza-2'-deoxycytidine, a DNA hypomethylating agent, for the treatment of high-risk myelodysplastic syndrome: a multicenter phase II study in elderly patients. J Clin Oncol 2000;18:956–962.

86. Lubbert M, Wijermans P, Kunzmann R et al. Cytogenetic responses in high-risk myelodysplastic syndrome following low-dose treatment with the DNA methylation inhibitor 5-aza-2'-deoxycytidine. Br J Haematol 2001;114:349–357.

87. Wijermans PW, Luebbert M, Verhoef G. Low dose Decitabine for elderly high risk MDS patients: Who will respond? Blood 2002;100:96A–97A.

88. DeSimone J, Koshy M, Dorn L et al. Maintenance of elevated fetal hemoglobin levels by decitabine during dose interval treatment of sickle cell anemia. Blood 2002;99:3905–3908.

89. Koshy M, Dorn L, Bressler L et al. 2-deoxy 5-azacytidine and fetal hemoglobin induction in sickle cell anemia. Blood 2000;96:2379–2384.

90. Daskalakis M, Nguyen TT, Nguyen C et al. Demethylation of a hypermethylated P15/INK4B gene in patients with myelodysplastic syndrome by 5-Aza-2'-deoxycytidine (decitabine) treatment. Blood 2002;100:2957–2964.

91. Herman JG, Baylin SB. Gene silencing in cancer in association with promoter hypermethylation. N Engl J Med 2003;349:2042–2054.

92. Gonzalgo ML, Hayashida T, Bender CM et al. The role of DNA methylation in expression of the p19/p16 locus in human bladder cancer cell lines. Cancer Res 1998;58:1245–1252.

93. Issa JP. Decitabine. Curr Opin Oncol 2003;15:446–451.

94. Maio M, Coral S, Fratta E et al. Epigenetic targets for immune intervention in human malignancies. Oncogene 2003;22:6484–6488.

95. Zaharko DS, Covey JM, Muneses CC. Experimental chemotherapy (L1210) with 5-aza-2'-deoxycytidine in combination with pyran copolymer (MVE-4), an immune adjuvant. J Natl Cancer Inst 1985;74:1319–1324.

96. Cameron EE, Bachman KE, Myohanen S et al. Synergy of demethylation and histone deacetylase inhibition in the re- expression of genes silenced in cancer. Nat Genet 1999;21:103–107.

97. Primeau M, Gagnon J, Momparler RL. Synergistic antineoplastic action of DNA methylation inhibitor 5-AZA-2'-deoxycytidine and histone deacetylase inhibitor depsipeptide on human breast carcinoma cells. Int J Cancer 2003;103:177–184.

98. El Osta A, Kantharidis P, Zalcberg JR, Wolffe AP. Precipitous release of methyl-CpG binding protein 2 and histone deacetylase 1 from the methylated human multidrug resistance gene (MDR1) on activation. Mol Cell Biol 2002;22:1844–1857.

99. Plumb JA, Strathdee G, Sludden J et al. Reversal of drug resistance in human tumor xenografts by 2'-deoxy-5-azacytidine-induced demethylation of the hMLH1 gene promoter. Cancer Res 2000;60:6039–6044.

100. Conway KE, McConnell BB, Bowring CE et al. TMS1, a novel proapoptotic caspase recruitment domain protein, is a target of methylation-induced gene silencing in human breast cancers. Cancer Res 2000;60:6236–6242.

101. Obata T, Toyota M, Satoh A et al. Identification of HRK as a Target of Epigenetic Inactivation in Colorectal and Gastric Cancer. Clin Cancer Res 2003;9:6410–6418.

102. Jones PA. Cancer. Death and methylation. Nature 2001;409:141:143–141, 144.

103. Karpf AR, Jones DA. Reactivating the expression of methylation silenced genes in human cancer. Oncogene 2002;21:5496–5503.

104. Anzai H, Frost P, Abbruzzese JL. Synergistic cytotoxicity with 2′-deoxy-5-azacytidine and topotecan in vitro and in vivo. Cancer Res 1992;52:2180–2185.

105. Zlatanova JS, van Holde KE. Chromatin loops and transcriptional regulation. Crit Rev Eukaryot Gene Expr 1992;2:211–224.

106. Razin SV, Petrov P, Hancock R. Precise localization of the alpha-globin gene cluster within one of the 20- to 300-kilobase DNA fragments released by cleavage of chicken chromosomal DNA at topoisomerase II sites in vivo: evidence that the fragments are DNA loops or domains. Proc Natl Acad Sci USA 1991;88:8515–8519.

107. Von Hoff DD, Slavik M, Muggia FM. 5-Azacytidine. A new anticancer drug with effectiveness in acute myelogenous leukemia. Ann Intern Med 1976;85:237–245.

108. Pinto A, Zagonel V. 5-Aza-2′-deoxycytidine (Decitabine) and 5-azacytidine in the treatment of acute myeloid leukemias and myelodysplastic syndromes: past, present and future trends. Leukemia 1993;7(Suppl 1):51–60.

109. Cheson BD, Zwiebel JA, Dancey J, Murgo A. Novel therapeutic agents for the treatment of myelodysplastic syndromes. Semin Oncol 2000;27:560–577.

110. Leone G, Teofili L, Voso MT, Lubbert M. DNA methylation and demethylating drugs in myelodysplastic syndromes and secondary leukemias. Haematologica 2002;87:1324–1341.

111. Silverman LR, Holland JF, Weinberg RS et al. Effects of treatment with 5-azacytidine on the in vivo and in vitro hematopoiesis in patients with myelodysplastic syndromes. Leukemia 1993;7(Suppl 1):21–29.

112. Leone G, Voso MT, Teofili L, Lubbert M. Inhibitors of DNA methylation in the treatment of hematological malignancies and MDS. Clin Immunol 2003;109:89–102.

113. Silverman LR, Demakos EP, Peterson BL et al. Randomized controlled trial of azacitidine in patients with the myelodysplastic syndrome: a study of the cancer and leukemia group B. J Clin Oncol 2002;20:2429–2440.

114. Amacher DE, Turner GN. The mutagenicity of 5-azacytidine and other inhibitors of replicative DNA synthesis in the L5178Y mouse lymphoma cell. Mutat Res 1987;176:123–131.

115. Rosen MB, Chernoff N. 5-Aza-2′-deoxycytidine-induced cytotoxicity and limb reduction defects in the mouse. Teratology 2002;65:180–190.

116. Rogers JM, Francis BM, Sulik KK et al. Cell death and cell cycle perturbation in the developmental toxicity of the demethylating agent, 5-aza-2′-deoxycytidine. Teratology 1994;50:332–339.

117. Rimoldi D, Srikantan V, Wilson VL, et al. Increased sensitivity of nontumorigenic fibroblasts expressing ras or myc oncogenes to malignant transformation induced by 5-aza-2′-deoxycytidine. Cancer Res 1991;51:324–330.

118. Ehrlich M. DNA methylation in cancer: too much, but also too little. Oncogene 2002;21:5400–5413.

119. Laird PW, Jackson-Grusby L, Fazeli A et al. Suppression of intestinal neoplasia by DNA hypomethylation. Cell 1995;81:197–205.

120. Trinh BN, Long TI, Nickel AE, et al. DNA methyltransferase deficiency modifies cancer susceptibility in mice lacking DNA mismatch repair. Mol Cell Biol 2002;22:2906–2917.

121. Gaudet F, Hodgson JG, Eden A et al. Induction of tumors in mice by genomic hypomethylation. Science 2003;300:489–492.

122. Bender CM, Pao MM, Jones PA. Inhibition of DNA methylation by 5-aza-2′-deoxycytidine suppresses the growth of human tumor cell lines. Cancer Res 1998;58:95–101.

123. Reid GK, Besterman JM, MacLeod AR. Selective inhibition of DNA methyltransferase enzymes as a novel strategy for cancer treatment. Curr Opin Mol Ther 2002;4:130–137.

124. Rhee I, Jair KW, Yen RW et al. CpG methylation is maintained in human cancer cells lacking DNMT1. Nature 2000;404:1003–1007.

125. Robert MF, Morin S, Beaulieu N et al. DNMT1 is required to maintain CpG methylation and aberrant gene silencing in human cancer cells. Nat Genet 2003;33:61–65.

126. Stewart DJ, Donehower RC, Eisenhauer EA et al. A phase I pharmacokinetic and pharmacodynamic study of the DNA methyltransferase 1 inhibitor MG98 administered twice weekly. Ann Oncol 2003;14:766–774.

127. Davis AJ, Gelmon KA, Siu LL et al. Phase I and pharmacologic study of the human DNA methyltransferase antisense oligodeoxynucleotide MG98 given as a 21-day continuous infusion every 4 weeks. Invest New Drugs 2003;21:85–97.

128. Leu YW, Rahmatpanah F, Shi H et al. Double RNA interference of DNMT3b and DNMT1 enhances DNA demethylation and gene reactivation. Cancer Res 2003;63:6110–6115.

129. Beaulieu N, Morin S, Chute IC, et al. An essential role for DNA methyltransferase DNMT3B in cancer cell survival. J Biol Chem 2002;277:28176–28181.

130. Laliberte J, Marquez VE, Momparler RL. Potent inhibitors for the deamination of cytosine arabinoside and 5-aza-2′-deoxycytidine by human cytidine deaminase. Cancer Chemother Pharmacol 1992;30:7–11.

131. Cheng JC, Matsen CB, Gonzales FA et al. Inhibition of DNA methylation and reactivation of silenced genes by zebularine. J Natl Cancer Inst 2003;95:399–409.

132. Cheng JC, Weisenberger DJ, Gonzales FA et al. Continuous zebularine treatment effectively sustains demethylation in human bladder cancer cells. Mol Cell Biol 2004;24:1270–1278.

133. Richardson BC. Role of DNA methylation in the regulation of cell function: autoimmunity, aging and cancer. J Nutr 2002;132(Suppl 8):2401S–2405S.

134. Lin X, Asgari K, Putzi MJ et al. Reversal of GSTP1 CpG island hypermethylation and reactivation of pi-class glutathione S-transferase (GSTP1) expression in human prostate cancer cells by treatment with procainamide. Cancer Res 2001;61:8611–8616.

135. Fang MZ, Wang Y, Ai N et al. Tea polyphenol (-)-epigallocatechin-3-gallate inhibits DNA methyltransferase and reactivates methylation-silenced genes in cancer cell lines. Cancer Res 2003;63:7563–7570.

136. Marks PA, Miller T, Richon VM. Histone deacetylases. Curr Opin Pharmacol 2003;3:344–351.

137. Piekarz RL, Robey R, Sandor V et al. Inhibitor of histone deacetylation, depsipeptide (FR901228), in the treatment of peripheral and cutaneous T-cell lymphoma: a case report. Blood 2001;98:2865–2868.

138. Saito A, Yamashita T, Mariko Y et al. A synthetic inhibitor of histone deacetylase, MS-27-275, with marked in vivo antitumor activity against human tumors. Proc Natl Acad Sci USA 1999;96:4592–4597.

139. Patnaik A, Rowinsky EK, Villalona MA et al. A phase I study of pivaloyloxymethyl butyrate, a prodrug of the differentiating agent butyric acid, in patients with advanced solid malignancies. Clin Cancer Res 2002;8:2142–2148.

140. Remiszewski SW. The discovery of NVP-LAQ824: from concept to clinic. Curr Med Chem 2003;10:2393–2402.

141. Phiel CJ, Zhang F, Huang EY, et al. Histone deacetylase is a direct target of valproic acid, a potent anticonvulsant, mood stabilizer, and teratogen. J Biol Chem 2001;276:36734–36741.

142. Kosugi H, Towatari M, Hatano S et al. Histone deacetylase inhibitors are the potent inducer/enhancer of differentiation in acute myeloid leukemia: a new approach to anti-leukemia therapy. Leukemia 1999;13:1316–1324.

143. Kim MS, Blake M, Baek JH et al. Inhibition of histone deacetylase increases cytotoxicity to anticancer drugs targeting DNA. Cancer Res 2003;63:7291–7300.

Chapter 7

New Applications for Thalidomide in the Treatment of Patients with Solid Cancer

Robert J. Amato

Thalidomide was first introduced in Europe in the mid-1950s as a non-barbiturate sedative/hypnotic and used to treat pregnancy-associated morning sickness.[1,2] Its use, however, was soon associated with stunted limb growth and other birth defects, prompting its withdrawal from world markets by the end of 1961. Subsequently, thalidomide was available for strictly defined research purposes. In 1965, thalidomide was shown to markedly reduce symptoms of erythema nodosum leprosum, an inflammatory manifestation of leprosy.[3] This observation ultimately led the United States Food and Drug Administration to approve the use of thalidomide in 1998 for the short-term treatment of the cutaneous manifestations of moderate to severe erythema nodosum leprosum and as maintenance therapy to prevent and suppress the manifestations of erythema nodosum leprosum recurrence.[1]

The potential of thalidomide in cancer therapy was first suggested in the mid-1960s. Disease stabilization was reported with thalidomide in a sarcoma patient, prompting further evaluation of this agent in patients with a variety of advanced cancers.[4] Palliative effects were noted in some patients, but an objective response was achieved by a patient with renal cell carcinoma whose pulmonary lesion disappeared after treatment.[5] In the 1990s, experimental studies revealed that thalidomide has antiangiogenic and immunomodulatory activities. Thalidomide was shown to inhibit angiogenesis induced by basic fibroblast growth factor (bFGF) in a rabbit corneal micropocket assay[6] and by bFGF and vascular endothelial growth factor (VEGF) in a murine corneal neovascularization model.[7] Thalidomide also was shown to inhibit tumor necrosis factor-α (TNF-α) production,[8] modulate cell adhesion molecule expression,[9] and modulate immune responses.[10] In addition to inhibiting TNF-α, thalidomide inhibited interferon (IFN)-γ and increased production of interleukin (IL) -4 and IL-5, thus shifting cytokine production from a Th1 to Th2 pattern.[11] Depending on the stimulus, thalidomide either inhibited or enhanced production of IL-12, a key cytokine in cellular immune responses.[10] More recently, thalidomide was shown to inhibit the transcription factor nuclear factor-κB (NF-κB), which regulates genes expressed during immune and inflammatory responses as well as those involved in oncogenic processes, such as cell growth, apoptosis suppression, and metastasis.[12] A schematic showing the possible sites of thalidomide action is shown in Figure 7.1.

These observations coincided with the emerging role of angiogenesis in cancer pathogenesis and fueled interest in reevaluating thalidomide in treatment of various malignancies. Thalidomide was initially considered for salvage therapy of

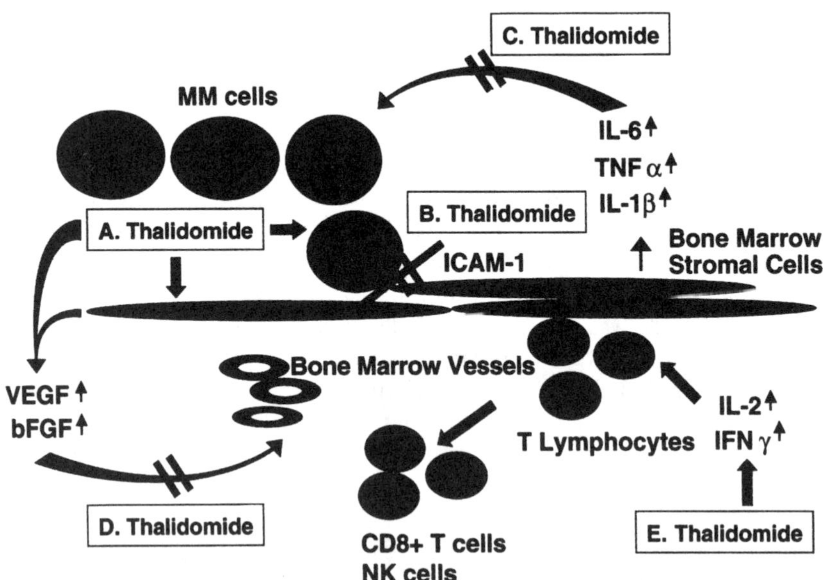

FIGURE 7.1 Mechanisms of action of thalidomide with possible relevance to cancer treatment. Multiple myeloma is used as an example. Thalidomide directly inhibits myeloma cell growth (**A**), blocks myeloma cell adhesion to bone marrow stromal cells (**B**), inhibits cytokine production (**C**), reduce growth factor-induced angiogenesis (**D**), and modulates T cell responses (**E**). Reprinted with permission from Richardson P, Hideshima T, Anderson K. *Biomedicine & Pharmacotherapy*, 2002;56:115–128.

multiple myeloma based on the association between survival and the degree of angiogenesis in the bone marrow of these patients.[13] Positive results were obtained initially with thalidomide monotherapy and subsequently with combination therapy in patients with relapsed and refractory myeloma, and this spurred evaluation of thalidomide in other malignancies.[14–17] This chapter reviews the progress realized with thalidomide in several solid tumors, initially in monotherapy and more recently in combination with other treatment modalities.

THALIDOMIDE IN BRAIN CANCER

Brain tumors are the leading cause of cancer deaths in children and the fourth leading cause in young adults.[18] More than 20 years ago, fractionated radiation therapy was shown to extend survival, but further progress in treating these tumors has been slow. Chemotherapy shows some activity in certain histologic subtypes, such as anaplastic astrocytomas, but it provides only a small survival benefit in those with the most common and most malignant form of brain cancer, glioblastoma multiforme.[19,20] High-grade gliomas undergo genetic alterations that result in overexpression of inducers of tumor angiogenesis and down-regulation of natural inhibitors of this process.[21] Thus, angiogenesis inhibition was viewed as an attractive approach for treating these brain tumors.

Monotherapy

Thalidomide showed promising activity in several phase II studies of patients with recurrent high-grade gliomas, producing objective response rates of 5% to 6% (Table 7.1). The doses of thalidomide used in these studies varied considerably; however, in general, the drug was well tolerated. Sedation/fatigue and constipation were the most common toxicities but were easily manageable.[22–24] Investigators at the National Cancer Institute (NCI) administered thalidomide at doses of 800 mg/day initially with escalation to a maximum of 1200 mg/day to 36 patients, most of whom had either recurrent glioblastoma multiforme (64%) or anaplastic astrocytomas (31%). All patients had previously received standard external-beam radiation therapy, and about half had received prior chemotherapy. Thalidomide produced objective radiographic partial responses in two (6%) patients and minor responses in two (6%) patients, and in addition, 12 (33%) others had stable disease. The median time to progression (TTP) was 10 weeks for the entire group, but 33 weeks for those with radiographic responses, whereas median survival from the start of thalidomide therapy was 28 weeks overall and 74 weeks for those with radiographic responses. Interestingly, changes in serum levels of bFGF were inversely correlated with TTP and overall survival. It is unclear, however, whether this observation reflects a direct antiangiogenic effect of thalidomide.[22]

TABLE 7.1 Activity of Thalidomide in High-Grade Gliomas

Study	Dose	Patients	Response Rate	Median TTP	Median Survival	Grade 3/4 Toxicity
Monotherapy						
Fine et al, 2000[22]	T 800 → 1,200 mg/d	39 recurrent (25 GBM; 12 AA; 2 AMG)	PR: 6% MR: 6% SD: 33%	10 wks	28 wks (1-year: 22%)	Somnolence (17%), cortical toxicity (11%), motor toxicity (8%)
Marx et al 2001[24]	T 100 → 500 mg/d	42 recurrent GBM	PR: 5% SD: 42%	~11 wks	31 wks (1-year: 35%)	Fatigue (8%), constipation (5%), rash (3%), xerostomia (3%)
Short et al 2001[23]	T 100 mg/d	18 recurrent	PR: 6% SD: 11%	NR	2.5 mos	Lethargy, somnolence, peripheral sensory neuropathy
Combination therapy						
Fine et al 2003[18]	Carmustine 600 mg/m² on d1 q 6 weeks + T 800 → 1,200 mg/day	40 recurrent (38 GBM; 2 AA)	CR: 3% PR: 21% SD: 24%	34 wks (CR/PR) 25 wks (SD) 8 wks (PD)	43 wks (CR/PR) 33 wks (SD) 19 wks (PD)	Thromboembolic events (30%), seizure (18%), cortical toxicity (13%), neutropenia (8%)
Bjeljac et al 2003[25]	Temozolomide 200 mg/m² x 5 d + T 200 mg/day q month vs. T 200 mg/day[a]	25 GBM vs. 19 GBM (after surgery and radiation)	—	36 wks vs. 17 wks (P<0.06)	103 wks vs. 63 wks (P<0.01)	None reported
Capparella et al 2003[26]	Temozolomide 75 mg/m²/d + T 400 mg/d x 6 weeks	7 GBM (after surgery but before radiation)	No PR or SD	5.3 wks	6 mos	Transaminitis (14%)

Abbreviations: T, thalidomide; GBM, glioblastoma multiforme; AA, anaplastic astrocytoma; AMG, anaplastic mixed glioma; CR, complete response; PR, partial response; MR, minor response; SD, stable disease; TTP, time to progression; NR, not reported.

[a]Median doses

In the other two studies of thalidomide monotherapy, lower drug doses were used. Investigators in Australia administered thalidomide 100 mg/day with dose escalation to 500 mg/day to 42 patients with recurrent glioblastoma multiforme. Among 38 evaluable patients, thalidomide produced partial responses in two (5%) patients and stable disease in 16 (42%) others. The median survival was 31 weeks, and one-year survival was 35%. Patients with partial responses or stable disease generally had their quality of life or performance status either improved or stabilized.[24] Finally, Short and colleagues administered thalidomide at 100 mg/day to 18 patients with recurrent gliomas who had failed previous radiation therapy and chemotherapy with packed-cell volume (PCV) and/or temozolomide. Twelve patients received treatment for more than four weeks, whereas the other six deteriorated before treatment responses could be assessed. One (6%) patient achieved a clinical and radiological partial response and 2 (11%) others had stable disease for two and four months, respectively. Median survival from the start of thalidomide therapy was 2.5 months.[23]

Combination Therapy

On the basis of the positive findings with thalidomide monotherapy and preclinical evidence showing synergism between thalidomide and cytotoxic agents, Fine and colleagues at NCI initiated a phase II trial of thalidomide in combination with carmustine (BCNU), the traditional cytotoxic drug used to treat gliomas. Forty patients with recurrent high-grade gliomas after standard surgery and radiation were treated with carmustine 200 mg/m^2 every six weeks and thalidomide 800 mg/day escalated to 1,200 mg/day as tolerated. All but two patients had glioblassurgery and radiationoma multiforme. Half had received prior chemotherapy. The objective radiographic response rate among 38 evaluable patients was 24%, which included one patient with a complete response and eight patients with partial responses. An additional nine (24%) patients had stable disease. The median progression-free survival was 100 days, which compared favorably with historic data for each drug alone. Median overall survival was 298 and 230 days for those with objective responses and stable disease, respectively, as compared to 133 days for those with progressive disease ($P < .0001$). Thromboembolic events occurred in 12 patients, including eight with deep vein thrombosis and seven with pulmonary emboli. These complications are common in patients with advanced gliomas, and therefore it is uncertain whether the carmustine-thalidomide regimen increased the underlying risk. Grade 4 hematologic toxicity consisted of three cases of neutropenia and one case of thrombocytopenia. The results of this study show that combination carmustine-thalidomide therapy has significant antitumor activity against recurrent high-grade gliomas. The activity compares favorably with each drug alone and with other agents and combinations reported in the literature.[18]

Preliminary results from two phase II studies of thalidomide in combination with temozolomide were recently reported. In the first study, 44 patients with glioblastoma multiforme underwent microsurgery and radiation therapy, and then received thalidomide either alone (n = 19) or with temozolomide (n = 25) for up to one year. The median dose of thalidomide was 200 mg daily, whereas the median dose of temozolomide was 200 mg/m^2 daily for five days each month. Median survival was significantly longer with combination temozolomide-thalidomide therapy (103 vs. 63 weeks; P <.01), whereas median TTP showed a trend in favor of the combination regimen (P <.06). On neuroradiological assessment, two (5%) patients showed tumor regression and 20 (45%) others had stable disease. The combination regimen was well tolerated, with toxicities reported to be mild or moderate.[25] In the other study, combination temozolomide-thalidomide was evaluated in newly diagnosed patients with glioblastoma multiforme after surgery but before radiation therapy. Temozolomide was administered daily at 75 mg/m^2 for six weeks in combination with thalidomide at a maximum dose of 400 mg/day. The study was terminated when an interim analysis showed that none of the first seven patients responded or stabilized with treatment.[26] Thus, these studies suggest that the activity of temozolomide-thalidomide in glioblastoma multiforme depends on the treatment setting: it may prolong survival in selected patients when given after surgery and radiation,[25] but short-term use before radiation therapy does not appear to be active.[26]

The feasibility of combining thalidomide with irinotecan, an agent that is active in treating primary brain tumors, is being evaluated in a phase I study of patients with recurrent anaplastic oligodendrogliomas or astrocytomas. Irinotecan 300 mg/m^2 was administered intravenously over 30 minutes on day 1 of a three-week cycle, and thalidomide was given at bedtime on days 3 to 19. The thalidomide dose was started at 200 mg orally and then escalated weekly in 100-mg increments to the maximum tolerated dose. In the preliminary report, three of the first four patients showed radiographic evidence of treatment responses. One of these patients completed 15 cycles of treatment and showed marked reduction in tumor size with improvement in clinical status, but required lengthening of the treatment cycle to four to five weeks due to neutropenia. The regimen was generally well tolerated with none of the patients showing evidence of irinotecan-associated diarrhea.[27]

THALIDOMIDE IN METASTATIC MELANOMA

Melanoma accounts for 3% to 4% of all new cancers in the United States.[28] Surgical excision is the treatment of choice for primary tumors and for locoregional recurrence. For patients with unresectable disease, dacarbazine-based chemotherapy is the standard treatment. Objective responses, however, are achieved in only 10% to 20% of patients and persist for a median of five to six months.[29] Temozolomide, an oral congener of dacarbazine, offers better progression-free survival (PFS) and quality of life, but overall survival is not improved significantly.[30] The switch of melanoma from a horizontal to vertical growth phase is accompanied by VEGF expression and angiogenesis, thus providing a rationale for considering thalidomide in this malignancy.[31]

Monotherapy

Mixed results have been reported with thalidomide monotherapy in metastatic melanoma. In an early investigation, Eisen et al administered thalidomide 100 mg/day to 17 patients with advanced melanoma, but did not observe any objective responses. One (6%) patient had stable disease and experienced symptomatic improvement.[32] Similarly, investigators in Brazil did not see any objective responses in 14 patients with metastatic melanoma when thalidomide was administered at a starting dose of 200 mg/day and then escalated in 200-mg increments every two weeks to a maximum of 800 mg/day.[33] However, thalidomide 200 mg daily produced a complete response in a 63-year-old male patient with recurrent melanoma who had failed immunotherapy and was not a candidate for aggressive surgery or chemotherapy. At the time of the report, the patient remained in complete remission while continuing to receive thalidomide 100 mg/day.[34]

Combination Therapy

Thalidomide showed synergistic effects with dacarbazine and temozolomide in animal models of melanoma, prompting its evaluation as part of combination therapy.[35] The temozolomide-thalidomide combination has been evaluated in several studies of advanced melanoma (Table 7.2). A dose-finding study was conducted at the Memorial Sloan-Kettering Cancer Center (MSKCC) in patients with unresectable stage III/IV melanoma without brain metastases. Five (55%) of nine patients who received temozolomide at a dose level of 75 mg/m^2/day for six weeks (followed by breaks of 2–4 weeks) and thalidomide 200 to 400 mg/day achieved objective responses, including one complete response. The median duration of response was six months. Notably, three of the responding patients were over age 70.[29] In a subsequent phase II study conducted at MSKCC, temozolomide-thalidomide was administered to 24 melanoma patients with measurable and progressive intracranial metastases. All but one patient also had extensive extra-cranial metastases. Overall 13 patients completed at least one cycle of therapy (range 1–4). Of 11 patients who were evaluable for brain responses, two achieved complete responses, one had a partial response, and five had stable disease. Nevertheless, seven of these patients showed progression of extra-cranial disease.[36] Thus, these results suggest that the activity of temozolomide-thalidomide may differ on intracranial versus extra-cranial disease.

Danson and colleagues evaluated combination temozolomide-thalidomide as part of a randomized phase II study. A total of 181 patients with metastatic melanoma were randomly assigned to receive one of three treatments: temozolo-

TABLE 7.2 Activity of Thalidomide in Metastatic Melanoma

Study	Dose	Patients	Response Rate	Median TTP	Median Survival	Grade 3/4 Toxicity
Monotherapy						
Eisen et al, 2000[32]	T 100 mg/d	17	PR: 0% SD: 16%	NR	NR	None
Reiriz et al 2003[33]	T 200 → 800 mg/d	14	PR: 0%	NR	NR	Toxicity grade NR
Combination therapy						
Hwu et al 2002[29]	Temozolomide 50-75 mg/m²/d x 6 weeks followed by 2-4 week breaks + T 200 → 400 mg/d	12 (no BM)	CR: 8%[a] PR: 33% SD: 25%	NR	12.3 months	Thromboembolic events (17%), neuropathy (17%), constipation (8%), rash (8%)
Hwu et al 2003[36]	Temozolomide 75 mg/m²/d x 6 weeks followed by 2-week break + T 200 → 400 mg/d[b]	24 (with BM)	IC sites[c]: CR: 18% PR: 9% SD: 45%	NR	5 months	Intracranial hemorrhage (29%), thromboembolic events (13%), rash (4%)
Danson et al 2002[35]	Temozolomide 200 mg/m² q 8h x 5 Temozolomide 200 mg/m²/d x 5d + IFN-α-2b 5 mIU 3x/wk	59 (5 with BM) 62 (2 with BM) 60 (4 with BM) 10	CR: 0% PR: 9% SD: 11% CR: 3% PR: 15% SD: 3%	NR	5.3 months (1-y: 18%; 2-y: 7%) 7.7 months (1-y: 26%; 2-y: 9%) 7.3 months (1-y: 24%; 2-y: 17%)	Thrombocytopenia (34% vs. 23% vs. 0%, P<0.05), neutropenia (28% vs. 21% vs. 2%, P<0.05), infection (16% vs. 7% vs. 0%, P< 0.05), nausea (6% vs. 5% vs. 5%), vomiting (6% vs. 2% vs. 4%), pulmonary toxicity (0% vs. 7% vs. 4%), lethargy (4% vs. 2% vs. 2%)
	Temozolomide 150-200 mg/m²/d x 5d + T 100 mg/d[d]		CR: 3% PR: 12% SD 10%	NR		

Pavlick et al 2003[37]	Dacarbazine 1 g/m^2 q 3 wks + T 200 → 400 mg/d	PR: 30% SD: 10%	NR	Neutropenia (50%), thrombocytopenia (20%), constipation (50%), rash (10%)

Abbreviations: T, thalidomide; BM, brain metastases; IC, intracranial; CR, complete response; PR, partial response; MR, minor response; SD, stable disease; TTP, time to progression; NR, not reported.

[a]All objective responses were achieved at the temozolomide 75-mg/m^2/day dose level.

[b]For patients 70 years or older, thalidomide was started at 100 mg and increased in 50-mg increments to a maximum of 250 mg/day.

[c]Responses are shown for intracranial sites only. In 7 of the 8 patients with responses or stable disease at intracranial sites, disease progression was seen at extra-cranial sites.

[d]Temozolomide was administered at a dose of 150 mg/m^2/day in the first cycle and then 200 mg/m^2/day in subsequent cycles in this group only.

mide 200 mg/m^2 every eight hours for five doses; temozolomide 200 mg/m^2/day for five days plus interferon alpha-2b (IFN-α–2b; 5 mIU) three times per week; or temozolomide 150 mg/m^2/day (increased to 200 mg/m^2 after the first cycle) for five days plus thalidomide 100 mg/day. Each regimen was repeated every four weeks for up to six cycles. Objective responses occurred at similar rates in the three treatment arms: 5 (9%) of 55 patients receiving 8-hourly temozolomide, 11 (18%) of 62 patients receiving temozolomide-IFN-α–2b, and 9 (15%) of 60 patients receiving temozolomide-thalidomide. Median overall survival (5.3, 7.7, and 7.3 months, respectively), one-year survival (18%, 26%, and 24%, respectively), and two-year survival (7%, 9%, and 17%, respectively) rates were comparable in the three groups. Hematologic toxicity was infrequent with temozolomide-thalidomide and occurred at a significantly lower rate than with the other two regimens. Nonhematologic toxicities did not differ across groups. The authors concluded that temozolomide-thalidomide is the most promising of the three regimens for future study.[35]

A combination of dacarbazine and thalidomide was evaluated in 10 patients with metastatic melanoma who had not received prior chemotherapy. Patients received dacarbazine 1,000 mg/m^2 intravenously every three weeks, whereas thalidomide was initiated at 200 mg at bedtime and escalated to a maximum dose of 400 mg. Patients received a median of five cycles of this regimen (range, 1–18). Toxicity attributed to thalidomide in this regimen included severe constipation in five patients and grade 2-3 peripheral neuropathy in four patients. Three (30%) patients achieved partial responses, and another patient had stable disease.[37]

Thalidomide also has been evaluated in combination with IFN-α–2b and with SU5416, a tyrosine kinase inhibitor of the VEGF receptor. In a preliminary report, seven patients with metastatic melanoma who failed first-line treatment received low-dose thalidomide (200 mg/day) plus IFN-α–2b (3 mIU 3 times/week started 2 weeks after thalidomide). Two patients completed four months of treatment and achieved stable disease and a mixed response, respectively. Myelosuppression and neuropathy were the dose-limiting toxicities of this regimen.[38] In the other phase II study, SU5416 was injected intravenously at a dose of 145 mg/m^2 twice weekly and thalidomide was started at 200 mg/day and escalated to a maximum of 400 mg as tolerated. Of 12 metastatic melanoma patients, one (8%) achieved a partial response lasting 11 months, and four others had stable disease for three to six months.[39]

THALIDOMIDE IN ANDROGEN-INDEPENDENT PROSTATE CANCER

Prostate cancer is the most common malignancy affecting men in the United States.[28] Most cases are diagnosed when the disease is localized and can be treated successfully by surgery or radiation therapy. In advanced disease, hormone ablation is the cornerstone of therapy, but ultimately, the tumor cells become independent of hormonal control and treatment becomes problematic.[40] Some chemotherapeutic regimens provide palliative benefit in androgen-independent prostate cancer, but none are curative. Although the progression of prostate cancer from hormone sensitive to hormone independent involves multiple steps, the presence of elevated levels of angiogenic factors such as VEGF in patients with androgen-independent prostate cancer implicates neovascularization in this process.[40–42]

Monotherapy

Investigators at NCI reported encouraging results with thalidomide monotherapy in men with androgen-independent prostate cancer. Patients received either low-dose (200 mg/day) or high-dose (200 mg/day escalated to 1,200 mg/day) thalidomide, with most continuing to receive luteinizing hormone-releasing hormone (LH-RH) therapy during the study. The high-dose arm was terminated early after 13 patients were enrolled, because none showed greater than 50% declines in PSA and few could tolerate doses higher than 200 mg. The size of the low-dose arm was subsequently expanded to 50 patients. In this latter group, 9 (18%) patients achieved PSA declines greater than or equal to 50% with thalidomide monotherapy. However, none of the patients achieved a partial response based on computed tomography (CT) or bone scan, although five patients did have minor responses. Median survival was 15.8 months.[43] Electrophysiological assessment showed that most men who received treatment for six months developed axonal neuropathy, which was characterized clinically by tingling paresthesias in a stocking-glove pattern.[44]

In another phase II study, investigators in England administered thalidomide 100 mg/day for up to six months to 20 men with androgen-independent prostate cancer.[45] Seven men completed six months of treatment, and of these, three achieved at least 50% reductions in PSA that were sustained throughout treatment, but then PSA increased after withdrawing thalidomide. Radiographic evaluations of response were not conducted in this study. Serum bFGF and VEGF declined in most men with falling PSA levels, whereas increasing levels of these angiogenic factors were associated with progressive disease.[45]

Combination Therapy

Several chemotherapeutic agents, including taxanes and anthracyclines, provide palliative effects in patients with androgen-independent prostate cancer, but none have been shown to prolong survival.[46] In an effort to produce more sustained control of PSA levels, improve quality of life, and possibly improve survival as well, several groups have evaluated thalidomide in combination with chemotherapy (Table 7.3). Interim results from a phase II study conducted at the NCI suggested that adding thalidomide to docetaxel may improve PSA response rates.[46] In

TABLE 7.3 Activity of Thalidomide in Androgen-Independent Prostate Cancer

Study	Dose	Patients	≥50% PSA Reduction	Median TTP	Median Survival	Grade 3/4 Toxicity
Monotherapy						
Figg et al 2001[43]	T 200 mg/d	50	18%	2.2 months	15.8 months (all patients)	18 events classified as =grade 3
	T 200 → 1,200 mg/d	13	0%	2.1 months		
Drake et al 2003[45]	T 100 mg/d Combination therapy	20	15%	NR	NR	Toxicity grade NR
Combination therapy						
Dahut et al 2002[47]	Docetaxel 30 mg/m^2 weekly x 3 wks q 4 wks	24	37%	NR	NR	Thromboembolic events in combination group (23%)[a]
	Docetaxel 30 mg/m^2 weekly x 3 wks + T 200 mg/d x 3 wks q 4 wks	49	51%			
Shevrin 2003[48]	Mitoxantrone 12 mg/m^2 q 3 wks + prednisone 10 mg/d + T 200 → 600 mg/d	15	PR: 33%	NR	NR	Venous thrombosis (13%), somnolence (7%), rash (7%)
Sarao et al 2003[49]	Paclitaxel 100 mg/m^2 + doxorubicin 20 mg/m^2 weekly x 3 wks q 5 wks + T 300 mg/d	12	44%	NR	NR	Constipation (100%), fatigue (100%), nausea (100%), neutropenia (81%), leukopenia (63%)

Abbreviations: T, thalidomide; PR, partial response; TTP, time to progression; NR, not reported.

[a]Thrombolic events occurred in 10 of first 43 patients receiving combination, but in none after starting prophylactic low molecular weight heparin.

this study, 75 patients with chemotherapy-naive androgen-independent prostate cancer were randomly assigned to receive weekly docetaxel 30 mg/m^2 given intravenously either alone or in combination with thalidomide 200 mg at bedtime.[46,47] Both treatments were administered for three weeks of a four-week cycle. Overall, 25 (51%) of 49 evaluable patients in the docetaxel–thalidomide group achieved greater than 50% reductions in PSA as compared to 9 (37%) of 24 patients receiving docetaxel alone. Thromboembolic events occurred in 10 patients who received combination therapy, but prophylactic low-molecular weight heparin prevented this complication in subsequent patients. Pleural effusions occurred at the similar rates in both groups: 16% with docetaxel alone and 14% with combination therapy. These findings suggest that thalidomide may enhance the activity of docetaxel in men with androgen-independent prostate cancer.[47]

In contrast, the addition of thalidomide to a regimen of mitoxantrone/prednisone did not appear to enhance activity. In a phase II study, 15 men with metastatic androgen-independent prostate cancer received mitoxantrone 12 mg/m^2 every three weeks in combination with prednisone 10 mg/day. Thalidomide was administered at bedtime starting at 200 mg and escalated in 200-mg increments every three weeks to either 400 mg or 600 mg. Five (33%) patients achieved partial responses, including three patients with greater than 80% reductions in PSA. One patient had resolution of pelvic adenopathy. The response rates achieved in this study were comparable to historic values with mitoxantrone-prednisone alone. However, the inclusion of thalidomide appeared to result in additional toxicity, some of which was significant. In addition to the expected constipation and somnolence, two patients had venous thrombosis and three patients experienced peripheral neuropathy.[48]

The feasibility of administering thalidomide with paclitaxel and doxorubicin was evaluated in a phase I study of 12 men with androgen-independent prostate cancer and median PSA levels of 30 ng/mL.[49,50] Patients received paclitaxel 100 mg/m^2 by a one-hour infusion and doxorubicin 20 mg/m^2 by a continuous 24-hour infusion weekly for three weeks of a five-week cycle.[50] Thalidomide 200-600 mg was administered at bedtime throughout each cycle. Patients were premedicated with dexamethasone, cimetidine, and diphenhydramine before each paclitaxel infusion. Nine of the 10 patients who completed at least one cycle of treatment showed PSA reductions. All patients had grade 3 constipation, fatigue, and nausea, and almost all had grade 3/4 neutropenia. A phase II study with the paclitaxel-doxorubicin-thalidomide regimen is in progress.[49]

In addition to chemotherapy, daily corticosteroid therapy offers palliative benefit in androgen-independent prostate cancer. Investigators at the H. Lee Moffitt Cancer Center and Research Institute evaluated thalidomide in combination with dexamethasone in a phase II study of men with androgen-independent prostate cancer who had been treated previously with cytotoxic chemotherapy. Patients received thalidomide 200 mg/day initially and then the dose was titrated to a target of 400 mg. Dexamethasone was administered orally at a dose of 0.75 mg twice daily. Interim results showed that all evaluable patients had PSA reductions after 28 days of treatment (range, 7–97%). Patients remained on treatment for a median of 84 days. Three patients had confirmed PSA reductions greater than 90%, and two of them also had evidence of disease regression on bone scan. Deep vein thrombosis was reported in 3 of the 16 patients without a previous history of it. Other toxicities were consistent with previous studies of thalidomide, including three patients with grade 3 constipation and one patient with grade 3 neuropathy. Planned accrual in this study is 40 patients.[51]

THALIDOMIDE IN RENAL CELL CARCINOMA

Renal cancer is diagnosed in nearly 32,000 people each year in the United States, most of which are characterized as renal cell carcinoma.[28,52] Approximately one-third to one-half of patients with renal cell carcinoma present with metastatic disease, and about 20% to 30% of those who underwent radical nephrectomy for early-stage renal cell carcinoma ultimately progress to metastatic disease. Once metastatic disease develops, median survival is only 7 to 11 months. Renal cell carcinoma is usually unresponsive to cytotoxic chemotherapy or radiation therapy, with no regimen consistently producing response rates above 10%.[52] IL-2 and IFN-α produce response rates of 10% to 15% and appear to improve survival relative to chemotherapy.[52–55] Combination of these biological response modifiers with chemotherapy further increases response rates to 15% to 30%, but demonstrating a survival advantage relative to IL-2 or IFN-α has been problematic.[52,53]

Monotherapy

Thalidomide is active in patients with advanced renal cell carcinoma producing response rates of 0% to 17% across eight studies (Table 7.4). In addition, 17% to 64% of patients in these studies achieved stable disease. Investigators at the Royal Marsden Hospital and University College in London initially showed the activity of thalidomide in renal cell carcinoma in consecutive studies using two different dose levels. In the first study, 18 patients with advanced renal cell carcinoma received thalidomide 100 mg at bedtime.[32] After a median follow-up of 36 months, three (17%) patients achieved partial responses and 3 (17%) others had stable disease lasting more than three months.[56] In the other study, thalidomide was started at 100 mg/day and the dose was escalated in 100-mg increments over five weeks to a target of 600 mg/day given in divided doses in the morning and at bedtime. In most patients (77%), the thalidomide dose was not titrated to 600 mg or had to be reduced due to toxicity, most commonly lethargy, constipation, and neuropathy. A daily dose of 400 mg was generally well tolerated. After a median follow-up of 20 months, 2 (9%) of 22 evaluable patients had partial re-

TABLE 7.4 Activity of Thalidomide Monotherapy in Renal Cell Carcinoma

Study	Dose	Patients	Response Rate	Median TTP	Median Survival	Grade 3/4 Toxicity
Eisen et al 2000[32]	T 100 mg/d	18	R: 17% SD: 17%	NR	NR[a]	None
Stebbbing et al 2001[56]	T 200 → 600 mg/d	25	PR: 9% SD: 55%	NR	9 months[a]	Lethargy (8%), constipation (4%), neuropathy (4%)
Novik et al 2001[57]	T 100 → 1,000 mg/d	27	PR: 0% SD: 26%	NR	NR	Deep vein thrombosis (7%)
Srinivas & Guardino 2002[58]	T 200 or 800 → 1,200 mg/d	14	PR: 0% SD: 46%	NR	NR	Somnolence (23%), fatigue (15%), constipation (8%), neuropathy (8%)
Motzer et al 2002[59]	T 200 → 800 mg/d	26	PR: 0% SD: 64%	4 months	6-mo PFS: 32%; 1-y OS: 57%	Dyspnea (12%), cardiovascular toxicity (8%), neurotoxicity (4%)
Daliani et al 2002[60]	T 200 → 1200 mg/d	20	PR: 11% SD: 47%	NR	PFS: 4.7 months OS: 18.1 months	Thromboembolic events (15%), fatigue (15%), somnolence (15%), neuropathy (5%)
Minor et al 2002[61]	T 400 → 1,200 mg/d	29	PR: 4% SD: 13%	2.3 months	3.5 months	Constipation (25%), venous thrombosis (8%), somnolence (4%), poor wound healing (4%)
Escudier et al 2002[62]	T 400 → 1,200 mg/d	40	PR: 5% SD: 23%	NR	10 months (1-y OS: 38%)	Fatigue (26%), lethargy (15%), neuropathy (10%), thromboembolism (10%), constipation (10%)
Eisen, 2003[63]	T 100 → 400 mg/d vs. MP 300 mg/d	59	SD: 5% SD: 0%	NR	12.2 months 4.8 months (P=0.37)	Constipation (13%), fatigue (6%), neuropathy (6%)

Abbreviations: T, thalidomide; MP, medroxyprogesterone; PR, partial response; SD, stable disease; TTP, time to progression; OS, overall survival; PFS, progression-free survival; NR, not reported.

[a]Median survival of 40 evaluable patients in combined studies of Eisen et al[32] and Stebbing et al[56].

sponses and 12 (55%) patients had stable disease for more than three months. Median survival for evaluable patients in these two studies combined was nine months (range: 1 to greater than 22 months).[56]

Thalidomide was recently compared with medroxyprogesterone in a randomized phase II study of patients with metastatic renal cell carcinoma who progressed after immunotherapy or were not candidates for immunotherapy. Thalidomide was administered at 100 mg/day for two weeks, and then the dose was escalated in 100-mg increments every two weeks to a maximum of 400 mg/day. Medroxyprogesterone was given at 300 mg/day. Both treatments were continued until disease progression. One (5%) of 19 evaluable patients in the thalidomide group had stable disease for at least three months, whereas all 24 patients in the medroxyprogesterone group progressed. Median survival was numerically longer in the thalidomide group (12.2 vs. 4.8 months), but the difference was not statistically significant ($P = .37$).[57]

Combination Therapy

Thalidomide has shown promising activity when combined with biological response modifiers and/or chemotherapy in some but not all studies of metastatic renal cell carcinoma (Table 7.5).

Thalidomide and IFN-α Investigators in London evaluated thalidomide plus IFN-α in 13 patients with metastatic renal cell carcinoma.[64] IFN-α was administered subcutaneously three times per week at a dose of 9 mIU, and then two weeks later, thalidomide was started at 100 mg at bedtime and increased in 100-mg increments each month to a maximum dose of 400 mg. None of the patients achieved objective responses to combination IFN-α/thalidomide treatment. Four (31%) patients experienced visual disturbances, but CT scans excluded cerebrovascular events or malignancy as the cause. One other patient had Stevens-Johnson reaction, which resolved on withdrawal of study drugs and treatment with corticosteroids.[64,71] The study investigators concluded that the IFN-α/thalidomide regimen was associated with "far greater" neurological toxicity than would be expected with either drug alone.[71]

In another phase II study, Israeli and Italian investigators administered IFN-α 3 mIU/day and thalidomide 100 mg/day to 19 patients with metastatic renal cell carcinoma. Six of the patients in this study had been treated previously with IFN-α. The IFN-α dose was reduced in 10 patients due to grade 3 toxicities, most commonly asthenia. Two patients discontinued therapy due to a mild visual disturbance and persistent headache, respectively. Of 14 evaluable patients, three (21%) patients achieved partial responses and seven (50%) patients had stable disease. At the time of the study report, 16 patients were still alive. The investigators of this study concluded that combination IFN-α/thalidomide is active in metastatic disease. Further patient accrual is continuing in this study using an initial IFN-α dose of 2 mIU.[65]

TABLE 7.5 Activity of Thalidomide in Combination Therapy of Renal Cell Carcinoma

Study	Dose	Patients	Response Rate	Median TTP	Median Survival	Grade 3/4 Toxicity
Sella et al 2003[65]	IFN-α (9 mIU 3x/wk) + T 100 → 400 mg/d	13	PR: 0%	NR	NR[a]	Visual disturbances (31%), Stevens-Johnson reaction (8%)
Nathan et al 2001[64]	IFN-α (3 mIU/d) + T 100 mg/d	19	PR: 21% SD: 50%	NR	17.4 months[a]	Asthenia (38%); gastrointestinal toxicity (11%)
Olencki et al 2003[66]	IL-2 (4.5 or 9 mIU/m²/d x 5d/wk) + T 100 or 200 mg/d	31	CR: 3% PR: 3%	NR	NR	Neutropenia (13%); thromboembolic events (6%); neuropathy (3%)
Amato et al submitted[67]	IL-2 (7 mIU/m²/d x 5d/wk x 4 wk q 6 wk) + T 200-600 mg/d[b]	52	CR: 6% PR: 31% SD: 16%	NR	NR	NR
Desai et al 2002[68]	Gemcitabine (600 mg/m² on d 1,8,15 q 4 wks); infusional 5-FU (150 mg/m²/d x 21 d) + T 200 → 400 mg/d	21	PR: 10% SD: 43%	NR	NR	Thromboembolic events (43%)
Amato et al submitted[69]	Capecitabine (1,900 mg/d x 2 wks q 3 wks), IFN-α (1 mIU/d), + T 400 mg/d	27	PR: 20% SD: 52%[c]	NR	>19 mo (pts with PR), 14 mo (SD), 1 mo (PD)	Hand-foot syndrome (40%), deep vein thrombosis (16%), paresthesias (16%), hemoptysis/epistaxis (12%), shortness of breath (12%)
Rabinowitz et al 2003[70]	5-FU (1,750 mg/m² on d1), IFN-α (6 mIU/m²/d on d 1,3,5), IL-2 (6 mIU/m² on d 2-5 weekly x 4 wks) q 6 wks + T 200 → 1,200 mg/d	8	CR: 13%	NR	NR	Fatigue (25%), paresthesias (13%), neutropenia (13%), hand-foot syndrome (13%), mucositis (13%), hypotension (13%)

Abbreviations: T, thalidomide; PR, partial response; SD, stable disease; TTP, time to progression; OS, overall survival; PFS, progression-free survival; PD, progressive disease; NR, not reported.

[a]Mean overall survival (range 1.4 + to 20.3 months).

[b]Thalidomide was evaluated at 3 dose levels (200, 400, and 600 mg/day in the phase I study and at 400 mg/day in the phase II study).

[c]Includes 1 patient with a minor response.

The Eastern Cooperative Oncology Group is conducting a randomized phase III trial (ECOG 2898) of combination IFN-α/thalidomide versus IFN-α in patients with previously untreated metastatic or unresectable renal cell carcinoma. The study is designed to compare the two regimens on PFS and quality of life. IFN-α is being administered subcutaneously at a dose of 1 mIU twice daily, and thalidomide is being started at 200 mg and then escalated as tolerated to a maximum of 1,000 mg/day. The accrual goal is 340 patients.[52]

Thalidomide and IL-2 Thalidomide also has been administered in combination with IL-2 in a phase I study conducted at the Cleveland Clinic Foundation and in a phase I/II study at Baylor College of Medicine. The Cleveland Clinic evaluated four different dose levels: IL-2 was administered subcutaneously five days per week at 4.5 or 9 mIU/m^2 with thalidomide 100 mg/day, or at 9 or 13.5 (week 1 only; then 9) mIU/m^2 with thalidomide 200 mg/day. Toxicity was termed moderate to severe and related to dose level. Dose-limiting toxicity was noted at the highest dose levels, which consisted primarily of grade 3 neutropenia lasting at least seven days. The maximum tolerated dose (MTD) was IL-2 at 9 mIU/m^2 plus thalidomide at 100 mg/day. Patients received a median of one six-week cycle (range 1–7). Two of 31 patients responded to treatment, including one patient who had been treated previously with IL-2. This study shows that combination IL-2/thalidomide is feasible and active, but the investigators noted that thalidomide appeared to increase the toxicity of IL-2. A phase II study is underway.[66]

The Baylor study enrolled 15 patients with metastatic renal cell carcinoma in the phase I portion and 37 previously untreated patients in the phase II portion. In both phases, IL-2 was administered at a fixed dose of 7 mIU/m^2 given subcutaneously on days 1 to 5 for four weeks of a six-week cycle. Thalidomide was started one week before IL-2 and administered daily throughout each cycle. The starting dose was 200 mg; it was increased in 200-mg increments every 48 hours to the target dose (200 to 600 mg in phase I and 400 mg in phase II). Of the 51 evaluable patients overall, three (6%) achieved complete responses and 16 (31%) had partial responses for an objective response rate of 37%. An additional 8 (16%) patients had stable disease. Survival in these studies ranged from four weeks to greater than 24 months, with 18 (35%) patients continuing to receive IL-2/thalidomide therapy at the time of the study report. The IL-2/thalidomide regimen was generally well tolerated. Most toxicities were mild and commonly associated with either thalidomide (somnolence, constipation, rash, and neuropathy) or IL-2 (flu-like symptoms, fluid retention, hypotension, and hypothyroidism). Two patients experienced deep vein thrombosis.[67]

A randomized phase III study of IL-2/thalidomide versus each drug alone is being planned in patients with previously untreated metastatic renal cell carcinoma. Thalidomide will be started at 200 mg/day and then increased to 400 mg/day as tolerated.[52]

Thalidomide and Chemotherapy Thalidomide was administered orally in combination with intravenous gemcitabine and continuous infusional 5-fluorouracil (5-FU) in a phase II study of patients with metastatic renal cell carcinoma. Each four-week cycle consisted of gemcitabine 600 mg/m^2 on days 1, 8, and 15, and 5-FU 150 mg/m^2/day intravenously continuously on days 1 to 21. Thalidomide was started at 200 mg/day and increased in 100-mg increments each week to a maximum of 400 mg/day. Nine of the 21 patients had received prior immunotherapy. Two (10%) patients had partial responses and nine (43%) had disease stabilization lasting for at least six months, but nine (43%) patients experienced venous thromboembolism. Thus, the addition of thalidomide to gemcitabine/5-FU did not improve response rates relative to historic values with the chemotherapy regimen alone, but it was associated with higher vascular toxicity.[68]

At Baylor College of Medicine, the feasibility of using thalidomide in combination with IFN-α and capecitabine was evaluated in 27 patients with metastatic renal cell carcinoma. Capecitabine 1,900 mg/m^2 was administered orally in divided doses each day for two weeks followed by one week of rest; IFN-α was given subcutaneously at 1 mIU/day and thalidomide orally at 400 mg/day, both without interruption. Five (20%) of 25 evaluable patients achieved partial responses, one (4%) patient had a minor response, and 12 (48%) others had stable disease. Patients with partial responses had median overall survival of greater than 19 months as compared to 14 months for those with stable disease and one month for those with progressive disease. Grade 3/4 toxicities were common, with the most common being hand-foot syndrome (40%), deep vein thrombosis (16%), and paresthesias (16%). The activity of the thalidomide/IFN-α/capecitabine regimen is notable given the patient population in this study was heavily pretreated and had poor performance status. Further evaluation of this regimen appears warranted.[69]

At the University of New Mexico, thalidomide was evaluated in combination with 5-FU, IFN-α, and IL-2 in eight patients with metastatic renal cell carcinoma. Each six-week cycle consisted of 5-FU at 1,750 mg/m^2 via continuous 24-hour infusion on day 1, IFN-α via subcutaneous injection at 6 mIU/m^2 on days 1, 3, and 5, and IL-2 at 6 mIU/m^2 via continuous infusion on days two to five weekly for four weeks. Thalidomide was started at 200 mg/day and then increased by 200-mg increments every two weeks to a target dose of 1,200 mg/day. One patient had a radiographic complete response of bone and pulmonary lesions after 10 cycles and at the time of the report was still alive without evidence of recurrence. There were no other objective responses. Toxicity was common but manageable, with grade 4 neutropenia and hypotension and grade 3 hand-foot syndrome, mucositis, and paresthesias each occurring in one patient. Further evaluation of this regimen is needed to elucidate the response rate.[70]

THALIDOMIDE IN OTHER SOLID TUMORS

Less clinical information about thalidomide is available in other solid malignancies. In metastatic colorectal cancer, thalidomide has been shown to reduce the gastrointestinal toxicity associated with second-line irinotecan therapy, thus allowing patients to complete chemotherapy.[72,73] In a group of 30 patients who had failed first-line 5-FU therapy, the combination of irinotecan 300 to 350 mg/m^2 every three weeks and thalidomide 400 mg at bedtime produced complete responses in three patients, partial responses in four patients, and stable disease in 11 others. After a median follow-up of 22 months, median PFS and overall survival appeared longer than historic data with irinotecan alone.[74] Randomized studies will be needed to determine whether thalidomide actually improves survival of patients with metastatic colorectal cancer. Preliminary evidence also has been obtained that the administration of thalidomide 400 mg at bedtime in combination with capecitabine may be active in patients with unresectable, recurrent, or metastatic hepatocellular carcinoma.[75]

Despite the encouraging activity of thalidomide in many solid malignancies, it has shown little activity in metastatic breast cancer and squamous cell carcinoma of the head and neck. None of 12 patients with metastatic breast cancer had objective responses or disease stabilization when treated with a dose of 100 mg/day.[32] In a randomized phase II study, none of 28 heavily pretreated patients with metastatic breast cancer responded to low-dose (200 mg/day) or high-dose (800 mg/day escalated to 1,200 mg/day) thalidomide. Disease stabilized in two patients in the low-dose group, but it was short-lived for one patient and the other discontinued therapy due to grade 3 peripheral neuropathy.[76] In a phase II study of 21 heavily pretreated patients with recurrent or metastatic squamous cell carcinoma of the head and neck, thalidomide monotherapy (200 mg/day increased to 1,000 mg/day) did not show any activity. After eight weeks of treatment, all patients had progressive disease based on standard criteria.[77]

FUTURE DIRECTIONS: IMiDs

The activity of thalidomide in multiple myeloma and solid tumors led to the design of novel analogs that optimize its immunological and antiangiogenic properties while minimizing side effects.[78] Two drug classes have been identified. The IMiDs™ (immunomodulatory drugs) are thalidomide derivatives with potent anti-inflammatory, T cell co-stimulatory, and antiangiogenic activities, which do not inhibit phosphodiesterase (PDE) type 4. In comparison, the SelCIDs™ (selective cytokine inhibitory drugs) are PDE 4 inhibitors that are chemically distinct from thalidomide but functionally linked by their ability to inhibit TNF-a production, angiogenesis, and tumor growth.[78,79]

Early clinical studies with the lead IMiD CC-5013 appear promising. In a phase I study of patients with relapsed and refractory multiple myeloma, CC-5013 was well tolerated and did not produce significant somnolence, constipation, or neuropathy. Myelosuppression developed after four weeks of treatment at the highest dose tested (50 mg/day), but the drug was well tolerated when administered at 25 mg/day. Overall, 17 (71%) of 24 evaluable patients demonstrated benefit from CC-5013, including 11 (69%) of 16 patients treated previously with thalidomide.[80] CC-5013 also was well tolerated when administered once daily for 21 days of a 28-day cycle to patients with recurrent brain malignancies. No sedation, constipation, peripheral neuropathy, or rash was seen, and only one drug-related toxicity greater than grade 1 was observed (grade 2 myelosuppression in a patient who had undergone previous bone marrow transplantation). Two patients with rapidly progressive glioblastoma had disease stabilization for five and seven months, respectively. A patient with a rapidly progressive spinal hemangioblastoma had disease stabilization for six months.[81] CC-5013 was administered to patients with metastatic androgen-independent prostate cancer at doses of 5 to 20 mg/day and continued until disease progression or unacceptable toxicity. Two of six patients treated with the highest dose had dose-limiting toxicities (grade 3 thrombosis and hypotension, respectively), but other toxicities were mild. Six (50%) of the 12 treated patients had stable PSA levels for at least eight weeks.[82]

CC-5013 is entering phase III clinical trials for multiple myeloma and metastatic melanoma, and it is also being evaluated in other malignancies.[78] At Baylor College of Medicine, CC-5013 is being evaluated in patients with metastatic renal cell carcinoma who may have failed one prior treatment. An interim analysis is scheduled after accrual of 17 patients. Another IMiD, CC-4047, is currently undergoing phase II testing in multiple myeloma and androgen-independent prostate cancer.[78] At Baylor, CC-4047 is being tested in androgen-independent prostate cancer patients who have failed up to one prior treatment. An interim analysis is planned after accrual of 19 patients.

CONCLUSION

Thalidomide is active in many solid tumors when administered as a single agent. Armed with greater knowledge about its preclinical and clinical activity, investigators are now looking at thalidomide as part of combination therapy. Recent studies show that thalidomide in combination with chemotherapy or immunotherapy improves treatment responses in several solid malignancies, including high-grade gliomas, metastatic melanoma, androgen-independent prostate cancer, and advanced renal cell carcinoma.[18,25,29,37,47,67,69] In the future, it will be important to evaluate thalidomide in combination with other angiogenesis inhibitors and other treatment approaches, such as vaccine therapy. Thalidomide trials will continue to be developed while the activity of several IMiDs are explored. Early studies suggest that the lead IMiD is not associated with the common side effects that sometimes limit thalidomide use.[80–82] Further investigation of thalidomide as well as the IMiDs is clearly warranted.

REFERENCES

1. Richardson P, Hideshima T, Anderson K. Thalidomide: emerging role in cancer medicine. Annu Rev Med 2002;53:629–657.

2. Amato RJ. Thalidomide: an antineoplastic agent. Curr Oncol Rep 2002;4:56–62.
3. Sheskin J. Further observation with thalidomide in lepra reactions. Lepr Rev 1965;36:183–187.
4. Olson KB, Hall TC, Horton J et al. Thalidomide (*N*-phthaloylglutamimide) in the treatment of advanced cancer. Clin Pharmacol Ther 1965;6:292–297.
5. Grabstald H, Golbey R. Clinical experiences with thalidomide in patients with cancer. Clin Pharmacol Ther 1965;6:298–302.
6. D'Amato RJ, Loughnan MS, Flynn E, Folkman J. Thalidomide is an inhibitor of angiogenesis. Proc Natl Acad Sci USA 1994;91:4082–4085.
7. Kenyon BM, Browne F, D'Amato RJ. Effects of thalidomide and related metabolites in a mouse corneal model of neovascularization. Exp Eye Res 1997;64:971–978.
8. Moreira AL, Sampaio EP, Zmuidzinas A et al. Thalidomide exerts its inhibitory action on tumor necrosis factor a by enhancing mRNA degradation. J Exp Med 1993;177:1675–1680.
9. Geitz H, Handt S, Zwingenberger K. Thalidomide selectively modulates the density of cell surface molecules involved in the adhesion cascade. Immunopharmacology 1996;31:213–221.
10. Gordon JN, Goggin PM. Thalidomide and its derivatives: emerging from the wilderness. Postgrad Med J 2003;79:127–132.
11. McHugh SM, Rifkin IR, Deighton J et al. The immunosuppressive drug thalidomide induces T helper cell type 2 (Th2) and concomitantly inhibits Th1 cytokine production in mitogen- and antigen-stimulated human peripheral blood mononuclear cell cultures. Clin Exp Immunol 1995;99:160–167.
12. Dredge K, Marriott JB, Dalgleish AG. Immunological effects of thalidomide and its chemical and functional analogs. Crit Rev Immunol 2002;22:425–437.
13. Rajkumar SV, Leong T, Roche PC et al. Prognostic value of bone marrow angiogenesis in multiple myeloma. Clin Cancer Res 2000;6:3111–3116.
14. Singhal S, Mehta J, Desikan R et al. Antitumor activity of thalidomide in refractory multiple myeloma. N Engl J Med 1999;341:1565–1571.
15. Barlogie B, Desikan R, Eddlemon P et al. Extended survival in advanced and refractory multiple myeloma after single-agent thalidomide: identification of prognostic factors in a phase 2 study of 169 patients. Blood 2001;98:492–494.
16. Palumbo A, Giaccone L, Bertola A et al. Low-dose thalidomide plus dexamethasone is an effective salvage therapy for advanced myeloma. Haematologica 2001;86:399–403.
17. Moehler TM, Neben K, Benner A et al. Salvage therapy for multiple myeloma with thalidomide and CED chemotherapy. Blood 2001;98:3846–3848.
18. Fine HA, Wen PY, Maher EA et al. Phase II trial of thalidomide and carmustine for patients with recurrent high-grade gliomas. J Clin Oncol 2003;21:2299–2304.
19. Yung WKA, Prados MD, Yaya-Tur R et al. Multicenter phase II trial of temozolomide in patients with anaplastic astrocytoma or anaplastic oligoastrocytoma at first relapse. J Clin Oncol 1999; 17:2762–2771.
20. Glioma Meta-analysis Trialists (GMT) Group. Chemotherapy in adult high-grade glioma: a systematic review and meta-analysis of individual patient data from 12 randomised trials. Lancet 2002;359:1011–1018.
21. Plate KH, Breier G, Weich HA, Risau W. Vascular endothelial growth factor is a potential tumor angiogenesis factor in human gliomas *in vivo*. Nature 1992;359:845–848.
22. Fine HA, Figg WD, Jaeckle K et al. Phase II trial of the antiangiogenic agent thalidomide in patients with recurrent high-grade gliomas. J Clin Oncol 2000;18:708–715.
23. Short SC, Traish D, Dowe A et al. Thalidomide as an anti-angiogenic agent in relapsed gliomas. J Neurooncol 2001;51:41–45.

24. Marx GM, Pavlakis N, McCowatt S et al. Phase II study of thalidomide in the treatment of recurrent glioblastoma multiforme. J Neurooncol 2001;54:31–38.

25. Bjeljac M, Baumann F, Bernays R. Combined thalidomide and temozolomide treatment in patients with glioblastoma multiforme [abstract #451]. Proc Am Soc Clin Oncol 2003;22:113.

26. Capparella JN, Johnson VM, Maestri-Moden X et al. Phase II trial of daily oral temozolomide and thalidomide in newly diagnosed glioblastoma multiforme before radiation therapy [abstract #483]. Proc Am Soc Clin Oncol 2003;22:121.

27. Adler W, Lee FC. A phase I trial using combination irinotecan and thalidomide for recurrent CNS tumors [abstract #489]. Proc Am Soc Clin Oncol 2003;22:122.

28. American Cancer Society. Cancer Facts & Figures 2003. Atlanta, GA: American Cancer Society, 2003.

29. Hwu W-J, Krown SE, Panageas KS et al. Temozolomide plus thalidomide in patients with advanced melanoma: results of a dose-finding trial. J Clin Oncol 2002;20:2610–2615.

30. Middleton MR, Grob JJ, Aaronson N et al. Randomized phase III study of temozolomide versus dacarbazine in the treatment of patients with advanced metastatic malignant melanoma. J Clin Oncol 2000;18:158–166.

31. Erhard H, Rietveld FJR, van Altena MC et al. Transition of horizontal to vertical growth phase melanoma is accompanied by induction of vascular endothelial growth factor expression and angiogenesis. Melanoma Res 1997;[suppl 2]:S19–S26.

32. Eisen T, Boshoff C, Mak I et al. Continuous low dose thalidomide: a phase II study in advanced melanoma, renal cell, ovarian and breast cancer. Br J Cancer 2000;82:812–817.

33. Reiriz AB, Richter M, Fernandes S et al. A phase II study of thalidomide in patients with metastatic malignant melanoma [abstract #2895]. Proc Am Soc Clin Oncol 2003;22:720.

34. Kudva GC, Collins BT, Dunphy FR II. Thalidomide for malignant melanoma. N Engl J Med 2001;345:1214–1215.

35. Danson S, Lorigan P, Arance A et al. Randomized phase II study of temozolomide given every 8 hours or daily with either interferon alfa-2b or thalidomide in metastatic malignant melanoma. J Clin Oncol 2003;21:2551–2557.

36. Hwu W-J, Krown SE, Lis E et al. Phase II study of temozolomide (TMZ) plus thalidomide in patients with brain metastasis from malignant melanoma [abstract #2894]. Proc Am Soc Clin Oncol 2003;22:720.

37. Pavlick AC, Oratz R, Bailes A et al. A phase II trial of DTIC with thalidomide in metastatic melanoma [abstract #1393]. Proc Am Soc Clin Oncol 2002;21:349a.

38. Solti M, Mastrangelo MJ, Berd D et al. Phase II study of low-dose thalidomide and interferon-alpha-2b (IFN) in patients with metastatic melanoma: preliminary results [abstract #2914]. Proc Am Soc Clin Oncol 2003;22:725.

39. Forero L, Rowinsky EK, Izbicka E et al. A phase II, pharmacokinetic (PK) and biologic study of SU5416 and thalidomide in patients with metastatic melanoma [abstract #2872]. Proc Am Soc Clin Oncol 2003;22:714.

40. Feldman BJ, Feldman D. The development of androgen-independent prostate cancer. Nat Rev Cancer 2001;1:34–45.

41. Ferrer FA, Miller LJ, Andrawis RI et al. Angiogenesis and prostate cancer: in vivo and in vitro expression of angiogenesis factors by prostate cancer cells. Urology 1998;51:161–167.

42. Duque JLF, Loughlin KR, Adam RM et al. Plasma levels of vascular endothelial growth factor are increased in patients with metastatic prostate cancer. Urology 1999;54:523–527.

43. Figg WD, Dahut W, Duray P et al. A randomized phase II trial of thalidomide, an angiogenesis inhibitor, in patients with androgen-independent prostate cancer. Clin Cancer Res 2001;7:1888–1893.

44. Molloy FM, Floeter MK, Syed NA et al. Thalidomide neuropathy in patients treated for metastatic prostate cancer. Muscle Nerve 2001;1050–1057.

45. Drake MJ, Robson W, Mehta P et al. An open-label phase II study of low-dose thalidomide in androgen-independent prostate cancer. Br J Cancer 2003;88:822–827.

46. Figg WD, Arlen P, Gulley J et al. A randomized phase II trial of docetaxel (Taxotere) plus thalidomide in androgen-independent prostate cancer. Semin Oncol 2001;28[suppl 15]:62–66.

47. Dahut WL, Arlen PM, Gulley J et al. A randomized phase II trial of docetaxel plus thalidomide in androgen-independent prostate cancer [abstract #730]. Proc Am Soc Clin Oncol 2002;21: 183a.

48. Shevrin DH. Phase II study of thalidomide and mitoxantrone/prednisone with hormone refractory prostate cancer [abstract #1787]. Proc Am Soc Clin Oncol 2003;22:445.

49. Sarao H, Lindsey S, Amato RJ. Phase I/II study of weekly paclitaxel, thalidomide, and doxorubicin in patients with androgen-independent prostate cancer [abstract #1761]. Proc Am Soc Clin Oncol 2003;22:438.

50. Amato RJ, Sarao H, Lindsay S. A phase I study of weekly paclitaxel, thalidomide, and doxorubicin in patients with androgen-independent prostate cancer. (submitted for publication).

51. Patterson SG, Fishman M, Kish J et al. Thalidomide plus daily oral dexamethasone for metastatic hormone refractory prostate cancer (HRPC) in patients previously treated with cytotoxic chemotherapy [abstract 1783]. Proc Am Soc Clin Oncol 2003;22:444.

52. Amato RJ. Thalidomide therapy for renal cell carcinoma. Crit Rev Oncol Hematol 2003;46: S59–S65.

53. Fossa SD, Martinelli G, Otto U et al. Recombinant interferon alfa-2a with or without vinblastine in metastatic renal cell carcinoma: results of a European multi-center phase III study. Ann Oncol 1992;3:301–305.

54. Minasian LM, Motzer RJ, Gluck L et al. Interferon alfa-2a in advanced renal cell carcinoma: treatment results and survival in 159 patients with long-term follow-up. J Clin Oncol 1993;11: 1368–1375.

55. Motzer RJ, Mazumdar M, Bacik J et al. Effect of cytokine therapy on survival for patients with advanced renal cell carcinoma. J Clin Oncol 2000;18:1928–1935.

56. Stebbing J, Benson C, Eisen T et al. The treatment of advanced renal cell cancer with high-dose oral thalidomide. Br J Cancer 2001;85:953–958.

57. Novik Y, Dutcher JP, Larkin M, Wiernik PH. Phase II study of thalidomide (T) in advanced refractory metastatic renal cell cancer (MRCC): a single institution experience [abstract #1057]. Proc Am Soc Clin Oncol 2001;20:265a.

58. Srinivas S, Guardino AE. Randomized trial of high and low dose thalidomide in metastatic renal cell carcinoma [abstract #2403]. Proc Am Soc Clin Oncol 2002;20:147b.

59. Motzer RJ, Berg W, Ginsburg M et al. Phase II trial of thalidomide for patients with advanced renal cell carcinoma. J Clin Oncol 2002;20:302–306.

60. Daliani DD, Papandreou CN, Thall PF et al. A pilot study of thalidomide in patients with advanced metastatic renal cell carcinoma. Cancer 2002;95:758–765.

61. Minor DR, Monroe D, Damico LA et al. A phase II study of thalidomide in advanced metastatic renal cell carcinoma. Invest New Drugs 2002;20:389–393.

62. Escudier B, Lassau N, Couanet D et al. Phase II trial of thalidomide in renal-cell carcinoma. Ann Oncol 2002;13:1029–1035.

63. Eisen T. Phase II results of a phase II/III study comparing thalidomide with medroxyprogesterone in patients with metastatic renal cell carcinoma [abstract 1606]. Proc Am Soc Clin Oncol 2003;22:400.

64. Nathan PD, Walker D, Bridle H et al. A phase II study investigating the use of thalidomide in conjunction with interferon-a in patients with metastatic renal cell carcinoma [abstract 1058]. Proc Am Soc Clin Oncol 2001;20:265a.

65. Sella A, Sternberg C, Yarom N et al. Phase II study of low dose thalidomide and interferon-alfa in metastatic renal cell carcinoma (RCC) [abstract #1614]. Proc Am Soc Clin Oncol 2003;22:402.

66. Olencki T, Malhi S, Mekhail T et al. Phase I trial of thalidomide and interleukin-2 (IL-2) in patients with metastatic renal cell carcinoma (RCC) [abstract #1554]. Proc Am Soc Clin Oncol 2003;22:387.

67. Amato RJ, Neveed F, Rawat A. Phase I/II study of thalidomide in combination with interleukin-2 in patients with metastatic renal cell carcinoma. (submitted for publication).

68. Desai AA, Vogelzang NJ, Rini BI et al. A high rate of venous thromboembolism in a multi-institutional phase II trial of weekly intravenous gemcitabine with continuous infusion fluorouracil and daily thalidomide in patients with metastatic renal cell carcinoma. Cancer 2002; 95:1629–1636.

69. Amato RJ, Thompson N, Neveed F. Interferon-a plus capecitabine and thalidomide in patients with metastatic renal cell carcinoma: a pilot study. (submitted for publication).

70. Rabinowitz M, Elias L, Lee F-C. Phase I/II trial of 5-fluorouracil, interferon-a, interleukin-2, and thalidomide for metastatic renal cell carcinoma [abstract #1788]. Proc Am Soc Clin Oncol 2003;22:445.

71. Nathan PD, Gore ME, Eisen TG. Unexpected toxicity of combination thalidomide and interferon alfa-2a treatment in metastatic renal cell carcinoma. J Clin Oncol 2002;20:1429–1430.

72. Govindarajan R, Heaton KM, Broadwater R et al. Effect of thalidomide on gastrointestinal toxic effects of irinotecan. Lancet 2000;356:566–567.

73. Govindarajan R. Irinotecan and thalidomide in metastatic colorectal cancer. Oncology 2000;14[suppl 13]:29–32.

74. Govindarajan R, Safar AM, Maddox A-M, Hutchins LF. Irinotecan and thalidomide prolong disease free and overall survival in 5FU refractory and metastatic colorectal cancer [abstract #997]. Proc Am Soc Clin Oncol 2003;22:249.

75. Chun HG, Waheed F, Iqbal A et al. A combination of capecitabine and thalidomide in patients with unresectable, recurrent or metastatic hepatocellular carcinoma [abstract #1407]. Proc Am Soc Clin Oncol 2003;22:350.

76. Baidas SM, Winer EP, Fleming GF et al. Phase II evaluation of thalidomide in patients with metastatic breast cancer. J Clin Oncol 2000;18:2710–2717.

77. Tseng JE, Glisson BS, Khuri FR et al. Phase II study of the antiangiogenesis agent thalidomide in recurrent or metastatic squamous cell carcinoma of the head and neck. Cancer 2001;92: 2364–2373.

78. Dredge K, Dalgleish AG, Marriott JB. Thalidomide analogs as emerging anti-cancer drugs. Anti-Cancer Drugs 2003;14:331–335.

79. Dredge K, Marriott JB, Macdonald CD et al. Novel thalidomide analogues display anti-angiogenic activity independently of immunomodulatory effects. Br J Cancer 2002;87:1166–1172.

80. Richardson PG, Schlossman RL, Weller E et al. Immunomodulatory drug CC-5013 overcomes drug resistance and is well tolerated in patients with relapsed multiple myeloma. Blood 2002;100:3063–3067.

81. Fine HA, Kim L, Royce C et al. A phase I trial of CC-5013, a potent thalidomide analog, in patients with recurrent high-grade gliomas and other refractory CNS malignancies [abstract #418]. Proc Am Soc Clin Oncol 2003;22:105.

82. Liu Y, Tohnya TM, Figg WD et al. Phase I study of CC-5013 (Revimid), a thalidomide derivative in patients with refractory metastatic cancer [abstract #927]. Proc Am Soc Clin Oncol 2003;22:231.

Chapter 8

New Approaches to Allografting in Non-Hodgkin's Lymphoma

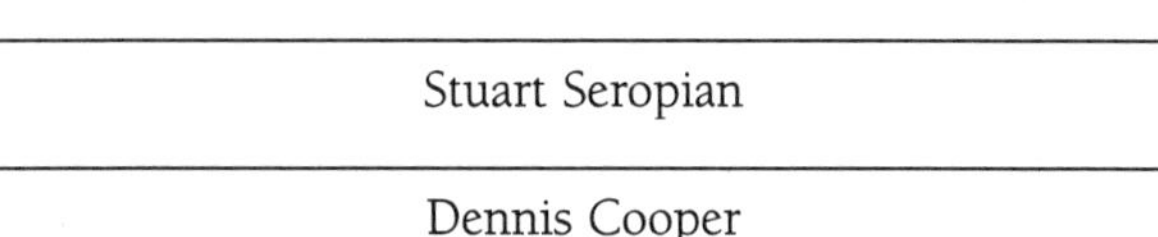

Stuart Seropian

Dennis Cooper

Despite an increasing number of therapeutic options for patients with non-Hodgkin's lymphoma (NHL), the overall results of treatment remain disappointing. Years of experimentation with combination chemotherapy regimens in varying doses and treatment schedules failed to improve survival, and it is only in recent years that new therapies such as humanized monoclonal antibodies have begun to favorably impact on outcome. Although autologous transplantation cures a fraction of patients with recurrent aggressive, chemosensitive lymphomas, it seems likely that alternative approaches will be necessary to substantially improve cure rates in patients with poor prognosis and/or resistant disease. With respect to the use of "up front" high-dose therapy in unfavorable patients, the failure thus far to confirm the superiority of high-dose therapy in prospective clinical trials suggests that any overall benefit for this approach is likely to be incremental rather than dramatic.

Stimulated by the lack of progress with standard treatment as well as new developments in transplant biology, allogeneic transplantation is being more intensively studied in NHL. The curative potential of allogeneic transplantation resides both in the efficacy of pretransplant conditioning regimens supported by tumor-free stem cell grafts and in the putative graft-versus-lymphoma (GVL) effect, wherein donor immune cells eradicate malignant lymphocytes. Nevertheless, enthusiasm for allografting patients with NHL has been tempered by the inability to identify subsets of patients in whom the superiority of allogeneic compared to autologous transplant is sufficient to justify a considerably higher rate of morbidity and mortality.

Over the past year several publications have further defined the role of allogeneic transplant in patients with NHL. Some of these studies suggest that much—if not all—of the apparent improvement in relapse rates after allogeneic transplant may be due to the delivery of tumor-free hematopoietic progenitor cells. Other studies strongly if not irrefutably emphasize a GVL effect that might obviate the need for intensive preparative regimens, at least in patients with low-grade and mantle cell lymphoma. Finally, other studies, including functional imaging with PET scans, have identified patients who because of a low cure rate with autologous transplant may be appropriate for other treatment strategies, including allogeneic transplantation.

EFFICACY OF CONVENTIONAL ALLOGRAFTING FOR NHL

A number of studies have been published recently comparing allografting to autologous transplant for various lymphoma subtypes (Table 8.1). It should be noted that these studies include patients transplanted over long periods of time and therefore are not entirely representative of modern transplant techniques. For example, the European Group for Bone and Marrow Transplantation (EBMT) registry series by Peniket et al. includes a substantial number of patients transplanted prior to 1990, a time when both the methods of diagnosis and classification of NHL and the supportive care practices for allografting were quite different than current methods.[1] Although powerful in terms of statistical numbers, transplant registry data are typically confounded by heterogeneous treatment practices and patient selection criteria from center to center. Allogeneic transplant patients included in such series typically have more advanced and/or resistant disease and are more heavily pretreated than autologous transplant recipients, and are by definition a higher risk group. Despite these shortcomings, such comparative analyses shed some light on the benefits and limitations of both autologous and allogeneic transplantation.

Two studies have dealt specifically with indolent lymphomas and reveal similar results. Investigators from the M.D. Anderson Cancer center reported on 112 patients with indolent NHL undergoing autologous or allogeneic transplant for refractory or recurrent disease between 1991 and 2000.[2] The majority of patients had a diagnosis of grade I or II follicular lymphoma and few had small lymphocytic lymphoma or grade III follicular lymphoma. Conventional chemotherapy

TABLE 8.1 Comparisons of Allogeneic and Autologous Transplant

Study	Source	Study Period	*N*	NHL Type	Results/Comments
Hosing et al.[2]	MD Anderson; single institution	1991–2000	Auto = 68 Allo = 44	Indolent histologies	Long-term results favor allografting
Van Besien et al.[3]	IBMTR/ABMTR registry study	1990–1999	Auto = 597 Auto-Purged-131 Allo = 176	Follicular NHL	Reduced relapse rates for allograft patients offset by higher TRM. TRM declined in later half of decade.
Peniket et al.[1]	EBMT Registry	1982–1998	Allo = 1018 Auto = 3054	Low grade = 231 Int. grade = 402 High grade = 385 3 autologous patients matched to each allo patient	Matched case analysis Relapse rates for most lymphoma subtypes lower than autografting despite higher risk disease. Higher TRM with allografts; 80% of allograft pts received BM grafts.
Levine et al.	IBMTR/ABMTR	1989–1998	Allo = 76 Auto = 128	Lymphoblastic Lymphoma	Lower relapse rates after allograft offset by higher TRM so OS equivalent at 5 years
Bierman et al.[4]	IBMTR/EBMT	1985–1998	Allo = 891 Auto = 2018 Auto-P = 376 Syngeneic = 89	Low grade = 762 Int grade = 1779 High-grade = 669	No GVL effect demonstrated. Low pt numbers for syngeneic transplant by NHL subtype

Abbreviations: NHL, non-Hodgkin's lymphoma; IBMTR, International Bone Marrow Transplant Registry; ABMTR, Autologous Blood and Marrow Transplant Registry; EBMT, European Bone Marrow Transplant Registry; TRM, treatment related mortality; OS, overall survival; GVL, graft-versus-lymphoma; BM, bone marrow. Levine JE, Harris RE, Loberiza FR, Jr, et al. A comparison of allogeneic and autologous bone marrow transplantation for lymphoblastic lymphoma. Blood 2003;101:2476–2482.

had failed in all cases. Patients were preferentially selected for autologous transplant if they had chemosensitive disease and less than 10% marrow involvement. Forty-three percent of patients in the allogeneic group had resistant disease at the time of transplant. Despite the fact that patients in the autologous group were more likely to have chemosensitive disease and to be in remission at the time of transplant, the overall survival (OS) and disease-free survival (DFS) were only 34% and 17%, respectively, at a median follow-up of 71 months. This contrasted to an OS and DFS of 49% and 45%, respectively, in the allogeneic group. The follow-up for the allogeneic patients is shorter because allogeneic transplant was not offered uniformly to patients until 1995, when the efficacy of allografting for disease control became more apparent. Treatment related mortality in the allogeneic group was high with 15 of 44 (34%) patients dying within 100 days of transplant, in contrast to a 6% day-100 mortality in the autologous group. Allotransplant was associated with a 45% risk of chronic graft-versus-host disease (GVHD) in surviving patients. Autologous transplant was associated with a 6% incidence of fatal myelodysplasia. Statistical analysis showed a significant advantage in DFS for allotransplant, but OS was of borderline significance (P = .05). Of note, no late relapses were observed in the allogeneic group whereas relapses as late as eight years out were noted in the autologous group.

In a similar analysis, investigators from the International Bone Marrow Transplant Registry (IBMTR) reported on 904 patients with follicular NHL undergoing allogeneic or autologous transplant from 1990 to 1999.[3] A subset of the patients undergoing an autograft in this series had a purging procedure to remove tumor cells from the graft. Purged autografts were used earlier in the decade and allografts later in the decade. As in the previously mentioned series, allogeneic patients were more likely to have advanced disease, bone marrow involvement, poor performance status, or chemo-resistant disease. Patients with follicular large cell lymphoma were included in this series and were more likely to undergo autologous transplant. Consequently, follow-up was again shorter for allogeneic patients at 36 months versus 49 months for purged and 41 months for unpurged autologous transplant patients. Not surprisingly, treatment-related mortality (TRM) was higher with allografts, with 24% TRM at one year and 30% at five years, but the relapse rate of 19% at one year, with few relapses thereafter, compared favorably to one and five year relapse rates of 36% and 58% after unpurged autologous and 25% and 43% relapse rates after purged autologous transplant, respectively. The early TRM but lower late relapse risk in allogeneic patients resulted in almost identical survival times in comparison to autotransplant. Notably, in this study an analysis of the effect of the date of transplant (early 90s vs. late 90s) revealed that mortality related to transplant declined significantly over the decade, particularly for allogeneic transplantation, most likely attributable to better patient and donor selection and supportive care practices.[3]

An EBMT registry study of 1185 allogeneic transplants for lymphoma between 1982 and 1998 compared results to autografts by first examining variables associated with outcome for specific NHL subtypes and then performing a 1:3 matched analysis.[1] In this study all lymphoma subtypes were included although the long duration of time over which patients were included raises questions as to the accuracy of disease classification, since lymphoma classification evolved significantly during the period in question. With striking similarity to the previously mentioned studies, relapse rates were lower with allografting (Burkitt's lymphoma was the one clear exception to this rule) but survival was not, due to higher mortality rates with allografting.

ALLOGENEIC TRANSPLANT: LOWER RELAPSE RATES BECAUSE OF GVL OR TUMOR-FREE STEM CELL GRAFTS?

Lower relapse rates after allogeneic transplant generally have been attributed to a graft-versus-tumor effect analogous to that observed in patients with acute myelogenous leukemia. Recently, this belief has been challenged by a large retrospective investigation. Bierman et al. analyzed registry data from the IBMTR and the EBMT and compared relapse rates after syngeneic, autologous, and allogeneic transplants.[4] Patients who received purged autografts and T-cell depleted allografts were included also in order to further study the role of tumor cell contamination and GVL effects on relapse, respectively. The major findings of this study were that in all histologies the relapse rates were similar after syngeneic and allogeneic transplants, and that T-cell depletion was not associated with a higher relapse rate than T-cell–replete grafts. These data suggest that the major advantage of allogeneic transplant was that it provided a tumor-free stem cell source. This hypothesis also is strengthened by the failure to show a favorable impact of acute or chronic GVHD on relapse rates. Syngeneic transplants were associated with a lower relapse rate than purged autografts in patients with low-grade lymphoma, suggesting that some of the autografts were incompletely purged or that there was another benefit of receiving a syngeneic transplant such as improved immune reconstitution.

The most important implication of this study is that enthusiasm for reduced-intensity regimens, which rely primarily upon a GVL effect, may be unwarranted. In fact, as described below, some of the recent results observed with reduced-intensity regimens are the strongest evidence of a GVL effect.

Reduced Intensity Allogeneic Transplant

Growing recognition in the past decade of the immunotherapeutic potential of allografts has led to a reconsideration of the necessity of high-dose myeloablative conditioning regimens traditionally administered prior to transplantation. Several clinical trials presented in the late 1990s established the ability to achieve donor engraftment following less-than-ablative conditioning regimens, giving rise to the new sub-field of nonmyeloablative transplantation.[5-9] Several terms have been applied to such regimens, the most broadly used of which is reduced intensity conditioning; others include nonmyeloablative, "mini" transplant, and "transplant-lite". A spectrum of regimens of varying intensity exists, but the most commonly used consist of fludarabine combined with an alkylating agent such as busulfan, cyclophosphamide or melphalan at an intermediate dose (Table 8.2). The potent T-lympholytic effects of fludarabine generally provide sufficient immunosuppression to prevent graft rejection, although the establishment of full donor-derived hematopoiesis and eradication of recipient cells, termed full donor chimerism, is not guaranteed.

Such regimens retain modest antitumor activity against most hematologic malignancies and are associated with significant myelosuppression; however, they do not generally cause excessive rates of mucositis or end-organ toxicity, and the length and depth of neutropenia/trhombocytopenia may be attenuated in comparison to traditional ablative regimens. Patients who are very elderly or in poor medical condition may be treated with even less intensive regimens such as that developed by the Seattle transplant team wherein immunosuppression, in the form of cyclosporine plus mycophenolate and low doses of fludarabine are combined with single fraction low-dose total body irradiation. This regimen may be administered on an outpatient basis and a significant portion of patients may not develop neutropenia or significant thrombocytopenia. While this regimen has been delivered safely even to patients at the extremes of age or medical condition, it lacks significant immediate antineoplastic activity and reliance is placed entirely on graft-versus-tumor (GVT) effects to control disease. The reduction in intensity of this approach also may result in higher rates of mixed hematopoietic chimerism, a development that theoretically hamper GVT effects.

In many respects, nonmyeloablative transplantation is an ideal therapy for selected patients with NHL. Indolent and mantle cell lymphomas appear susceptible to GVT effects and primarily affect an older age population not usually eligible to receive traditional ablative therapies.[10] The growth rate of such tumors may allow sufficient time for GVL effects to occur. Patients with aggressive lymphomas, in contrast, may be less likely to benefit from a reduced intensity approach if their disease is not in remission at the time of transplant or is kinetically active. In either case, a reduction in the treatment-related toxicity attributed to high-dose conditioning regimens in lymphoma patients could be expected to decrease treatment-related mortality. During the last five years, significant clinical research has been conducted using reduced intensity regimens for multiple tumor types and mature data on lymphoma patients participating in such studies are now becoming available.

In a large retrospective review, the EBMT reported results of reduced intensity allografting in188 patients between 1996 and 2000.[11] Included in this series were 52 patients with indolent lymphomas, 62 patients with typical aggressive histologies, and 22 patients with mantle cell lymphoma. Data were collected from 51 transplant centers, and therefore treatment methods, in-

TABLE 8.2 Reduced Intensity Regimens

Conditioning Regimen	Ref.	GVHD Prophylaxis	Mucositis	Myelosuppression	Chimerism	GVHD	Comments
TBI +/– Flu	6, 9	CsA/MMF	None	Minimal	Variable	46% Grade II-IV Acute GVHD	May be performed as outpatient. Addition of fludaribine lowers risk of rejection or mixed chimerism
Flu/Bu/ATG	5	CsA with early taper	Minimal	Modest	Transient mixed chimerism in minority of patients	25% Grade III/IV Acute GVHD	Severe acute GVHD associated with early withdrawal of CsA.
Flu/cyclophosphamide	7	Tacrolimus + methotrexate	Minimal	Modest	Transient mixed chimerism in minority of patients	20% Grade II-IV Acute GVHD	T cell engraftment precedes myeloid engraftment
Flu/Mel/Campath	8	Tacrolimus + methotrexate	NR	Modest	Transient mixed chimerism in minority of patients	29% Grade III/IV Acute GVHD	Includes unrelated donor transplants

Abbreviations: TBI, total body irradiation; Flu, fludarabine; Bu, busulfan; Mel, melphalan; BEAM, BCNU, etoposide, ara-C, melphalan; CsA, cyclosporine; MMF, mycophenolate mofetil; GVHD, graft–versus-host disease; NR, not reported.

cluding conditioning regimens and GVHD prophylaxis, were heterogeneous. The median age of patients in this series was 40 years, significantly less than the median age of lymphoma patients. Of note, almost half of the patients had undergone prior high dose therapy and autologous transplant, a group that is traditionally considered to be at risk for very high rates of TRM if a second transplant is performed. The majority of patients were treated with a fludarabine-based conditioning regimen and over a third of the patients also received alemtuzamab (Campath 1-A), an antiCD52 antibody capable of depleting T-lymphocytes in vivo. The administration of Campath is of importance, as this therapy results in a partial in vivo depletion of transplanted T-lymphocytes and lessens the risk for GVHD, but it also may reduce the chances of achieving a GVL effect. Estimated overall survival at two years was 50%. By multivariate analysis only chemosensitivity was associated with improved survival. The rate of progression of disease was particularly high for patients with aggressive histologies (78% at 2 years) and mantle cell NHL (100% at 2 years). Treatment related mortality for patients with a previous transplant was 30% at one year. Twenty-two patients received donor lymphocyte infusions to treat persistent or progressive disease after transplant. Fourteen of these patients received donor lymphocyte infusions (DLI) as the sole therapy and 10 showed evidence of response with six achieving complete remission (CR). The results of DLI in this study are encouraging and support the presence of a GVL effect. The poor results in aggressive NHL and mantle cell lymphoma (MCL) may reflect the inability of less intensive regimens to control such diseases for an adequate time period for GVL effects to develop; however, the high proportion of patients receiving in vivo T-cell depletion in the form of alemtuzumab and the consequent low rate of GVHD suggest that the GVL effect likely was abrogated by this modification of the reduced intensity approach.

In contrast to the poor results of MCL in the latter investigation, two separate studies have shown a more potent GVL effect with T-cell replete grafts in patients with MCL. Among a larger series of patients with different lymphoma histologies, Seropian et al. described three patients with relapsed MCL after autologous transplant who have remained disease-free for more than three years after a reduced intensity allogeneic transplant.[12] All three patients had evidence of acute and chronic GVHD. In a separate study of 18 patients with relapsed MCL, including five who had relapsed after autologous transplant, Khouri et al. described a current-event-free survival of 82% at three years.[10] Most impressively, no patient developed greater than grade 2 GVHD, suggesting that a GVL effect could occur without GVHD. As it seems very unlikely that any patient in these two series was cured by the preparative regimen, the long-term disease-free survival provides indirect but strong evidence for a GVL effect. In addition, one of two relapsed patients in the Khouri et al. series experienced a durable (45+ months) CR after DLI infusion, further supporting a GVL effect. These data, if validated in larger studies, suggest that allogeneic transplant with reduced intensity conditioning could become an important therapy for relapsed MCL patients, particularly as autologous transplant in this setting has been relatively ineffective.

Reduced intensity allogeneic transplant also has recently been shown to be potentially curative in patients with chronic lymphocytic lymphoma (CLL) and, by inference, small lymphocytic lymphoma (SLL). In a study of the Cooperative German Transplant Study Group, 62% of 30 patients had progression-free survival at two years. The CR rate increased from 25% at one year to 66% at years, suggesting an ongoing GVL effect that can clearly not be explained by the preparative regimen.[13] Six of 12 patients who had CR were refractory to fludarabine and none of the patients who achieved at least a partial remission (PR) died of progressive CLL. These results provide great hope for patients with fludarabine-refractory disease and provide support for further investigation of allogeneic transplant in patients with recurrent poor prognosis disease.

Despite the impressive data for reduced-intensity transplant in patients with low-grade and mantle cell lymphoma, the available information is not as encouraging for patients with more aggressive histologies with active disease. In the EBMT study discussed above, 78% of patients showed disease progression at two years. Tanimoto et al. reported more encouraging results, but with a high rate of GVHD and only brief follow-up.[14] More encouraging preliminary results were presented recently in patients who relapsed after a prior autologous transplant and then achieved a good remission prior to reduced-intensity allogeneic transplant. In a series of 20 patients, including nine patients with diffuse large cell lymphoma, all 20 patients achieved a CR after allogeneic transplant and only one patient died (non-relapse mortality). The low TRM stands in marked contrast with the unacceptably high rates of TRM reported with standard conditioning, which suggests that relapse after autologous transplant is not necessarily fatal.[15] However, it should be noted that this group appeared to have disease more favorable than that usually observed following relapse.

Ablative Transplants in Patients with Aggressive Histologies

High-dose chemotherapy and autologous stem cell transplant are recognized as the treatments of choice for patients with relapsed chemosensitive aggressive lymphoma. As a result, and because of a considerably higher TRM, ablative allogeneic transplant has not been extensively studied recently in this group despite retrospective analyses suggesting a lower relapse rate. In the series by Seropian et al., 8 of 13 patients with aggressive histology not felt to be curable with autologous transplant (including 3 of 5 patients who had a prior autologous transplant) experienced prolonged disease-free survival and probable cure after ablative allogeneic transplant. These results suggest that allogeneic transplant should be studied further in poor prognosis patients. Two different types of studies have helped to clarify the population of patients who may be most appropriate for clinical investigation. Hamlin et al. found that the age-adjusted International Prognostic Index at the time of disease recurrence (sAAIPI) successfully predicted outcome of autologous transplant and found that high risk patients had a less than 20% cure rate.[16] Importantly, the outcome in high risk patients was poor even in those who responded to salvage chemotherapy. Alternatively, functional imaging with the PET scan appears to separate patients who have a good chance of cure with an autologous transplant from those with a dismal prognosis. Three different studies published in 2003 have found that patients with persistently positive PET scans after two to three courses of salvage therapy have a greater than 70% risk of disease progression after autologous transplant.[17-19] These data suggest that a poor risk group can be identified even among chemosensitive patients who would be appropriate candidates for innovative transplant approaches.

Treatment of Persistent or Recurrent NHL After Transplant

A limited number of reports in the past have suggested that recurrent lymphoma following allogeneic transplantation may be treated in the same fashion as other hematologic malignancies, with attempts at inducing graft-versus-tumor effects by withdrawing immunosuppression and/or administering donor lymphocytes. Such approaches have met with mixed success and may be dependent on factors such as disease burden and histologic classification. Since GVL effects are somewhat time-dependent, it has been suggested that aggressive lymphomas may be less susceptible to such maneuvers based solely on a kinetic basis. Adjunctive treatments capable of controlling post-transplant disease, without causing undue toxicity or interference with the development of donor-derived immune function, therefore might be expected to improve the odds of successfully inducing GVL effects. In the EBMT registry series of reduced intensity transplantation reported by Robinson et al., the rate of response to DLI was encouraging and was not limited to patients with indolent lymphoma.[11]

In an interesting study from Israel, patients at particularly high risk for recurrence after a transplant procedure on the basis of chemo-refractory disease and multiple relapse were treated with a planned post-transplant course of rituximab following hematopoietic engraftment.[20] Twenty eight patients were included in this study, 12 of whom received an allogeneic transplant. Seven patients in PR after transplant were converted to a CR after rituximab therapy. Two additional patients who relapsed after transplant received a second course of rituximab along with other attempts to induce a GVL response that appeared to be successful. Because there was no comparator arm, the relative contributions of rituximab therapy and other therapies (such as DLI) on outcome is difficult to discern. The investigators documented a high rate of neutropenia and severe hypogammaglobulinemia in the allogeneic transplant recipients receiving rituximab in this study. Fever occurred in association with these side effects in some patients, though no mortality occurred. These effects appeared to be readily treated with growth factors and immune globulin replacement.

In the Yale series mentioned previously,[12] 10 patients had persistent or recurrent disease following allograft and received further therapy that was tailored to the patients prior history and clinical situation. Seven patients were treated with the hope of inducing a GVL effect by withdrawing immunosuppression and, in six cases, administering donor lymphocytes (DLI). Additional therapies administered at the time of recurrence to some patients also included rituximab, interferon and radiotherapy to isolated sites of disease. Four patients responded to this strategy, all of whom developed GVHD. Two of these patients, with aggressive histologies, remain in complete remission at 46 and 58 months post-transplant. One patient died of disease progression and one died in continued remission at 37 months post-transplant of sequelae of chronic GVHD.

A small study from England assessed the use of BEAM-Campath for patients with follicular lymphoma with molecular monitoring for bcl-2/IgH translocations.[21] A goal of this study was to examine the utility of monitoring of minimal residual disease, with respect to post-transplant modifications of immunosuppression and administration of donor lymphocytes. Patients received a lower dose of etoposide than is ordinarily administered for allografting with BEAM and, therefore, the conditioning regimen was referred to as reduced intensity. Patients received rituximab prior to transplant followed by conditioning and then cyclosporine as a single agent for a short period of time and then tapered at day +58. Three patients in this study received DLI to treat disease progression and/or declining donor chimerism and DLI was effective. Rituximab was also used post-transplant to treat persistent disease and appeared effective in treating marrow but not nodal disease.

Additional case reports continue to appear documenting such phenomenon. Wong et al. reported a patient with diffuse large B cell NHL with recurrent disease four months following an allograft from a matched unrelated donor.[22] Withdrawal of immunosuppression and rituximab (1000 mg/m^2) weekly resulted in a second CR.[22] Espanol et al. reported a patient with CLL who developed Richter's syndrome post-matched sibling donor allograft treated with withdrawal of immunosuppression and donor lymphocyte infusion. The patient remained in complete remission 18 months later.[23]

To summarize, the above experiences provide further evidence for the presence of a GVL effect and suggest that allografting, whether performed following full ablative conditioning or reduced intensity programs, may be combined with additional therapies to induce durable remissions.

Allografting for Unusual Diseases

The advent of tools capable of reducing the morbidity of allografting such as reduced intensity programs, better antibiotics, and new treatments for GVHD has renewed interest in attempts at allografts for patients with specific NHL subtypes who might benefit from a graft versus lymphoma, but who traditionally have been felt to be at too high a risk for the procedure.

In a study of three patients with advanced mycosis Fungoides, Soligo et al. reported the results of reduced intensity transplant following low-dose total body irradiation with short duration cyclosporine A (CsA) and mycophenolate mofetil (MMF) as the GVHD prophylaxis.[24] All three patients had poor prognosis refractory advanced stage disease and achieved CR following allograft concomitant with the development of GVHD. One patient died of infectious complications.

A report from Japan discussed the feasibility of allogeneic transplant in 11 patients with HTLV-I–associated adult T-cell leukemia/lymphoma transplanted with conventional or reduced intensity approaches.[25] Four of six patients transplanted in CR survived and are in CR at a median of 25 months from transplant. Seven deaths were due to transplant related complications including GVHD, gastrointestinal bleeding and interstitial pneumonitis. Of note, two patients with recurrent disease after transplant achieved CR after withdrawal of immunosuppression and administration of DLI.

SUMMARY

Allografting appears to be a potentially curative procedure for several "incurable lymphomas" including relapsed mantle cell lymphoma and the various small cell lymphomas (CLL/SLL, follicular lymphoma, marginal cell lymphoma). Because of transplant-related complications, especially GVHD, as well as the development of newer highly effective, non-toxic but ultimately palliative treatments (e.g., Zevalin and Bexxar), the timing of allografting remains a crucial question. Reduced intensity allogeneic transplants appear to be highly effective in small cell and mantle cell lymphomas, and appear to be feasible and effective in patients who have exhausted other treatments including autologous transplant. Moreover, reduced intensity allografting has allowed an older generation a chance for a cure that was not previously available. Reduced-intensity transplants have not yet proved to be effective in intermediate grade lymphomas with active disease, but require further investigation in patients who have obtained a remission or near CR but who are very likely to relapse (e.g., patients in second or third response). Functional imaging studies will facilitate the study of allogeneic transplants in chemosensitive but high-risk patients who are unlikely to be cured with autologous transplant.

REFERENCES

1. Peniket AJ, Ruiz de Elvira MC, Taghipour G, et al. An EBMT registry matched study of allogeneic stem cell transplants for lymphoma: allogeneic transplantation is associated with a lower relapse rate but a higher procedure-related mortality rate than autologous transplantation. Bone Marrow Transplant 2003;31:667–678.
2. Hosing C, Saliba RM, McLaughlin P, et al. Long-term results favor allogeneic over autologous

hematopoietic stem cell transplantation in patients with refractory or recurrent indolent non-Hodgkin's lymphoma. Ann Oncol 2003;14:737–744.

3. Van Besien K, Loberiza FR, Bajorunaite R, et al. Comparison of autologous and allogeneic hematopoietic stem cell transplantation for follicular lymphoma. Blood 2003;102:3521-3529.
4. Bierman PJ, Sweetenham JW, Loberiza FR Jr, et al. Syngeneic hematopoietic stem-cell transplantation for non-Hodgkin's lymphoma: a comparison with allogeneic and autologous transplantation—The Lymphoma Working Committee of the International Bone Marrow Transplant Registry and the European Group for Blood and Marrow Transplantation. J Clin Oncol 2003;21:3744–3753.
5. Slavin S, Nagler A, Naparstek E, et al. Nonmyeloablative stem cell transplantation and cell therapy as an alternative to conventional bone marrow transplantation with lethal cytoreduction for the treatment of malignant and nonmalignant hematologic diseases. Blood 1998;91: 756–763.
6. McSweeney P, Niederwieser D, Shizuru J, et al. Outpatient allografting with minimally myelosuppressive, immunosuppressive conditioning of low-dose TBI and postgrafting cyclosporine (CSP) and mycophenolate mofetil (MMF). Blood 1999;94:393a.
7. Childs R, Clave E, Contentin N, et al. Engraftment kinetics after nonmyeloablative allogeneic peripheral blood stem cell transplantation: full donor T-cell chimerism precedes alloimmune responses. Blood 1999;94:3234–3241.
8. Giralt S, Estey E, Albitar M, et al. Engraftment of allogeneic hematopoietic progenitor cells with purine analog-containing chemotherapy: harnessing graft-versus-leukemia without myeloablative therapy. Blood 1997;89:4531–4536.
9. Sandmaier B, Maloney D, Gooley T, et al. Low dose TBI conditioning for hematopoietic stem cell transplants (HSCT) from HLA-matched related donors for patients with hematologic malignancies: influence of fludarabine or cytoreductive autografts on outcome. American Society of Hematology, Annual Meeting, 2002, pp 145a.
10. Khouri IF, Lee MS, Romaguera J, et al. Allogeneic hematopoietic transplantation for mantle-cell lymphoma: molecular remissions and evidence of graft-versus-malignancy. Ann Oncol 1999;10:1293–1299.
11. Robinson SP, Goldstone AH, Mackinnon S, et al. Chemoresistant or aggressive lymphoma predicts for a poor outcome following reduced-intensity allogeneic progenitor cell transplantation: an analysis from the Lymphoma Working Party of the European Group for Blood and Bone Marrow Transplantation. Blood 2002;100:4310–4316.
12. Seropian S, Bahceci F, Cooper DL. Allogeneic peripheral blood stem cell transplantation for high-risk non-Hodgkin's lymphoma. Bone Marrow Transplant 2003;32:763–769.
13. Schetelig J, Thiede C, Bornhauser M, et al. Evidence of a graft-versus-leukemia effect in chronic lymphocytic leukemia after reduced-intensity conditioning and allogeneic stem-cell transplantation: the Cooperative German Transplant Study Group. J Clin Oncol 2003;21:2747–2753.
14. Tanimoto TE, Kusumi E, Hamaki T, et al. High complete response rate after allogeneic hematopoietic stem cell transplantation with reduced-intensity conditioning regimens in advanced malignant lymphoma. Bone Marrow Transplant 2003;32:131–137.
15. Escalon M, Champlin R, Rima S, et al. Non-myeloablative allogeneic hematopoietic transplantation: a promising salvage therapy for patients with non-Hodgkin's lymphoma (NHL) whose disease has failed a prior autologous stem cell transplantation (ASCT). American Society of Hematology, Annual Meeting, 2003, pp 75a.
16. Hamlin PA, Zelenetz AD, Kewalramani T, et al. Age-adjusted International Prognostic Index predicts autologous stem cell transplantation outcome for patients with relapsed or primary refractory diffuse large B-cell lymphoma. Blood 2003;102:1989–1996.

17. Spaepen K, Stroobants S, Dupont P, et al. Prognostic value of pretransplantation positron emission tomography using fluorine 18-fluorodeoxyglucose in patients with aggressive lymphoma treated with high-dose chemotherapy and stem cell transplantation. Blood 2003;102:53–59.

18. Schot B, van Imhoff G, Pruim J, et al. Predictive value of early 18F-fluoro-deoxyglucose positron emission tomography in chemosensitive relapsed lymphoma. Br J Haematol 2003;123:282–287.

19. Filmont JE, Czernin J, Yap C, et al. Value of F-18 fluorodeoxyglucose positron emission tomography for predicting the clinical outcome of patients with aggressive lymphoma prior to and after autologous stem-cell transplantation. Chest 2003;124:608–613.

20. Shimoni A, Hardan I, Avigdor A, et al. Rituximab reduces relapse risk after allogeneic and autologous stem cell transplantation in patients with high-risk aggressive non-Hodgkin's lymphoma. Br J Haematol 2003;122:457–464.

21. Ho AY, Devereux S, Mufti GJ, et al. Reduced-intensity rituximab-BEAM-CAMPATH allogeneic haematopoietic stem cell transplantation for follicular lymphoma is feasible and induces durable molecular remissions. Bone Marrow Transplant 2003;31:551–557.

22. Wong R, de Lima M, Couriel D, et al. Treatment of relapsing refractory diffuse large cell lymphoma after matched unrelated donor bone marrow transplant with immunosuppression withdrawal and rituximab. Leuk Lymphoma 2003;44:829–832.

23. Espanol I, Buchler T, Ferra C, et al. Richter's syndrome after allogeneic stem cell transplantation for chronic lymphocytic leukaemia successfully treated by withdrawal of immunosuppression, and donor lymphocyte infusion. Bone Marrow Transplant 2003;31:215–218.

24. Soligo D, Ibatici A, Berti E, et al. Treatment of advanced mycosis fungoides by allogeneic stem-cell transplantation with a nonmyeloablative regimen. Bone Marrow Transplant 2003;31:663–666.

25. Kami M, Hamaki T, Miyakoshi S, et al. Allogeneic haematopoietic stem cell transplantation for the treatment of adult T-cell leukaemia/lymphoma. Br J Haematol 2003;120:304–309.

Chapter 9

Clinical Applications of Molecular Profiling in Lymphomas

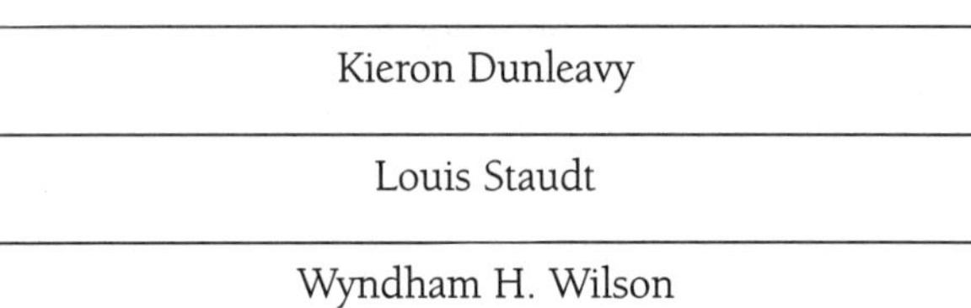

Kieron Dunleavy

Louis Staudt

Wyndham H. Wilson

Lymphomas are a heterogeneous group of diseases that vary from clinically indolent to aggressive and from incurable to curable. Histological classification schemes were initially developed in an attempt to organize these diseases into groups with shared pathogenesis and clinical behavior with an aim to guide treatment. Over the years, these classifications have evolved from exclusively morphological to the current ones that incorporate immunophenotype and genetic endpoints, such as the Revised European-American Classification of Lymphoid Neoplasms (REAL) and the World Health Organization (WHO) Classification of Neoplastic Diseases of Hematopoietic and Lymphoid Tissues.[1,2] This evolution is the direct result of insights into the molecular pathogenesis of lymphoma, including the identification of "hallmark" genetic abnormalities.

Although advances in molecular biology have helped identify expression of individual gene products important in cellular proliferation, differentiation and death, insights into large scale gene expression have not been possible until recently. A variety of complementary technologies are now available that can measure the expression of thousands of genes in parallel, termed molecular profiling, and can link biology to a genetic expression signature. The application of this technology to lymphoma is providing insights into unique molecular signatures of distinct types of B-cell malignancies. It can relate lymphoid neoplasms to normal stages in B-cell development and physiology, and may provide a new way to classify lymphomas, and to predict clinical outcome. Indeed, as the molecular analysis of tumors improves, the classification of human cancers is likely to become more refined and informative. In the present review, we briefly describe the genetic basis of lymphomas, and the science and application of genetic profiling in lymphomas.

MOLECULAR ABNORMALITIES IN LYMPHOMA

It is instructive to review what is known about the functional significance of genetic abnormalities in lymphomas, as they have an important relationship to molecular profiles. Indeed, a number of these genetic abnormalities are of prognostic value and have formed the basis for molecular predictors of clinical outcome. At a molecular level, the genetic lesions identified in lymphomas include oncogene activation or loss of tumor suppressor genes caused by chromosomal translocation, deletion or mutation, or by introduction of exogenous viral genomes into the human chromosome. The molecular cloning of genetic loci involved in the translocations most frequently associated with lymphomas has led to the identification of a number of protooncogenes involved in lymphomagenesis. Distinguishing immunologic and genetic features, presumably reflecting disease biology, have been identified for many lymphoma subtypes and are incorporated into the WHO classification. However, what is absent is an adequate understanding of the "ripple effect" of these genetic abnormalities on the cellular gene expression.

Due to the recent development of molecular profiling, the studies have focused primarily on the more common B-cell lymphomas, which are generally categorized as indolent or aggressive. The genetic hallmark of follicular lymphoma (FL), the most common indolent lymphoma subtype, is the t(14;18)(q32;q21) translocation with rearrangement of the *bcl-2* gene, present in 80% to 90% of cases, and overexpression of the *bcl-2* gene product (Table 9.1).[12,13] Inhibition of apoptosis by *bcl-2*, which occurs in normal germinal center cells, appears to play an important role in lymphomagenesis.[12,14] However, constitutive *bcl-2* expression is not necessarily required for survival as it may be turned off in FL cells that have undergone aggressive transformation.[15] The role of *p53* mutation/deletion observed in some transformed FLs is also uncertain, although loss of *p53* function is associated with decreased apoptosis and clinical drug resistance.[3,16] The functional significance of genetic abnormalities in small lymphocytic lymphoma/B-cell chronic lymphocytic leukemia (CLL) is more uncertain, although many of these have important clinical effects (Table 9.1). Clonal chromosomal abnormalities can be detected in nearly half of these patients with deletions of the long arm of chromosome 13 being the most common.[17] Trisomy 12 anomalies are frequent also, found in 10% to 30% of cases, followed by deletions in the long arm of chromosome 11, termed 11q-, in some 10% to 20% of cases; both anomalies are associated with more aggressive disease compared to patients harboring the more common del 13q14.[5,18] Abnormalities in the *p53* gene, located on the short arm of chromosome 17, at 17p13, also has been associated with a poor clinical outcome in CLL and is found in half of patients with a Richter's transformation.[19,20] Of developmental and clinical relevance is the mutational status of the immunoglobulin variable heavy (VH) region in CLL.[21] Normal developmental biology suggests that CLL cells with or without VH somatic mutations correspond to antigen-dependent and independent phases, respectively, and in the former case is associated with longer survival.[21]

Among aggressive lymphomas, diffuse large B-cell lymphoma (DLBCL) is the most common type, comprising a third of all lymphomas.[22] This histological category is likely to contain multiple disease entities as suggested by its variable clinical presentation, natural history, morphologic variants and molecular characteristics.[23] The diverse morphological variants of DLBCL, which include centroblastic, immunoblastic, T-cell/histiocyte rich and anaplastic types, have some known molecular correlates, but alone, cannot reliably be distinguished as distinct diseases.[23] Other DLBCL subtypes such as primary mediastinal B cell lymphoma (PMBL) and intravascular large B cell lymphoma have been identified as distinct subtypes of DLBCL based on a combination of clinical, histological and molecular findings.[23] It is also important to recognize that large cell "transformation" of an indolent B-cell lymphoma/leukemia, a relatively common occurrence, involves pathways of lymphomagenesis distinct from de novo DLBCL. These entities, however, may share histological, immunophenotypic and oncogenetic characteristics.[24]

Within DLBCL, a common molecular abnormality seen in over half of cases involves the deregulation of *bcl-6*, either through promoter substitution or by multiple, often bi-allelic mutation clustering in its 5′ non-coding region; up to 35% of cases show abnormalities of the 3q27 region (Table 9.1).[25] Bcl-6 protein functions as a transcription factor that binds a specific DNA sequence and represses transcription from linked promoters. It is important in the normal functioning of the germinal center B cells and is required for germinal center cell formation during the antigen-driven immune response.[26] DLBCLs with high expression of *bcl-6* are usually of germinal center B-cell origin, and in part this may help distinguish them from other DLBCL subtypes.[27] The functional significance of *bcl-6* overexpression and/or deregulation on clinical outcome is uncertain, although some studies have found an improved survival in such patients, possibly related to their association with cells of germinal center origin.[28] Another common, albeit variable, finding is the overexpression of *bcl-2*, which is reported to be present in 24% to 55% of cases from two studies.[7,29] Interestingly, only 14% to 17% of these cases were found to harbor a *bcl-2* gene rearrangement from the t(14;18) translocation, suggesting the presence of variable molecular mechanisms of bcl-2 overexpression. Paradoxically, overexpression of the bcl-2 protein, but not the *bcl-2* gene rearrangement, is associated with decreased survival, suggesting that the anti-apoptotic effect of the bcl-2 protein is not the important determinant of outcome.[7,29] Microarray profiling studies, however, have shed light on this apparent paradox, as discussed below. Other variable molecular findings in DLBCL include mutation of the *p53* gene, found in approximately 20% of cases at initial diagnosis; this has also been associated with decreased survival and drug resistance, presumably through its anti-apoptotic effects.[9,16] Specific immunophenotypic and genotypic features also have been associated with the PMBL subtype of DLBCL, such as overexpression of the *MAL* gene, a finding that supports a unique biological heritage for this disease.[23,30,31]

Mantle cell lymphoma is considerably less common than DLBCL and only relatively recently was recognized as a distinct disease entity (Table 9.1).[23] Virtually all cases contain the t(11;14)(q13;q32) translocation between the immunoglobulin heavy chain and the *cyclin D1* (*PRAD1*, *bcl-1*) genes.[10] Deregulation of *bcl-1* leads to overexpression of its gene product cyclin-D1, which promotes progression from the G1 to S stages of the cell cycle.[32] Unlike DLBCL, most patients are incurable and have a relatively short median survival of three to five years.[33]

Despite our improved ability to subtype lymphomas based on morphology, immunophenotype and molecular abnormalities, we only have a limited ability to predict a patient's clinical course. This is well illustrated by DLBCL in which only one third of patients are cured with CHOP-based treatment.[34] The ability of single gene products such as *bcl-2* or *p53* by immunohistochemistry to identify patients at increased risk of failure suggests that gene expression arrays may provide significantly more information. Indeed, gene expression analysis may reveal the downstream targets of important transcription factors such as *bcl-6*.

TECHNIQUES OF MOLECULAR PROFILING

Molecular profiling relies on the differential transcription of genes into messenger RNA (mRNA) that depend on a multiplicity of factors, such as cell lineage and stage of differentiation, activity of intracellular pathways and external factors. Of course, proteins are the final conduit through which genes exert their biological effect and molecular profiling is an indirect reflection of their action. Nevertheless, molecular profiling provides a snap shot of the expression of thousands of genes, thereby generating a finger print of gene expression. Importantly, the molecular profile of a tumor biopsy is influenced not only by its unique genetic composition, but also by its microenvironment, which is comprised of multiple cell types.

Significant improvements and refinements have been made over the past several years in molecular microarray technology. The core technology entails the

TABLE 9.1 Chromosomal Translocations in Non-Hodgkin's Lymphoma

Lymphoma Subtype	Translocation	% of Cases Affected	Proto-oncogene	Putative Function	Clinical Correlate
Follicular Center Cell	t(14:18)(q32:q21)	75%–90%	bcl-2	Inhibits apoptosis	No association with prognosis
	17p13		p53	Confers resistance to chemotherapy	Large cell transformation and shorter time to disease progression[3]
Small Lymphocytic/ CLL	Trisomy 12	10%–30%		Loss of tumor suppressor function; Associated with Ig-unmutated type	Advanced disease, atypical morphology and resistant disease[4]
	13q14	50%		Putative tumor suppressor gene unknown	Improved survival[5]
	11q22-23	10%–20%		Unknown	Aggressive disease and worse prognosis[11]
	17p13	6%	p53	Confers resistance to chemotherapy	Shorter survival[11]
Diffuse Large B-cell	del (3)(q27)	35%	bcl-6	Transcription factor for germinal center formation	Extranodal DLBCL. Impact on treatment outcome controversial[6]
	t(14;18)(q32:q21)	20%–50%	bcl-2	Inhibition of apoptosis	Poor prognosis[7,8]
	17p13	20%	p53	Confers resistance to chemotherapy	Poor prognosis[8,9]
Mantle cell	t(11;14)(q13;q32)		bcl-1/ Cyclin D1	Cell cycle regulator. Promotes G_1 to S progression	Seen in 70% of cases with cytogenetics and virtually 100% with FISH[10]
	17p13	8%	p53	Confers resistance to chemotherapy	Worse prognosis and blastic morphology[11]

immobilization of thousands of DNA probes (the genes defined for inclusion in the array) on a solid surface that are hybridized against fluorophore labeled cDNA or mRNA targets from template RNA sources. The hybridization of a sample to an array is essentially a highly parallel search by each molecule for a matching partner on an affinity matrix, determined by the rules of molecular recognition. The two major types of arrays used in gene molecular profiling are "spotted arrays," where the probes are deposited onto glass slides by contact or ink jet printing and "in situ" arrays, where oligo probes are synthesized (in silico) via photolithographic synthesis as in Affymetrix Genechip arrays (Affymetrix, Santa Clara, CA). In the glass slide cDNA microarray, the sample mRNA, labeled with a red fluorochrome, is quantitated relative to the expression of a known mixture of mRNA, pooled from multiple cell lines, and labeled with a different (green) fluorochrome. The samples are combined and hybridized on the array. The overexpression of the sample RNA relative to the known RNA fluoresces red whereas a sample with under expression fluoresces green. The bound fluorescent probe to each spot on the microarray is quantified using a scanning confocal microscope coupled with a computerized image analyzer.[35]

An important component of microarray profiling is the analytical approach and interpretation of results. Analysis of the gene expression data may be performed using a variety of supervised and unsupervised approaches. With supervised approaches, gene expression is correlated with an endpoint such as patient survival, and a list of associated genes with variable probabilities is generated. Because of the large number of genes, however, spurious correlations are likely to occur. An unsupervised analysis looks for genes that show similar patterns of gene expression and organizes them into clusters. Clues to the biological significance of these clusters may be obtained from review of the associated genes, many of which may be known components of a biological pathway, and by comparison to similar patterns in normal cells.[36] These genes can be grouped into biological "signatures" that are coordinately expressed in a particular cell type or state of cellular activation. Large sample sizes and the use of discovery and validation sample sets all contribute to the increased accuracy of the scientific conclusions.

MOLECULAR PROFILING

Indolent B-cell Lymphomas

Follicular lymphomas are clinically heterogeneous with survival ranging from under one year to over 20 years following diagnosis. Although single molecular events such as *p53* mutation have been associated with histological transformation and shorter survival, broader insights into tumor biology and the molecular basis of clinical behavior only recently have been made using microarray profiling.[37] The proliferation signature, which includes genes more highly expressed in dividing than resting cells, is able to distinguish FL and CLL from the more highly proliferative DLBCLs, with the former clustered next to resting B cells.[38] Furthermore, genes characteristic of germinal center B cells were highly expressed in FL and distinguished FL from CLL. Indeed, the observations that FL cells undergo somatic mutation of the immunoglobulin (*IG*) genes has led to the suggestion that transformation of FL occurs within a germinal center B cell, a finding which is supported by the presence of a germinal center B-cell gene signature being virtually unchanged in the FL cases.[39] To help gain further insight into the clinical heterogeneity of FL, molecular profiling of 191 samples was performed using an Affymetrix U133 microarray and a molecular predictor of survival was developed.[40] Overall, 81 predictor genes were identified, which appeared to reflect infiltrating immune cells in the tumor mass and B cell differentiation genes, and these were used to construct a predictive model. This molecular model divided patients into quartiles based on their risk, and was able to identify a median survival of 3.9 years from >15 years at the highest and lowest quartiles, respectively. Importantly, the model could stratify patient survival even within good clinical risk groups.

In another approach, the gene expression of FL cases that responded to rituximab, a therapeutic chimeric IgG1 monoclonal antibody to the CD20 B-cell antigen, was compared to the gene expression of nonresponders.[41] Using a supervised approach, 71 genes were found to have a significantly higher expression in rituximab non-responders compared to responders. Many of these genes appear to be involved in inflammation and the immune response and included genes encoding complement proteins, T-cell receptor signaling proteins and cytokines. Furthermore, the gene expression patterns in these cases segregated into two groups with one group showing a gene expression pattern closer to that of normal lymphoid tissues than the other FL group. Interestingly, the rituximab nonresponders were more likely to show a gene expression pattern more characteristic of normal lymphoid tissues. It is provocative to speculate that the immune microenvironment plays an important role in the clinical heterogeneity of FL, possibly in its capacity to regulate FL cell replication and death. It is perhaps less likely that the microenvironment reflects the biological characteristics of the FL.

Several studies also have examined matched biopsy pairs to examine changes in gene expression associated with histological transformation of FL to DLBCL, an occurrence found in up to 60% of cases.[42–44] In one study, Lossos et al analyzed sequential biopsy specimens from 12 patients and observed two different gene expression patterns associated with histological transformation.[43] One group showed an increase in the expression of *c-myc* and its regulated genes, whereas the other group showed a decrease in the expression of these genes. As *c-myc* is associated with cell growth and proliferation, increased expression of relevant genes could be secondary to the change in cell size, like cytoskeleton and ribosomal genes, and cellular replication, both of which are associated with the transformed phenotype. On the other hand, if the expression of *c-myc* and/or its target genes, which are reported to promote apoptosis, are decreased, this in turn may lead to decreased apoptosis and contribute to transformation. Interestingly, a comparison of the molecular profiles of transformed and de novo DLBCL revealed significant differences, with the former showing a greater similarity to FL, suggesting that they have variable pathways of lymphomagenesis.[43]

CLL, like FL, has a broad survival range and is incurable with standard treatments. In CLL, however, there is a molecular correlate of outcome based on the mutational state of the immunoglobulin (*Ig*) variable gene.[21] The observation that somatic hypermutation of *Ig* genes occurs in B cells at the germinal center stage of differentiation and that *Ig*-mutated CLL has a distinct (favorable) outcome compared to *Ig*-unmutated CLL, led to the hypothesis that CLL may be two diseases arising at different stages of differentiation. To help assess this hypothesis, a molecular profile of CLL was constructed using the NCI Lymphochip.[45] This specialized chip contains 17,850 cDNA clones selected from genes preferentially expressed by lymphoid cells or with known or suspected roles in immunology or cancer.[35] Genes from a germinal center B cell library comprised the majority of clones because of their suspected role in lymphomagenesis. To provide a comparative framework, cells from FL, DLBCL and normal B and T cell subpopulations were analyzed also.[45] An expression signature was constructed in which a broad category of genes distinguished CLL from other B cell malignancies and various normal B cells. Interestingly, the signature genes were not highly expressed in germinal center B cells or resting blood B cells, and included several named genes not previously known to be expressed in CLL. *Wnt3* in particular was highly and selectively expressed in CLL. The *Wnt* gene family encodes proteins that control development and mediate malignant transformation. The CLL cases also preferentially expressed genes that distinguished resting blood B cells from activated blood B cells and dividing germinal center B cells, findings consistent with the generally low proliferative nature of the disease. Additionally, genes preferentially expressed by B cells enriched in CD5+ expression, a subpopulation proposed as the normal counterpart of CLL, were not noticeably higher in the CLL cells. Such a finding does not support this hypothesis.

The characterization of a common gene expression signature for CLL, irrespective of *Ig* mutational status, suggests that CLL shares common pathways of transformation and/or cell of origin (Fig. 9.1A).[45,46] On the other hand, the influence of *Ig* mutational status on prognosis indicates an important biological effect (Fig. 9.1B). To help assess this, a supervised analysis of genes expressed in *Ig*-mutated and *Ig*-unmutated cases was performed and approximately 175 differentially expressed genes ($P < .001$) were identified. Among these genes, *ZAP-70* was the most discriminating, with an average 4.3-fold higher expression in *Ig*-unmutated compared to *Ig*-mutated cases (Fig. 9.1A). *ZAP-70* was highly correlated with *Ig*-unmutated CLL or nearly equivalent to somatic mutation analysis of the *IgVH* genes as a prognostic marker (Fig. 9.1B). *ZAP-70* encodes a crucial protein kinase found in normal T cells that transduces signals from the T-cell receptor antigen.[47] Interestingly, a *ZAP-70*-related kinase tranduces signals from the B cell receptor (BCR), raising the possibility that *ZAP-70* may alter BCR signaling in CLL cells.[48] Other differentially expressed genes in *Ig*-unmutated CLL included those induced during blood B-cell activation, many of which encode proteins involved in cell cycle control or cell cycle progression (Fig. 9.1A). Conversely, most genes expressed at lower levels in *Ig*-mutated cases are highly reduced during B cell activation. Indeed, the enrichment of genes modulated during BCR signaling in *Ig*-unmutated CLL raises the hypothesis that either these cells are undergoing continuous antigen stimulation, with gene expression reminiscent of BCR signaling, or that these cells are activating signaling pathways engaged during B cell activation due to other pathogenetic alterations.[45]

Aggressive B-cell Lymphomas

Although DLBCL is recognized as more than one disease in the WHO classification, it has been difficult to readily subdivide it into distinct disease entities because of overlapping morphology and variable pathogenetic features.[23] As a result, treatment strategies have primarily depended on clinical features such as stage and the International Prognostic Index (IPI), which are likely to be surrogates of tumor biology.[49] Large scale genomic profiling, however, has the potential to recognize new subtypes of DLBCL and to relate them to treatment outcome.

The initial studies in DLBCL were performed using the specialized Lymphochip microarray. To provide a comparative basis for the interpretation of DLBCL gene expression, arrays also were performed on samples from FL, CLL, lymphoma, and leukemia cell lines, and normal lymphocyte subpopulations obtained under a variety of activation conditions and tissue sites.[38]. Genes associated with cellular proliferation showed a clear distinction among the lymphoma types with DLBCL generally showing higher albeit variable expression, a finding that corresponds to the known variation in tumor proliferation index as measured by *MIB-1/Ki-67* antibodies.[16] The proliferation signature genes were a diverse group and included cell-cycle control and check-point genes, DNA synthesis and replication genes, as well as the *Ki-67* gene. Another prominent feature of DLBCL was a group of genes that defined a "lymph-node" signature that appeared to reflect the non-malignant cells in the biopsy samples. This signature was shared also by normal lymph nodes and tonsils and included genes associated with monocytes and macrophages (CD14, CD105, CSF-1 receptor), and genes involved in extracellular matrix remodeling (*MMP9* matrix metalloproteinase and *TIMP-3*). More variable was the presence of a T-cell expression signature that included components of the T cell receptor and downstream signaling genes.

Genes that distinguished germinal center (GC) B cells from other stages of B cell differentiation also were differentially expressed in the DLBCL cases, and

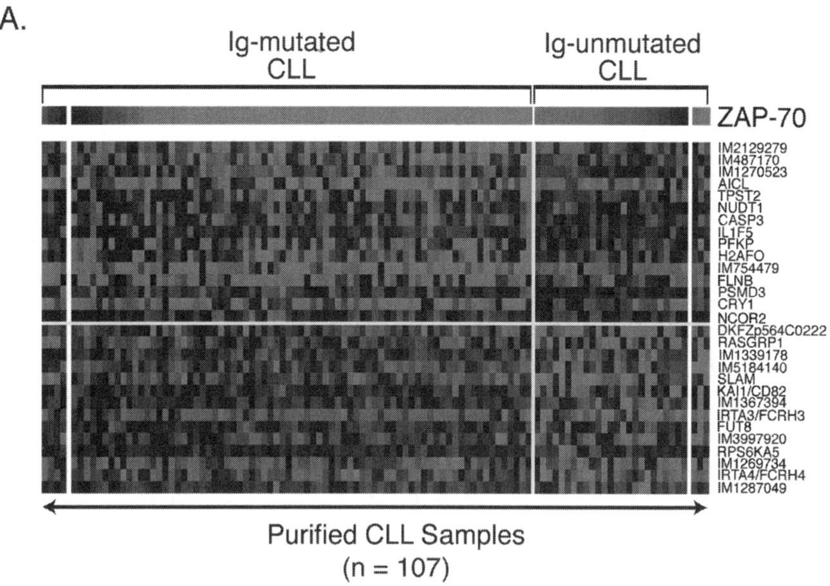

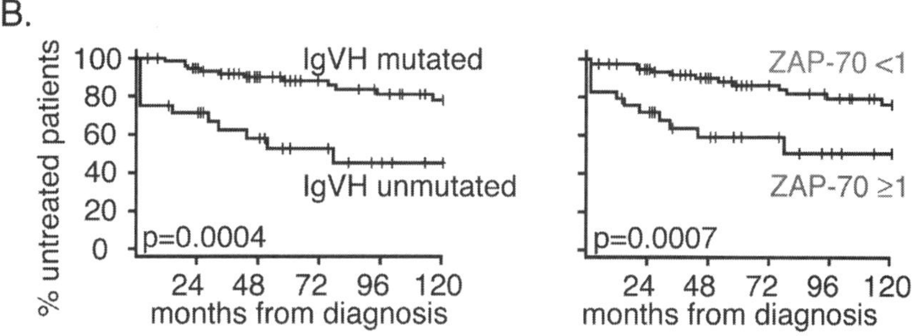

FIGURE 9.1 Genes that are differentially expressed between *Ig*-mutated and *Ig*-unmutated CLL and the effect of *ZAP-70* on prognosis. (A) The 30 most differentially expressed genes between *Ig*-mutated and *Ig*-unmutated CLL at a significance of $P < .00001$ are shown. Columns represent individual patients ($N = 107$) and rows represent individual genes. Patients are grouped by their *IgVH* mutational status and, within subtypes, are arranged by the relative expression level of *ZAP-70*, which is the best CLL subtype distinction gene. Patients discordant for *IgVH* mutation and *ZAP-70* expression appear at the left (*Ig*-mutated CLL, *ZAP-70* expression above cutoff) and right (*Ig*-unmutated CLL, *AZP-70* expression below cutoff) ends of the spectrum. Named genes are labeled with the gene symbols and IMAGE clone numbers (IM) are given for unnamed genes. The upper half contains genes more highly expressed in *Ig*-unmutated CLL and the lower half contains genes more highly expressed in *Ig*-mutated CLL. In each group, genes are arranged from top to bottom in descending order of statistical significance. (B) Effect of *IgVH* mutational status and *ZAP-70* expression on time to first treatment. *ZAP-70* expression was nearly equivalent to *IgVH* mutational status as a prognostic marker and may be developed as a diagnostic test.

were independent of other expression signatures, suggesting that they could be used to define different subsets (Fig. 9.2A).[38,46] To test this hypothesis, DCBCL cases were reclustered using only the GC B cell signature and this revealed two major branches that expressed to a varying degree, genes associated with germinal center B cells and activated B cells. These data suggested that DLBCL can be subdivided into cases derived from a germinal center B cell, termed a GC B cell-like (GCB), and an activated post-germinal center B cell, termed activated B cell-like (ABC) DLBCL. Genes associated with GCB DLBCL included known markers of germinal center differentiation such as *CD10* and the *bcl-6* genes, which may be translocated or mutated in DLBCL, as well as numerous new genes (Fig. 9.1A).[25] In contrast, most genes that defined ABC DLBCL were not expressed by normal GC B cells, but instead were induced during in vitro activation of peripheral B cells such as cyclin D2 and CD44. The ABC DLBCL signature also included the *IRF4* (*MUM1*) gene that is transiently induced during normal lymphocyte activation and is necessary for antigen receptor-driven B-cell proliferation (Fig. 9.1A).[50,51] A noteworthy feature of ABC DLBCL was the expression of two anti-apoptotic genes. These included *FLIP* (FLICE-like inhibitory protein), a dominant-negative mimic of caspase 8 that can block Fas-mediated apoptosis, and *bcl-2*, a prominent anti-apoptotic gene that is induced over 30-fold during peripheral B cell activation.[52] Indeed, most ABC DLBCLs had an over fourfold higher *bcl-2* expression than GCB DLBCLs, and there was no correlation with *bcl-2* translocation.[38]

These results suggest that the GCB and ABC DLBCL subtypes are derived from B cells at different stages of differentiation and are pathogenetically distinct. Support for this hypothesis comes from analysis of *IgVH* mutations, a process that occurs in B cells during the germinal center reaction. Although virtually all DLBCL cases harbor *IgVH* mutations, only the GCB cases exhibit ongoing somatic mutations, a characteristic of normal germinal center B cells, whereas the ABC cases do not carry intraclonal variations in their mutated *IgVH* genes, suggesting they are derived from normal B cells that have passed through the germinal center.[53] Furthermore, two recurrent oncogenic events, the t(14;18) translocation involving the *bcl-2* gene and amplification of the *c-rel* locus on chromosome 2p were exclusively found in the GCB subgroup, providing further evidence that the GCB and ABC subtypes represent different diseases with distinct mechanisms of lymphomagenesis. The association of t(14;18) translocation in DLBCL with the GCB subgroup was further validated by a study showing that 7 of 35 cases with the translocation had a GCB gene expression profile, and that six of these seven cases showed similar profiles among themselves.[54] There were also significant histological differences among the subgroups, with centroblastic monomorphic histology more common in the GCB subtype and centroblastic polymorphic and immunoblastic histologies more common in the ABC and type 3 subtypes.[55]

If this new taxonomy defines true DLBCL subtypes, one would also predict that it should have clinical prognostic value. Because all biopsies analyzed in this study were de novo DLBCL and came from untreated patients receiving doxorubicin-based chemotherapy, it was possible to correlate survival and the DLBCL subtype.[38,46] This analysis revealed a statistically significant difference in overall survival at five years of 59% in GCB and 31% in ABC subtypes of DLBCL (Fig. 9.2B). Furthermore, these subgroups were also statistically significant within each of the prognostic subgroups identified by the International Prognostic Index (IPI), indicating that the IPI and molecular profiling identify different features that influence survival. These results led to a larger study by Rosenwald et al in which samples from 240 patients with DLBCL were analyzed by molecular profiling and for the presence of genomic abnormalities.[55] This larger study reconfirmed the validity of the ABC and GCB taxonomy, and identified a third group, termed type 3, which did not highly express the genes associated with the former subtypes and did not appear to be a distinct DLBCL subtype. Using a supervised approach of the gene expression profiles from these cases, a molecular prognostic predictor was developed for DLBCL (Fig. 9.2C).[55] The final model combined four expression signatures that were defined by the GCB signature (favorable), MHC class II signature (favorable), lymph-node signature (favorable), and the proliferation signature (unfavorable) and expression of the bone morphogenetic protein 6 (*BMP6*) gene (unfavorable). To estimate survival outcome, each DLBCL case is assigned a score calculated from the weighted sum of these components and ranked in quartiles according to their scores (Fig. 9.2C). This model successfully predicted survival risk and was independent of the IPI.

Another study by Shipp et al undertook a similar goal to develop an outcome predictor using a different array chip that contained 6817 genes.[56] In this study of 58 patients, E2F and vascular endothelial grown factor (VEGF) were highly correlated with cured versus fatal/refractory disease, respectively; findings that are consistent with a previously known association with DLBCL outcome. Using a supervised approach, a highly accurate predictor containing 13 genes was able to discern patients likely to be cured from those who had fatal/refractory disease with a five-year overall survival of 70% versus 12%, respectively. This predictor, like the one described above, was independent of the IPI. Notably, three of the outcome predictor genes in this model, *NOR1*, *PDE4B*, and *PKC-β*, appear to play a role in chemotherapy response and cellular proliferation. The mitogen-inducible nuclear orphan receptor (NOR1) was overexpressed in cured patients, compared to fatal/refractory patients, and may increase the apoptotic response to chemotherapy.[57] In contrast, PDE4B, a cyclic AMP (cAMP)-specific phosphodiesterase, was increased in fatal/refractory patients. The *PDE4B* gene encodes for a protein that limits the inhibitory effects of cAMP protein kinase A (PKA) on cellular proliferation and cytokine release, and may be a useful therapeutic target.[58] PKC-β also was overexpressed in fatal/refractory patients and plays a central role in B cell signaling and survival.[59] Interestingly, Shipp et al were unable to validate the Rosenwald et al outcome prediction model (Fig. 9.2C) with their data set.[55,56] Although they identified the same two major clusters associated with cell of ori-

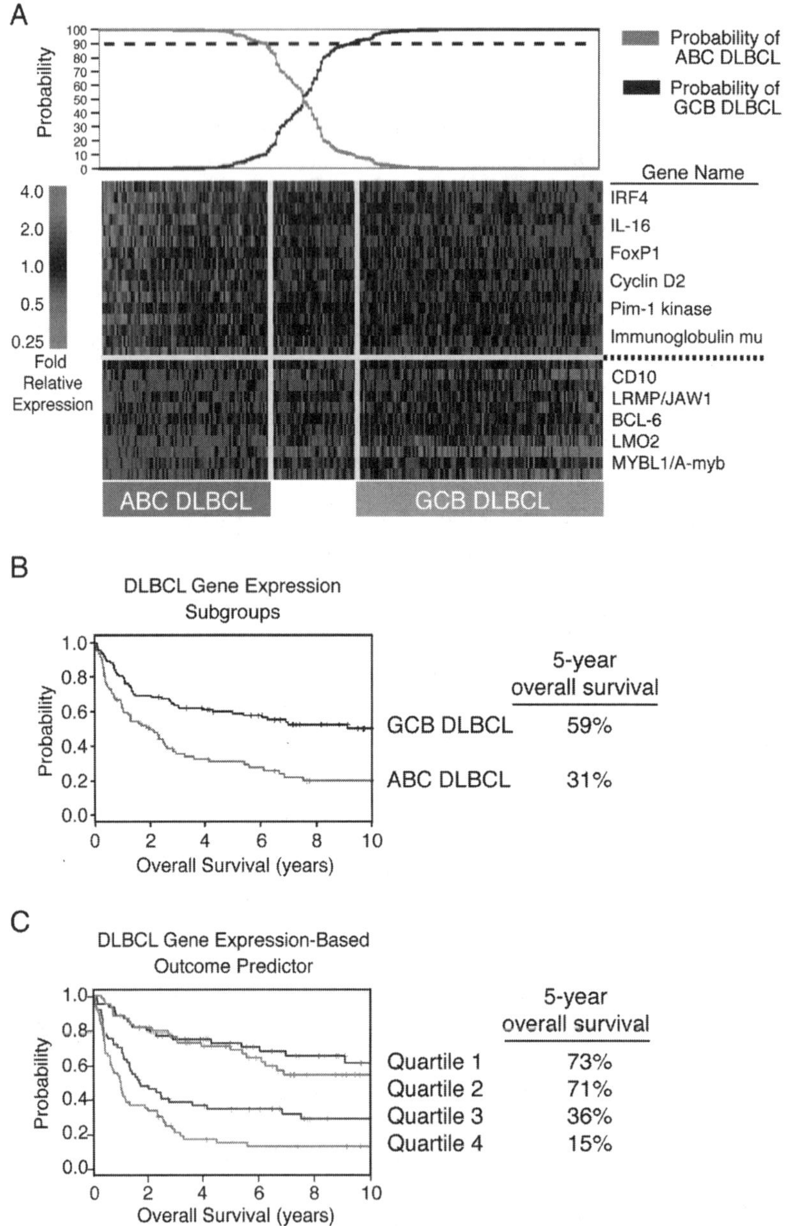

FIGURE 9.2 Diagnosis of DLBCL subtypes by gene expression and development of a molecular outcome predictor in previously untreated patients with DLBCL following chemotherapy. (A) The expression levels of 27 genes from the subgroup predictor in 274 DLBCL samples are shown according to the color scale at the left. Six named genes that showed increased expression in either the ABC or GCB subgroups are shown at the right. The likelihood that a DLBCL sample belongs to the ABC or GCB subgroup is shown on top and is arranged by probability. (B) Kaplan-Meier estimates of overall survival are shown according to GCB or ABC DLBCL subtype. (C) Kaplan-Meier estimates of overall survival according to the molecular outcome predictor are shown for each quartile.

gin, this distinction did not significantly correlate with patient outcome, calling into question the biological validity of the GCB and ABC DLBCL taxonomy. A reanalysis of this data set, however, using the most discriminating genes showed a significant correlation between the GCB and ABC DLBCL subtypes and outcome, and reconfirmed the validity of the original observation.[36,55]

Further confirmation for the cell of origin taxonomy for DLBCL was provided by a recent study employing tissue microarray (TMA).[60] In this study, 142 DLBCL cases were stained with antibodies associated with the germinal center, CD10, *bcl-6*, or post-germinal center, MUM1, and categorized as either of GCB or non-GCB origin. Overall, 42% of cases were considered GCB and 58% non-GCB, with five-year overall survivals of 76% and 34%, respectively. Notably, when compared to the molecular profiling classification, the sensitivity of TMA was 71% for the GCB and 88% for the non-GCB groups. Furthermore, within the non-GCB group, expression of *bcl-2* was an adverse predictor, a finding consistent with previous immunohistochemical studies and the gene expression predictor.[7,55] These results indicate that *bcl-2* overexpression is only unfavorable when associated with non-GCB DLBCL subtypes, suggesting that *bcl-2* is a surrogate marker for the unfavorable non-GCB subtypes and alone may not be a significant cause of treatment failure in DLBCL.

Molecular profiling also has been applied to primary mediastinal B cell lymphoma (PMBL), an important subtype of DLBCL that mostly occurs in young patients.[61] This subtype is defined by a combination of clinical and pathological features and some cases may have pathological features reminiscent of Hodgkin's lymphoma, all of which can confound an accurate diagnosis.[23,62] Two recent studies using molecular profiling have confirmed the unique biological identity of PMBL and have shown a strong relationship between PMBL and Hodgkin's lymphoma.[63,64] Cases of PMBL could be identified accurately by a model using 35 genes that were more highly expressed in PMBL and 11 genes that were more highly expressed in DLBCL.[63] When this model was applied to 46 patients with a diagnosis of PMBL, 76% were classified as PMBL. Of the remaining 11 cases, however, seven and four were classified as belonging to the GCB and ABC DLBCL subtypes, respectively, indicating that, although these latter cases predominantly involved the mediastinum, they were not PMBL. Clinically, cases identified as PMBL by gene expression appeared to have a relatively favorable five-year survival of 64% compared to 59% and 30%, respectively, for the GCB and ABC DLBCL subtypes.

Not surprisingly, the gene expression of PMBL revealed an intriguing relationship to Hodgkin's lymphoma. Over one third of the PMBL signature genes were more highly expressed by Hodgkin's lymphoma cell lines than by GCB DLBCL cell lines, and five of these signature genes, *MAL*, *SNFT*, *TNFRSF6*, *TARC*, and *CD30*, are expressed as proteins in Reed-Sternberg cells.[65,66] Furthermore, over half of PMBL cases and three Hodgkin's lymphoma cell lines had gains/amplifications in a region of chromosome 9p. There were, however, important differences between PMBL and Hodgkin's lymphoma. A subset of PMBL signature genes were not highly expressed in Hodgkin's lymphoma cell lines and the down-regulation of mature B-cell genes, characteristic of Hodgkin's lymphomas, was not observed in PMBL. This important molecular link between PMBL and Hodgkin's lymphoma has been demonstrated also by another recent study.[64] These studies clearly demonstrate that the clinical heterogeneity of DLBCL is reflected by important differences in gene expression profiles, and provide a new taxonomy in which at least three molecularly and clinical distinct subtypes, GCB, ABC, and PMBL, can be discerned.

Mantle cell lymphoma (MCL), while relatively uncommon, is both aggressive and incurable with a median survival of three to four years.[33] To help gain insights into its pathogenesis with an aim of identifying new therapeutic targets and of predicting survival outcome, a study of 101 cases was undertaken.[67] A supervised approach to discover genes associated with survival found that 58% of the predictor genes were associated with cellular proliferation, with higher expression of this signature being associated with worse overall survival (Fig. 9.3A). By using a quantitative measure of tumor cell proliferation, a predictive model was developed that subdivided patients into quartiles with median survival times of 0.8, 2.3, 3.3, and 6.7 years (Fig. 9.3B). To further elucidate molecular mechanisms of survival, a search for oncogenic events that might explain the variable proliferation was undertaken. In some of the more proliferative MCL cases, there were higher levels of *cyclin D1* mRNA due to the preferential expression of a more stable isoform, and more common deletions of the *INK4a/ARF* locus, which encodes the $p16^{INK4a}$ and $p14^{ARF}$ tumor suppressors. Although both of these oncogenic events were independently associated with shorter survival, they were not as predictive as the proliferation signature alone.[67,68] Deletions at the *p53* and ATM (ataxia telangiectasia mutation) loci also were noted in some cases, but were not correlated with the tumor proliferation signature.[68] Hence, the proliferation signature is a quantitative integrator of multiple oncogenic events that influences survival of MCL.

CLINICAL APPLICATION OF MOLECULAR PROFILING

Molecular profiling in lymphomas has numerous immediate clinical applications as well as an enormous potential to identify new therapeutic targets. The practical clinical application of this technology, however, is presently limited by the lack of appropriate "diagnostic" array chips and the routine collection and storage of fresh biopsy material. Additionally, there is a need for the validation of molecular profiling in prospective studies. Current applications include the following:

1. Molecular profiling may be used to improve the accuracy of pathological diagnoses. As the complexity of the pathological classification systems increases, the diagnostic error rate likely will rise. Indeed, the use of specialized "diagnostic" chips should significantly increase diagnostic reliability, both by serving as a diagnostic check and by assisting with borderline cases. In addi-

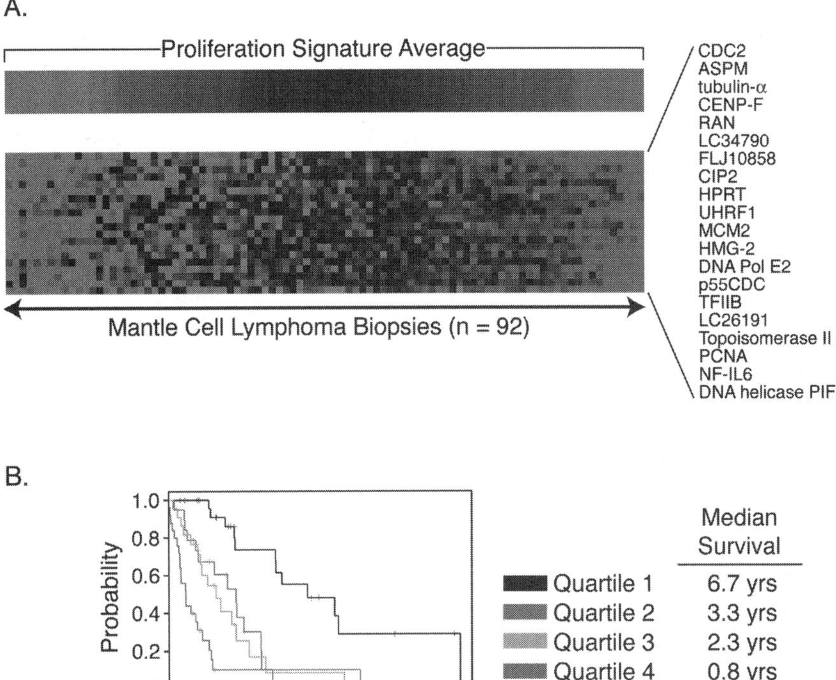

FIGURE 9.3 Gene expression-based predictor of survival in mantle cell lymphoma. (A) Expression of 20 proliferation signature genes used to compute the proliferation signature average is shown. Cases are ordered according to their proliferation signature average. The color scale depicts a fourfold range in gene expression. (B) Kaplan-Meier estimates of overall survival according to the molecular outcome predictor are shown for each quartile. Only the proliferation signature contributed to the outcome prediction.

tion, such chips will be required to identify diagnostic categories based on molecular profiling. Furthermore, microarray profiling has provided a new classification taxonomy, as exemplified by the GCB, ABC, and PMBL DLBCL subtypes, and this should be incorporated into new clinical trials.

2. Molecular profiling is a biologically based predictor of outcome, which is independent of clinical prognostic indices, as shown in Figures 9.1A, 9.2B, 9.2C, and 9.3B.[36,40,55,56,63,67] Unlike prognostic models based exclusively on clinical features, molecular profiling models are a direct measure of biological events. As such, when applied to new therapeutic regimens, molecular profiling models can provide insight into the molecular mechanisms of treatment outcome and identify future therapeutic targets. An example of its

potential application comes from several studies. Two recent reports found that the benefit of rituximab in DLBCL is primarily restricted to tumors expressing *bcl-2*, suggesting that rituximab may overcome the adverse effects of the ABC subtype, where the unfavorable effect of *bcl-2* is found.[69,70] In another study, it was found that the DLBCL proliferation rate, as measured by *Ki-67/MIB-1*, did not adversely affect outcome with the dose-adjusted (DA)-EPOCH infusional regimen, suggesting that infusional chemotherapy may overcome the adverse effects of the proliferation signature.[68] To test these findings and to prospectively validate the use of microarray profiling, a phase III randomized study is planned to compare bolus treatment with CHOP to infusional treatment with DA-EPOCH with the addition of rituximab in both arms. Tumor samples will be analyzed by microarray profiling to assess the molecular predictors of outcome in the hope of identifying regimen specific predictors and future therapeutic directions.

3. By elucidating pertinent pathways of lymphomagenesis, molecular profiling may identify clinically useful targets, including those for therapeutic development. For example, microarray profiling showed that *ZAP 70* expression was highly correlated with the Ig-unmutated CLL subtype (Fig. 9.1B).[46,71,72] This led to the validation of *ZAP 70* as a marker of Ig-unmutated CLL and its potential development as a diagnostic test.[71,72] Microarray profiling also has identified potential therapeutic targets. Shipp et al highlighted the potential importance of PKC-β as a therapeutic target in DLBCL.[56] Molecular profiling in DLBCL also revealed a high expression of *NF-κB* target genes in the ABC, but not the GCB DLBCL subtypes, as shown in Figure 9.4.[55,73] *NF-κB* signaling interferes with apoptotic cell death triggered by chemother-

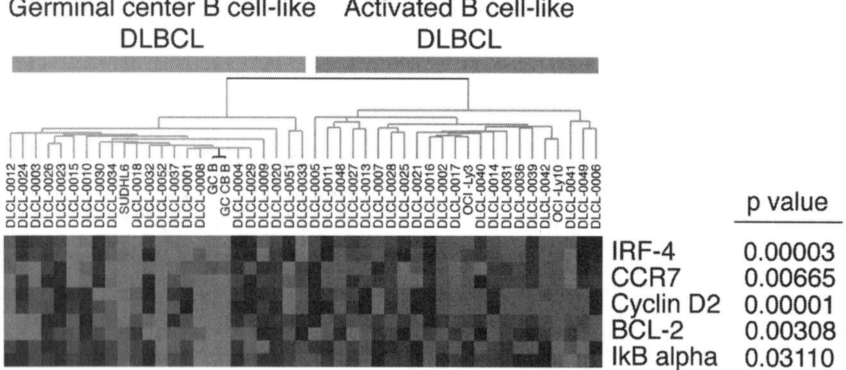

FIGURE 9.4 Gene expression analysis of NF-κB target genes according to GCB and ABC DLBCL subtype. The relative expression of the *bcl-2* gene is increased in the ABC subtype, along with other NF-kB target genes.

apeutic agents, and its inhibition in ABC-like DLBCL cell lines was cytotoxic, whereas GCB-like cell lines were unaffected.[73] *NF-κB* also is constitutively activated in mantle cell lymphoma and its inhibition leads to cell cycle arrest and apoptosis.[74] Bortezomib, a proteasome inhibitor, acts to downregulate the *NF-κB* pathway and may enhance the cytotoxicity of chemotherapy in ABC DLBCL and mantle cell lymphomas.[75] Clinical trials are in progress to evaluate bortezomib in these settings.

REFERENCES

1. Harris NL, Jaffe ES, Stein H et al. A revised European-American classification of lymphoid neoplasms: a proposal from the International Lymphoma Study Group. Blood 1994;84:1361–1392.
2. Jaffe ES, Harris NL, Diebold J, Muller-Hermelink HK. World Health Organization classification of neoplastic diseases of the hematopoietic and lymphoid tissues. A progress report. Am J Clin Pathol 1999;111:S8–S12.
3. Tilly H, Rossi A, Stamatoullas A et al. Prognostic value of chromosomal abnormalities in follicular lymphoma. Blood 1994;84:1043–1049.
4. Knauf WU, Knuutila S, Zeigmeister B, Thiel E. Trisomy 12 in B-cell chronic lymphocytic leukemia: correlation with advanced disease, atypical morphology, high levels of sCD25, and with refractoriness to treatment. Leuk Lymphoma 1995;19:289–294.
5. Dohner H, Stilgenbauer S, Dohner K et al. Chromosome aberrations in B-cell chronic lymphocytic leukemia: reassessment based on molecular cytogenetic analysis. J Mol Med 1999;77:266–281.
6. Ueda C, Akasaka T, Ohno H. Non-immunoglobulin/BCL6 gene fusion in diffuse large B-cell lymphoma: prognostic implications. Leuk Lymphoma 2002;43:1375–1381.
7. Gascoyne RD, Adomat SA, Krajewski S et al. Prognostic significance of Bcl-2 protein expression and Bcl-2 gene rearrangement in diffuse aggressive non-Hodgkin's lymphoma. Blood 1997;90:244–251.
8. Wilson WH, Grossbard ML, Pittaluga S et al. Dose-adjusted EPOCH chemotherapy for untreated large B-cell lymphomas: a pharmacodynamic approach with high efficacy. Blood 2002;99:2685–2693.
9. Ichikawa A, Kinoshita T, Watanabe T et al. Mutations of the p53 gene as a prognostic factor in aggressive B-cell lymphoma. N Engl J Med 1997;337:529–534.
10. Bosch F, Jares P, Campo E et al. PRAD-1/cyclin D1 gene overexpression in chronic lymphoproliferative disorders: a highly specific marker of mantle cell lymphoma. Blood 1994;84:2726–2732.
11. Raty R, Franssila K, Jansson SE et al. Predictive factors for blastoid transformation in the common variant of mantle cell lymphoma. Eur J Cancer 2003;39:321–329.
12. Cleary ML, Sklar J. Nucleotide sequence of a t(14;18) chromosomal breakpoint in follicular lymphoma and demonstration of a breakpoint-cluster region near a transcriptionally active locus on chromosome 18. Proc Natl Acad Sci USA 1985;82:7439–7443.
13. Weiss LM, Warnke RA, Sklar J, Cleary ML. Molecular analysis of the t(14;18) chromosomal translocation in malignant lymphomas. N Engl J Med 1987;317:1185–1189.
14. McDonnell TJ, Deane N, Platt FM et al. bcl-2-immunoglobulin transgenic mice demonstrate extended B cell survival and follicular lymphoproliferation. Cell 1989;57:79–88.
15. Lai R, Arber DA, Chang KL et al. Frequency of bcl-2 expression in non-Hodgkin's lymphoma: a study of 778 cases with comparison of marginal zone lymphoma and monocytoid B-cell hyperplasia. Mod Pathol 1998;11:864–869.

16. Wilson WH, Teruya-Feldstein J, Fest T et al. Relationship of p53, bcl-2, and tumor proliferation to clinical drug resistance in non-Hodgkin's lymphomas. Blood 1997;89:601–609.

17. Gaidano G, Newcomb EW, Gong JZ et al. Analysis of alterations of oncogenes and tumor suppressor genes in chronic lymphocytic leukemia. Am J Pathol 1994;144:1312–1319.

18. Matutes E, Oscier D, Garcia-Marco J et al. Trisomy 12 defines a group of CLL with atypical morphology: correlation between cytogenetic, clinical and laboratory features in 544 patients. Br J Haematol 1996;92:382–388.

19. Sturm I, Bosanquet AG, Hermann S et al. Mutation of p53 and consecutive selective drug resistance in B-CLL occurs as a consequence of prior DNA-damaging chemotherapy. Cell Death Differ 2003;10:477–484.

20. Nakamura N, Abe M. Richter syndrome in B-cell chronic lymphocytic leukemia. Pathol Int 2003;53:195–203.

21. Hamblin TJ, Davis Z, Gardiner A et al. Unmutated Ig V(H) genes are associated with a more aggressive form of chronic lymphocytic leukemia. Blood 1999;94:1848–1854.

22. A clinical evaluation of the International Lymphoma Study Group classification of non-Hodgkin's lymphoma. The Non-Hodgkin's Lymphoma Classification Project. Blood 1997;89: 3909–3918.

23. Jaffe ES, Harris NL, Stein H, Vardiman JW, eds. Tumours of haematopoietic and lymphoid tissues. In World Health Organization Classification of Tumours. Lyon, France: IARC Press, 2001.

24. Martinez-Climent JA, Alizadeh AA, Segraves R et al. Transformation of follicular lymphoma to diffuse large cell lymphoma is associated with a heterogeneous set of DNA copy number and gene expression alterations. Blood 2003;101:3109–3117.

25. Dalla-Favera R, Migliazza A, Chang CC et al. Molecular pathogenesis of B cell malignancy: the role of BCL-6. Curr Top Microbiol Immunol 1999;246:257–263; discussion 263–255.

26. Pasqualucci L, Migliazza A, Fracchiolla N et al. BCL-6 mutations in normal germinal center B cells: Evidence of somatic hypermutation acting outside Ig loci. PNAS 1998;95:11816–11821.

27. Colomo L, Lopez-Guillermo A, Perales M et al. Clinical impact of the differentiation profile assessed by immunophenotyping in patients with diffuse large B-cell lymphoma. Blood 2003; 101:78–84.

28. Barrans SL, Carter I, Owen RG et al. Germinal center phenotype and bcl-2 expression combined with the International Prognostic Index improves patient risk stratification in diffuse large B-cell lymphoma. Blood 2002;99:1136–1143.

29. Hill ME, MacLennan KA, Cunningham DC et al. Prognostic significance of BCL-2 expression and bcl-2 major breakpoint region rearrangement in diffuse large cell non-Hodgkin's lymphoma: a British National Lymphoma Investigation Study. Blood 1996;88:1046–1051.

30. Copie-Bergman C, Plonquet A, Alonso MA et al. MAL expression in lymphoid cells: further evidence for MAL as a distinct molecular marker of primary mediastinal large B-cell lymphomas. Mod Pathol 2002;15:1172–1180.

31. Joos S, Otano-Joos MI, Ziegler S et al. Primary mediastinal (thymic) B-cell lymphoma is characterized by gains of chromosomal material including 9p and amplification of the REL gene. Blood 1996;87:1571–1578.

32. Dreyling MH, Bullinger L, Ott G et al. Alterations of the cyclin D1/p16-pRB pathway in mantle cell lymphoma. Cancer Res 1997;57:4608–4614.

33. Barista I, Romaguera JE, Cabanillas F. Mantle-cell lymphoma. Lancet Oncol 2001;2:141–148.

34. Fisher RI, Gaynor ER, Dahlberg S et al. Comparison of a standard regimen (CHOP) with three intensive chemotherapy regimens for advanced non-Hodgkin's lymphoma. N Engl J Med 1993;328:1002–1006.

35. Alizadeh A, Eisen M, Botstein D et al. Probing lymphocyte biology by genomic-scale gene expression analysis. J Clin Immunol 1998;18:373–379.

36. Wright G, Tan B, Rosenwald A et al. A gene expression-based method to diagnose clinically distinct subgroups of diffuse large B cell lymphoma. Proc Natl Acad Sci USA 2003;100:9991–9996.

37. Sander CA, Yano T, Clark HM et al. p53 mutation is associated with progression in follicular lymphomas. Blood 1993;82:1994–2004.

38. Alizadeh AA, Eisen MB, Davis RE et al. Distinct types of diffuse large B-cell lymphoma identified by gene expression profiling. Nature 2000;403:503–511.

39. Bahler DW, Levy R. Clonal evolution of a follicular lymphoma: evidence for antigen selection. Proc Natl Acad Sci USA 1992;89:6770–6774.

40. Dave SS WG, Tan B, et al. A molecular predictor of survival following diagnosis of follicular lymphoma. Blood 2003;102:617a.

41. Bohen SP, Troyanskaya OG, Alter O et al. Variation in gene expression patterns in follicular lymphoma and the response to rituximab. Proc Natl Acad Sci USA 2003;100:1926–1930.

42. de Vos S, Hofmann WK, Grogan TM et al. Gene expression profile of serial samples of transformed B-cell lymphomas. Lab Invest 2003;83:271–285.

43. Lossos IS, Alizadeh AA, Diehn M et al. Transformation of follicular lymphoma to diffuse large-cell lymphoma: alternative patterns with increased or decreased expression of c-myc and its regulated genes. Proc Natl Acad Sci USA 2002;99:8886–8891.

44. Martinez-Climent JA, Alizadeh AA, Segraves R et al. Transformation of follicular lymphoma to diffuse large cell lymphoma is associated with a heterogeneous set of DNA copy number and gene expression alterations. Blood 2003;101:3109–3117.

45. Rosenwald A, Alizadeh AA, Widhopf G et al. Relation of gene expression phenotype to immunoglobulin mutation genotype in B cell chronic lymphocytic leukemia. J Exp Med 2001; 194:1639–1647.

46. Wiestner A, Staudt LM. Towards a molecular diagnosis and targeted therapy of lymphoid malignancies. Semin Hematol 2003;40:296–307.

47. Chu DH, Morita CT, Weiss A. The Syk family of protein tyrosine kinases in T-cell activation and development. Immunol Rev 1998;165:167–180.

48. Turner M, Schweighoffer E, Colucci F et al. Tyrosine kinase SYK: essential functions for immunoreceptor signalling. Immunol Today 2000;21:148–154.

49. The International Non-Hodgkin's Lymphoma Prognostic Factors Project. A predictive model for aggressive non-Hodgkin's lymphoma. N Engl J Med 1993;329:987–994.

50. Matsuyama T, Grossman A, Mittrucker HW et al. Molecular cloning of LSIRF, a lymphoid-specific member of the interferon regulatory factor family that binds the interferon-stimulated response element (ISRE). Nucl Acids Res 1995;23:2127–2136.

51. Mittrucker HW, Matsuyama T, Grossman A et al. Requirement for the transcription factor LSIRF/IRF4 for mature B and T lymphocyte function. Science 1997;275:540–543.

52. Tschopp J, Irmler M, Thome M. Inhibition of fas death signals by FLIPs. Curr Opin Immunol 1998;10:552–558.

53. Lossos IS, Alizadeh AA, Eisen MB et al. Ongoing immunoglobulin somatic mutation in germinal center B cell-like but not in activated B cell-like diffuse large cell lymphomas. Proc Natl Acad Sci USA 2000;97:10209–10213.

54. Huang JZ, Sanger WG, Greiner TC et al. The t(14;18) defines a unique subset of diffuse large B-cell lymphoma with a germinal center B-cell gene expression profile. Blood 2002;99:2285–2290.

55. Rosenwald A, Wright G, Chan WC et al. The use of molecular profiling to predict survival after chemotherapy for diffuse large-B-cell lymphoma. N Engl J Med 2002;346:1937–1947.

56. Shipp MA, Ross KN, Tamayo P et al. Diffuse large B-cell lymphoma outcome prediction by gene-expression profiling and supervised machine learning. Nat Med 2002;8:68–74.

57. Brenner C, Kroemer G. Apoptosis. Mitochondria—the death signal integrators. Science 2000; 289:1150–1151.

58. Manning CD, Burman M, Christensen SB et al. Suppression of human inflammatory cell function by subtype-selective PDE4 inhibitors correlates with inhibition of PDE4A and PDE4B. Br J Pharmacol 1999;128:1393–1398.

59. Leitges M, Schmedt C, Guinamard R et al. Immunodeficiency in protein kinase cbeta-deficient mice. Science 1996;273:788–791.

60. Hans CP, Weisenburger DD, Greiner TC et al. Confirmation of the molecular classification of diffuse large B-cell lymphoma by immunohistochemistry using a tissue microarray. Blood 2004;103:275–282.

61. Abou-Elella AA, Weisenburger DD, Vose JM et al. Primary mediastinal large B-cell lymphoma: a clinicopathologic study of 43 patients from the Nebraska Lymphoma Study Group. J Clin Oncol 1999;17:784–790.

62. Gonzalez CL, Medeiros LJ, Jaffe ES. Composite lymphoma. A clinicopathologic analysis of nine patients with Hodgkin's disease and B-cell non-Hodgkin's lymphoma. Am J Clin Pathol 1991;96:81–89.

63. Rosenwald A, Wright G, Leroy K et al. Molecular diagnosis of primary mediastinal B cell lymphoma identifies a clinically favorable subgroup of diffuse large B cell lymphoma related to Hodgkin lymphoma. J Exp Med 2003;198:851–862.

64. Savage KJ, Monti S, Kutok JL et al. The molecular signature of mediastinal large B-cell lymphoma differs from that of other diffuse large B-cell lymphomas and shares features with classical Hodgkin's lymphoma. Blood 2003;102:3871–3879.

65. Stein H, Gerdes J, Schwab U et al. Evidence for the detection of the normal counterpart of Hodgkin and Sternberg-Reed cells. Hematol Oncol 1983;1:21–29.

66. Peh SC, Kim LH, Poppema S. TARC, a CC chemokine, is frequently expressed in classic Hodgkin's lymphoma but not in NLP Hodgkin's lymphoma, T-cell-rich B-cell lymphoma, and most cases of anaplastic large cell lymphoma. Am J Surg Pathol 2001;25:925–929.

67. Rosenwald A, Wright G, Wiestner A et al. The proliferation gene expression signature is a quantitative integrator of oncogenic events that predicts survival in mantle cell lymphoma. Cancer Cell 2003;3:185–197.

68. Fang NY, Greiner TC, Weisenburger DD et al. Oligonucleotide microarrays demonstrate the highest frequency of ATM mutations in the mantle cell subtype of lymphoma. Proc Natl Acad Sci USA 2003;100:5372–5377.

69. Wilson W. PS, O'Connor P, Hegde U et al. Rituximab may overcome BCL-2-associated chemotherapy resistance in untreated diffuse large B-cell lymphomas. Proc Am Soc Hematol 99:2001.

70. Mounier N, Briere J, Gisselbrecht C et al. Rituximab plus CHOP (R-CHOP) overcomes bcl-2–associated resistance to chemotherapy in elderly patients with diffuse large B-cell lymphoma (DLBCL). Blood 2003;101:4279–4284.

71. Wiestner A, Rosenwald A, Barry TS et al. ZAP-70 expression identifies a chronic lymphocytic leukemia subtype with unmutated immunoglobulin genes, inferior clinical outcome, and distinct gene expression profile. Blood 2003;101:4944–4951.

72. Crespo M, Bosch F, Villamor N et al. ZAP-70 expression as a surrogate for immunoglobulin-variable-region mutations in chronic lymphocytic leukemia. N Engl J Med 2003;348:1764–1775.

73. Davis RE, Brown KD, Siebenlist U, Staudt LM. Constitutive nuclear factor kappaB activity is required for survival of activated B cell-like diffuse large B cell lymphoma cells. J Exp Med 2001;194:1861–1874.

74. Pham LV, Tamayo AT, Yoshimura LC et al. Inhibition of constitutive NF-kappa B activation in mantle cell lymphoma B cells leads to induction of cell cycle arrest and apoptosis. J Immunol 2003;171:88–95.

75. Adams J. Proteasome inhibition in cancer: development of PS-341. Semin Oncol 2001;28:613–619.

Chapter 10

Chemotherapy Combined with Monoclonal Antibodies in the Treatment of Patients with Diffuse Large B-cell Lymphoma

Bertrand Coiffier

The use of monoclonal antibodies (mAb) for the treatment of patients with lymphoma was initiated about seven years ago. They first were developed for the so-called "low-grade" or indolent lymphomas.[1] Murine antibodies have been used with toxin or isotopes attached to them[2–4] where the antibody is used to specifically transport the active agent, often a radionucleide, to lymphoma cells. In the case of unmodified, naked monoclonal antibodies, such as rituximab, the chimeric human-mouse antibody fixes the antigen on the membrane of lymphoma cells with the murine antibody part and stimulates the immune host mechanisms through the human Fc part. The action of fixing the antigen on the cell surface also may trigger a cascade of biologic events leading to the cell death through the apoptotic process.

Rituximab (Rituxan®, MabThera®) was the first monoclonal antibody developed with activity by itself and it has revolutionized the therapy of B-cell lymphomas. In vitro data have shown that this unconjugated antibody can induce lymphoma cell lysis through activation of the complement cascade (complement-dependent cytolysis or CDC) and/or activation of immune cells through the Fc fixation (antibody-dependent cell cytolysis or ADCC).[5,6] These immune mechanisms were thought to be effective only in low proliferating tumor; thus, the different phase I and phase II studies that were realized during the first five years only included patients with indolent lymphoma. However, this activity recently was demonstrated in more aggressive lymphomas such as mantle cell lymphoma (MCL) and diffuse large B-cell lymphoma (DLCL).[7,8] With such a good activity observed with rituximab, several mAb were developed for the treatment of patients with lymphoma (Table 10.1).

RATIONALE FOR THE USE OF MONOCLONAL ANTIBODIES IN LYMPHOMA PATIENTS

Three main approaches have been used in the development of mAb therapy. Unconjugated antibodies mediate cell death through different mechanisms related to the antigen and the antibodies. Conjugated antibodies act mainly through the toxin or the radioisotope attached to the antibody. The selection of a suitable antigen was the first step for these treatments. Criteria were that the antigen must not be shared by critical tissues such as hematopoietic stem cells, must not be associated with much toxicity if all target cells are eliminated, and be present only on lymphoma cells. Unfortunately, specific antigens for B or T lymphoma cells are unknown and all antigens currently known are shared by the normal B or T cells.

TABLE 10.1 Monoclonal Antibodies Used in the Treatment of Patients with Lymphoma

Antibody	Antigen	Conjugate	Major studies
Rituximab (MabThera, Rituxan)	CD20	None	Maloney et al[5] Coiffier et al[9]
Alemtuzumab (Campath)	CD52	None	Keating et al[10] Lundin et al[11]
Epratuzumab (Lymphocide)	CD22	None	Leonard et al[12]
Hu1D10	HLA-DR	None	Shi et al[13]
Ibritumomab tiuxetan (Zevalin)	CD20	Y-90	Gordon et al[14] Witzig et al[15]
Tositumomab (Bexxar)	CD20	^{131}I	Kaminski et al[16] Vose et al[17]
Denileukin diftitox (Ontak)	IL-2R	Diphtheria toxin	Olsen et al[18]

The target antigen must be present either on all lymphoma cells or on the self-renewing clonogenic population of lymphoma cells. Lymphoma cells should not be able to escape the antibody effect through the development of antigen variants, antigen-negative clones, or the modulation of the antigen on the cell surface. If mAb-toxin conjugates need to be internalized for the toxin to access the critical cellular processes, unconjugated mAb must remain on the cell surface to allow the Fc portion of the antibody to activate immunologic mechanisms or to activate internal mechanisms leading to cell death. Unconjugated mAb may have direct cytotoxic effects on tumor cells, either in blocking the binding of an endogenous ligand, which deprives the cell of a critical survival signal, or in mimicking it, which triggers growth arrest. These functions may potentiate the effects of chemotherapy.[19–23] Humanized mAb have a greater efficiency than mouse mAb for activating these immunologic mechanisms. Antigen density and mAb binding affinity may influence the cytotoxic efficacy for unconjugated antibodies but radioimmunoconjugates emit particles with enough energy to kill adjacent cells, cells with a low antigen density, or non-antigen-bearing cells. However, they may kill vital normal cells and increase the toxicity of the treatment.

The presence of circulating antigens may be a problem leading to the formation of antigen-antibody complexes and a rapid clearance of the mAb. The mAb must not be eliminated through immunologic mechanisms because of its own difference with the host. When xenophobic (mouse) antibodies are used, a rapid appearance of human anti-mouse antibodies (HAMA) may alter the pharmacokinetics of the mAb, particularly during the re-treatment phases. Genetic engineering has allowed the humanization of antibodies and has created chimeric proteins with a small antigen-binding mouse part and a large human constant Fc region. These chimeric mAb have substantially decreased their immunogenicity, and then prolonged their half-lives. They also improve the ability to mediate complement-dependent cytotoxicity (CDC) and antibody-dependent cell-mediated cytotoxicity (ADCC).

A large variety of antigens potentially can be chosen as the target (Table 10.1). If the early trials focused on Ig idiotype, the CD20 antigen is probably the ideal target for B-cell lymphomas, but other antigens are currently being tested, such as CD22 or CD52.[24,25] The CD20 antigen is not expressed on stem cells or precursor B-cells, but is found on normal mature B-cells and malignant B-cells, with the exception of plasma cells and myeloma cells. It is usually present on all cells of the tumor clone. It is expressed in high density in all B-cell lymphoma, but usually faintly on chronic lymphocytic leukemia cells. This antigen is stable in the membrane of B-cell, does not have any known variant, and does not modulate or internalize in response to antibody binding.

Currently, several mAb have been largely used clinically (Table 10.1): humanized chimeric antibody directed against CD20 antigen (rituximab), CD22 antigen (epratuzumab), or CD52 antigen (alemtuzumab), mouse antibodies conjugated with radioisotope, or immunotoxin. Tositumomab (previously referred to as anti-B1 antibody) is a mouse immunoglobulin G2a monoclonal antibody specific for CD20 labeled with iodine-131 (^{131}I tositumomab or Bexxar) and yttrium-90 ibritumomab tiuxetan (IDEC-Y2B8 or Zevalin) is a murine immunoglobulin G_1 kappa monoclonal antibody that covalently binds MX-DTPA (tiuxetan), which chelates the radioisotope yttrium-90. Denileukin diftitox (DAB_{389} IL-2, Ontak) is not really a monoclonal antibody, but a novel recombinant fusion protein consisting of peptide sequences of the membrane translocation domains of diphtheria toxin and human interleukin-2 (IL-2). This gene results in the production of a single polypeptide chain that is capable of inhibiting protein synthesis in cells that express the IL-2 receptor, resulting in cell death. This immunotoxin only has shown activity in cutaneous T-cell lymphomas. A few other monoclonal antibodies directed against other antigens such as ferritin, human lymphocyte antigen (HLA), or other B cell or T cell markers are currently in early testing, but it is too early to have significant results.

RITUXIMAB ALONE FOR THE TREATMENT OF LYMPHOMAS

The first studies with mAb were done on patients with relapsing or refractory indolent lymphomas, mostly follicular.[26] These data demonstrated the good efficacy of rituximab and its safety in patients already being treated with multiple chemotherapy regimens. For mantle cell lymphoma (MCL), two European studies with rituximab showed a response rate in naïve or pretreated patients between 35% and 40%, with 10% to 15% complete responses.[27,28] However, the median duration of the response was only 12 months, even in patients with a very good response.

The first study evaluating the response rate in patients with aggressive lymphoma (DLCL or MCL) patients was conducted in Europe in 1998.[8] This study included patients in first or second relapses with "intermediate or high-grade lymphoma" according to the Working Formulation.[29] Nine elderly patients not previously treated were included. Five patients reached a complete remission (CR) and 12 a partial remission (PR) for an overall response rate of 32%, without a difference between the two doses. The response rate was higher in patients in a first or second relapse than in primary refractory patients and in those with smaller tumors. This study showed that more aggressive lymphomas than follicular lymphoma may respond to rituximab therapy, and it opened the development of rituximab therapy in all types of B cell lymphomas. Recently, promising results were presented with rituximab alone in 17 patients with aggressive lymphoma who either failed or relapsed after high-dose therapy and autotransplant.[30] The median time from autotransplant to relapse was 10 months (range 2 to 48 months) and the median number of prior therapies was three (range 2–6). The overall response rate to rituximab was 53% with four CR (24%) and five PR

(29%), 54% in DLCL patients (3 CR, 4 PR), and 50% in MCL patients (1 CR, 1 PR). Median progression-free survival for all responders was 10 months. These encouraging results must be confirmed in a larger group of patients.

The experience with other unconjugated mAb is limited except for alemtuzumab, which has been widely used in chronic lymphocytic leukemia (CLL) and prolymphocytic leukemia.[10,11] Alemtuzumab is a humanized monoclonal antibody directed against CD52, a cell surface protein expressed at high density on most normal and malignant B and T lymphocytes, but not on hematopoietic stem cells. Its role in lymphoma is less known but may be interesting, particularly for T cell lymphoma where no other mAb is available.[31,32] Very few, if any, studies have been done in aggressive lymphoma and it is not currently recommended for this disease. Epratuzumab is a humanized mAb directed against CD22, which is present on nearly mature B-cells. CD22 is involved in B-cell activation and interaction with T cells. CD22 is rapidly internalized when bound with antibody. Epratuzumab is currently being tested in different settings, some of them involving DLCL patients.[12] Preliminary results have shown interesting activity, but these results have to be confirmed before any recommendation for its use in clinical practice can be made.

RADIOLABELED MONOCLONAL ANTIBODIES ALONE

Several phase II studies have demonstrated activity in radiolabeled mAb, either ^{90}Y-ibritumomab tiuxetan or ^{131}I-tositumomab, in relapsing patients with lymphoma, mostly follicular lymphoma.[4,17,33,34] The response rate in these studies was often greater than with rituximab in nearly identical patients, usually around 70%, and particularly the CR rate, which was approximately 30%. However, the duration of the response was not different from that observed with rituximab, that is, around 12 months. Very few data have been generated for aggressive lymphomas.

In one comparative study, ^{90}Y-ibritumomab showed a higher response rate for ^{90}Y-ibritumomab than for rituximab in relapsing patients with follicular lymphoma, but progression-free survival and time to next treatment were not statistically different between the two treatments.[15] If radiolabeled mAbs have the disadvantage of inducing more hematologic toxicity and of inducing HAMA, thus preventing their repeated use, they also seem to have efficacy in the case of rituximab failure.[34]

PHASE II STUDIES COMBINING RITUXIMAB AND CHEMOTHERAPY

The first phase II study of a combination of chemotherapy (CHOP) and rituximab was presented by Czuczman et al in patients with untreated follicular lymphoma.[35] In this study, because of a possible toxicity of the combination, rituximab was more interspersed with CHOP cycles than combined with them: two infusions were done before CHOP and two after CHOP, with only two infusions in the middle of CHOP cycles. Nevertheless, this schema showed a high efficacy, with 100% of the patients responding. The current median follow-up is longer than five years, but the median progression-free survival was not reached with 70% of the patients still in response at five years.[36] Since this study, numerous phase II studies have described the combination of rituximab with other drugs such as fludarabine or other regimens such as DHAP.[37] The common point between all these studies was the fact that the remission rate seemed higher and the duration of response longer than with historical patients treated with the same chemotherapy alone. However, the low number of patients in these studies did not permit definitive conclusions on the benefit of any combination.

In previously untreated MCL, CHOP plus rituximab was associated with a very good response (48% of CR and 48% of PR).[38] Half of the patients reached a molecular response. However, the duration of response was not improve in patients with a molecular response and seemed not to be any longer than usually observed with CHOP chemotherapy alone. Clearly, this regimen was insufficient to cure any patients, and researchers are currently improving on it by doing high-dose therapy and autologous transplant in responding patients after R-CHOP or another combination of chemotherapy and rituximab. Another regimen, the combination of rituximab and Hyper-CVAD, was presented as associated with a very high response rate, particularly in young patients, but these preliminary results are not yet published and the toxicity of Hyper-CVAD is generally considered to be too high.[39]

One important phase II study has been presented with the combination of CHOP and rituximab in aggressive B-cell lymphomas.[40] In this study, 33 patients with previously untreated advanced aggressive B-cell NHL received an infusion of rituximab (375 mg/m^2) on day –2 of each cycle of CHOP chemotherapy for six cycles. The overall response rate was 94% (31 out of 33 patients). Twenty patients reached a CR (61%), 11 patients a PR (33%), and two patients were classified as having progressive disease. The median duration of response and time to progression had not been reached after a median observation time of 26 months; 29 of the responding patients remained in remission during this period, including 15 of 16 patients with an IPI score >2. *bcl-2* gene rearrangement was present in 39% of the patients, who had either a follicular large cell lymphoma or a transformation of follicular lymphoma, but no difference in the response rate was observed for patients with or without a *bcl-2* rearrangement. Patients with a true DLCL or adverse prognostic parameters had a lower response rate. This combination of CHOP and rituximab did not increase the toxicity of both types of chemotherapy. In this first report of the safety and efficacy of rituximab in combination with standard-dose CHOP for the treatment of aggressive B-cell lymphoma, the responses were at least comparable to those that were achieved with CHOP alone with no significant added toxicity.

Several phase II studies with a combination of rituximab and different chemotherapy regimens such as DHAP, EPOCH, VNCOP-B, fludarabine-based regimens, and ICE have been presented.[41–43] However, most of these presentations were made during meetings and only abstracts are available. The constant findings of these studies were that the combination of chemotherapy plus rituximab did not seem to increase the toxicity of the chemotherapy regimen, and it seemed to allow a higher response rate and a longer duration of response than in historical controls. In this regard, the 55% response rate obtained with R-ICE in patients with DLCL and refractory to the first line therapy is demonstrative of the improvement of response.[44] R-EPOCH was associated also with a 71% response rate in these refractory patients.[43]

RANDOMIZED TRIALS COMBINING CHEMOTHERAPY AND RITUXIMAB FOR DIFFUSE LARGE CELL LYMPHOMAS

No study has presented a comparison of the efficacy of rituximab alone to chemotherapy in DLCL patients. However, the Groupe d'Etude des Lymphomes de l'Adulte (GELA) recently published their preliminary results of a study in elderly patients with DLCL comparing eight cycles of CHOP to eight cycles of CHOP plus rituximab (R-CHOP).[9] The classical doses of CHOP were given every three weeks and rituximab was given at the dose of 375 mg/m^2 on the same day of the CHOP. Granulocyte-colony stimulating factor (G-CSF) may be added if patients had febrile neutropenia or infection during the previous cycle, and it was given in 50% of the patients. Three hundred and ninety-nine newly diagnosed elderly patients were included in this trial, 197 in CHOP arm and 202 in R-CHOP arm. Patients were 60 to 80 years old, were stratified for Age-Adjusted International Prognostic Index (IPI) scores (0–1 vs. 2–3), had performance status (PS) less or equal to 2, and no contra-indication to doxorubicin. The primary endpoint was event-free survival (EFS), with events defined as disease progression or relapse, death, or initiation of new alternative treatment. Secondary endpoints were response rate, survival, and safety.

The median age of these patients was 69 years. Adverse prognostic parameters were equally distributed between arms: 64% of the patients had stage IV disease, 20% had PS >1, 38% had B symptoms, 66% had elevated lactate dehydrogenase (LDH), 28% had bone marrow involvement, 31% had bulky tumors, 28% had >1 extranodal disease sites, and 60% had an IPI score of 2 or 3. At the time of the analysis, 96% of cases were reviewed by an independent panel and DLCL histology was confirmed in 84%. No major difference between the two arms was observed for hematologic toxicity, or grade 3 or 4 infection, mucositis, vomiting, liver, cardiac, neurological, renal, or lung toxicity. Nineteen patients had a grade 3 or 4 infusion-related syndrome during the first rituximab infusion.

At the end of treatment, 75% of the patients had reached a CR or an undocumented CR (CRu) in the R-CHOP arm compared to 63% in the CHOP arm (P = .005). Twenty-two percent of the patients treated with CHOP had a progression during the treatment compared to 9% in the R-CHOP arm. With a median follow-up of two years, 120 events (61%) were observed in the CHOP arm and 86 (43%) in the R-CHOP arm, most of them being a progression during or after treatment (P = .002; Fig. 10.1).With a longer follow-up, more relapses were observed in the CHOP arm compared to R-CHOP arm.[45] This higher response rate and lower progression rate observed with the combination of CHOP and rituximab translated into statistically longer event-free survival, disease-free survival, and overall survival (Fig. 10.2). As patients were stratified for the age-adjusted International Prognostic Index,[46] an analysis for low-risk and high-risk patients was possible; it showed that a benefit was observed in both groups (Fig. 10.3). The benefit of the addition of rituximab to

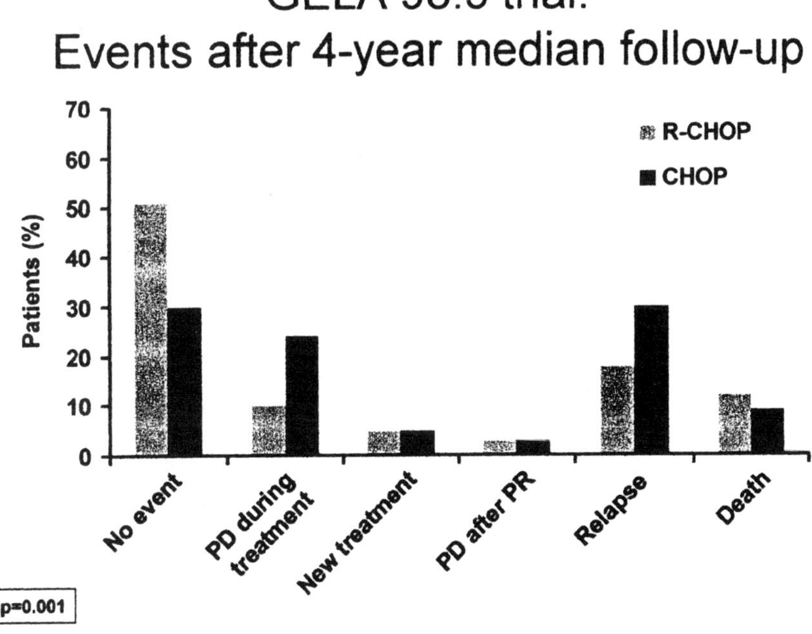

FIGURE 10.1 Events observed after a median two-year follow-up in the GELA study comparing R-CHOP and CHOP chemotherapy in elderly patients with untreated diffuse large B-cell lymphoma.[9]

4-year Update of the GELA Study

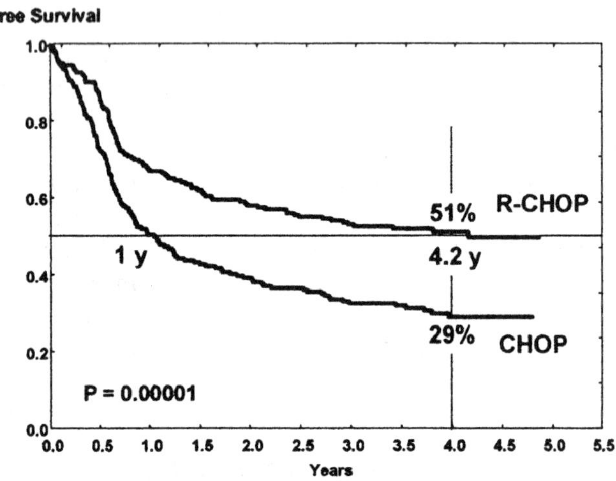

FIGURE 10.2 Event-free survival of the 399 patients of the GELA randomized study comparing CHOP and R-CHOP in elderly patients with diffuse large B-cell lymphoma.[9]

the CHOP chemotherapy was even more important in patients with low-risk disease according to the age-adjusted International Prognostic Index: the improvement over CHOP alone at two years was over 50% (71% of the patients event-free compared to 45%). This study demonstrated that the addition of rituximab to CHOP chemotherapy led to significant prolongation of event-free survival and overall survival in elderly patients with DLCL, without significant additional toxicity. The benefit of the combination was extremely important for patients expressing bcl-2 protein, an abnormality usually associated with chemoresistance, poor response to treatment, and shorter survival.[48,49] In this randomized study, patients treated with CHOP had a poorer outcome if they expressed bcl-2 protein. However, patients treated with R-CHOP had a similar outcome if they expressed bcl-2 protein or not.[50] This observation illustrates the fact that rituximab induces a sensitization to the activity of chemotherapy drugs by acting on the apoptosis mechanisms.[51]

Other randomized studies are in progress or have been completed using a similar setting that found elderly patients or younger patients with or without adverse prognostic parameters, but none has been published yet. In the intergroup study led by ECOG[52], elderly patients were randomized between CHOP and R-CHOP with a second randomization for responders between a consolidation with rituximab (4 injections every 6 months for 2 years) or nothing. The main differ-

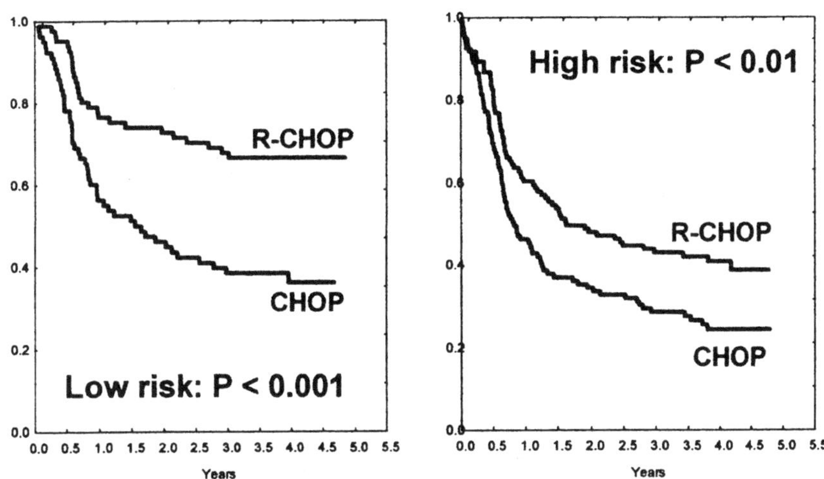

FIGURE 10.3 Event-free survival of the 399 patients of the GELA randomized study comparing CHOP and R-CHOP in elderly patients with diffuse large B-cell lymphoma according to the age-adjusted International Prognostic Index. Patients were divided into low-risk patients (A) with 0 or 1 adverse parameter and high-risk patients (B) with 2 or 3 adverse parameters.[47]

ences with the GELA study were the number of cycles of CHOP that may be reduced to six for patients responding quickly to the chemotherapy and the number of rituximab injections. Rituximab was given once every two cycles of CHOP, so patients received half of the dosage given the GELA study. While the results are yet immature, they confirmed the interest of R-CHOP in first line patients for improving duration of response. They also showed that rituximab in maintenance improves the disease-free survival in patients treated with CHOP only. However, the benefit of maintenance therapy for patients treated with R-CHOP was not clear. In fact, the efficacy of this combination was so effective that physicians recommended it and use it.[53,54]

RITUXIMAB PLUS CHEMOTHERAPY IN OTHER LYMPHOMAS

Numerous studies are ongoing to test the benefit of the addition of rituximab to chemotherapy in naïve or relapsing patients with different types of lymphoma. If some of them are closed for accrual, most are currently ongoing and a few have been published, even as abstracts. One German study compared the FCM regimen to FCM plus rituximab in relapsing patients with FL and MCL.[55,56] Response rates increased from 53% (15% CR) to 89% (36% CR) when rituximab was added to FCM (*P* <.001) and this was found in both types of lymphoma. For the 35 patients with MCL, the response rates were 33% (0% CR) and 64% (35% CR), respectively. Survival data were immature at time of preliminary presentation, but there was a trend in favor of a longer time-to-progression for patients treated with rituximab. Another German study compared mitoxantrone, chlorambucil, and prednisolone (MCP) plus rituximab versus chemotherapy (MCP) alone in previously untreated, advanced, treatment-demanding indolent lymphomas and MCL; it also found a higher response rate.[57]

An Italian study included 28 previously untreated MCL patients and treated them with three cycles of standard-dose debulking chemotherapy followed by a high-dose rituximab-supplemented sequence (R-HDS) including high-dose cyclophosphamide, high-dose cytarabine, high-dose melphalan, and high-dose Mitoxantrone plus Melphalan.[58] Except for one patient who died of toxicity, the 27 patients assessable for response achieved a CR and 24 remain in continuous complete remission after a median follow-up of 35 months.

COMBINATION OF OTHER MONOCLONAL ANTIBODIES WITH CHEMOTHERAPY

Other unconjugated mAb have not yet been associated with chemotherapy except alemtuzumab combined with fludarabine in CLL patients. Radiolabeled mAb were combined with chemotherapy at the time of high-dose therapy followed by autologous stem cell transplantation.[59] Studies are currently ongoing combining radiolabeled mAb and standard chemotherapy in a sequential setting, the mAb following the chemotherapy.[60] Such a combination has been presented only for follicular lymphoma: The SWOG conducted a phase II trial consisting of six cycles of CHOP followed by tositumomab/iodine ^{131}I tositumomab. The overall response rate to the entire treatment regimen was 90%, including 67% complete remissions. The two-year progression-free survival was estimated to be 81%. However, the benefit of this sequence only can be demonstrated by randomized studies and no results are available currently. This utilization is not very different from the maintenance therapy discussed in the next section, the only difference being that radiolabeled mAb are used only once and not several times after the chemotherapy.

RITUXIMAB AS MAINTENANCE THERAPY AFTER CHEMOTHERAPY

Because the efficacy of rituximab seems more important when the tumor mass is smaller, its efficacy theoretically may be higher in patients responding to chemotherapy either in first line or in relapse, and thus it should be used as a maintenance therapy to prevent recurrences. If studies are ongoing in this setting in patients with follicular lymphoma or DLCL, only studies done in indolent lymphoma have been presented to date.[41,61] Currently, there are no sufficient data to use rituximab as maintenance therapy in patients with aggressive lymphoma. Moreover, because of the possible synergism between chemotherapy and rituximab, if both had to be given to a patient, the combination of the two regimens during induction therapy probably would be better.

RITUXIMAB BEFORE HARVESTING STEM CELLS

In vivo purged with rituximab therapy has been shown to be effective in follicular lymphoma patients, most of them having a disappearance of bcl-2 rearranged cells in the harvest. No such marker exists in DLCL and the proportion of patients with circulating lymphoma cells is largely less than in indolent lymphoma. Thus, the value of such an in vivo purge is disputed and no study has been presented that has used such a setting. However, some DLCL are in fact a transformation of an unknown indolent lymphoma and, in this case, the advantages of treating the patients with rituximab alone or in combination with chemotherapy may be more obvious.

MONOCLONAL ANTIBODIES IN STEM CELL TRANSPLANTATION

Rituximab has been used either for improving the salvage chemotherapy or for purging the transplant (discussed earlier in this chapter). It also has been used after autologous or allogeneic transplant to decrease the relapse rate.[62,63] In this setting, it seems that rituximab may complete the response for patients with persisting abnormalities. However, the benefit may be demonstrated only by future randomized studies.[64]

Radiolabeled monoclonal antibodies have been used in combination with chemotherapy for increasing the effect of the conditioning regimen before autotransplant. Patients with relapsed or refractory mantle cell lymphoma received infusions of ^{131}I labeled tositumomab followed 10 days later by administration of high-dose etoposide, cyclophosphamide, and autologous stem cells.[65] Among the 11 patients with measurable disease, the respective complete and overall response rates were 91% and 100%, respectively. Overall survival at three years from transplantation was estimated at 93%, and progression-free survival was estimated at 61%. In another study, rituximab was labeled with ^{131}I and administered alone to patients with relapsing or refractory MCL.[66] Only six patients were included, however, which limits the result to describing its feasibility.

CONCLUSION

These different studies all showed that rituximab has some activity by itself in DLCL and, more importantly, that this activity is increased when it is combined with chemotherapy. Future studies will define the definition of the appropriate use of rituximab in combination with chemotherapy to answer the following questions: which regimen? How many infusions of rituximab should be used?

Can it be utilized for maintenance therapy? Because of the long half-life of rituximab, the day of the infusion in combination with chemotherapy does not matter and doing both on the same day is probably the easiest treatment for the patient. The place of other combinations or other mAbs is not yet well defined.

ACKNOWLEDGMENTS

The author has served as a consultant to Roche, Genentech or IDEC, the manufacturers of rituximab; has been a member of speakers bureaus sponsored by Roche, Genentech or IDEC; and has provided both services for other companies making anti-lymphoma drugs or other monoclonal antibodies.

REFERENCES

1. Grillo-Lopez AJ, White CA, Varns C et al. Overview of the clinical development of rituximab: First monoclonal antibody approved for the treatment of lymphoma. Semin Oncol 1999;26:66–73.
2. Grossbard ML, Fidias P, Kinsella J et al. Anti-B4-blocked ricin: A phase II trial of 7 day continuous infusion in patients with multiple myeloma. Br J Haematol 1998;102:509–515.
3. Kaminski MS, Zasadny KR, Francis IR et al. Iodine-131 – Anti-B1 radioimmunotherapy for B-cell lymphoma. J Clin Oncol 1996;14:1974–1981.
4. Witzig TE, White CA, Wiseman GA et al. Phase I/II trial of IDEC-Y2B8 radioimmunotherapy for treatment of relapsed or refractory CD20(+) B-cell non-Hodgkin's lymphoma. J Clin Oncol 1999;17:3793–3803.
5. Maloney DG, Liles TM, Czerwinski DK et al. Phase I clinical trial using escalating single-dose infusion of chimeric anti-CD20 monoclonal antibody (IDEC-C2B8) in patients with recurrent B-cell lymphoma. Blood 1994;84:2457–2466.
6. Maloney DG, Grillolopez AJ, Bodkin DJ et al. IDEC-C2B8: results of a phase I multiple-dose trial in patients with relapsed non-Hodgkin's lymphoma. J Clin Oncol 1997;15:3266–3274.
7. Foran JM, Rohatiner AZS, Coiffier B et al. Multicenter phase II study of fludarabine phosphate for patients with newly diagnosed lymphoplasmacytoid lymphoma, Waldenstrom's macroglobulinemia, and mantle-cell lymphoma. J Clin Oncol 1999;17:546–553.
8. Coiffier B, Haioun C, Ketterer N et al. Rituximab (anti-CD20 monoclonal antibody) for the treatment of patients with relapsing or refractory aggressive lymphoma. A multicenter phase II study. Blood 1998;92:1927–1932.
9. Coiffier B, Lepage E, Brière J et al. CHOP Chemotherapy plus rituximab compared with CHOP alone in elderly patients with diffuse large B-cell lymphoma. N Engl J Med 2002;346:235–242.
10. Keating MJ, Flinn I, Jain V et al. Therapeutic role of alemtuzumab (Campath-1H) in patients who have failed fludarabine: results of a large international study. Blood 2002;99:3554–3561.
11. Lundin J, Kimby E, Bjorkholm M et al. Phase II trial of subcutaneous anti-CD52 monoclonal antibody alemtuzumab (Campath-1H) as first-line treatment for patients with B-cell chronic lymphocytic leukemia (B-CLL). Blood 2002;100:768–773.
12. Leonard JP, Coleman M, Ketas JC et al. Phase I/II trial of epratuzumab (humanized anti-CD22 antibody) in indolent non-Hodgkin's lymphoma. J Clin Oncol 2003;21:3051–3059.
13. Shi JD, Bullock C, Hall WC et al. In vivo pharmacodynamic effects of Hu1D10 (Remitogen), a humanized antibody reactive against a polymorphic determinant of HLA-DR expressed on B cells. Leuk Lymph 2002;43:1303–1312.
14. Gordon LI, Witzig TE, Wiseman GA et al. Yttrium 90 ibritumomab tiuxetan radioimmunotherapy for relapsed or refractory low-grade non-Hodgkin's lymphoma. Semin Oncol 2002;29:87–92.

15. Witzig TE, Gordon LI, Cabanillas F et al. Randomized controlled trial of yttrium-90-labeled ibritumomab tiuxetan radioimmunotherapy versus rituximab immunotherapy for patients with relapsed or refractory low-grade, follicular, or transformed B-cell non-Hodgkin's lymphoma. J Clin Oncol 2002;20:2453–2463.

16. Kaminski MS, Estes J, Zasadny KR et al. Radioimmunotherapy with iodine I-131 tositumomab for relapsed or refractory B-cell non-Hodgkin lymphoma: updated results and long-term follow-up of the University of Michigan experience. Blood 2000;96:1259–1266.

17. Vose JM, Wahl RL, Saleh M et al. Multicenter phase II study of iodine-131 tositumomab for chemotherapy-relapsed/refractory low-grade and transformed low-grade B-cell non-Hodgkin's lymphomas. J Clin Oncol 2000;18:1316–1323.

18. Olsen E, Duvic M, Frankel A et al. Pivotal phase III trial of two dose levels of denileukin diftitox for the treatment of cutaneous T-cell lymphoma. J Clin Oncol 2001;19:376–388.

19. Demidem A, Lam T, Alas S et al. Chimeric anti-Cd20 (Idec-C2b8) monoclonal antibody sensitizes a B cell lymphoma cell line to cell killing by cytotoxic drugs. Cancer Biother Radiopharm 1997;12:177–186.

20. Shan D, Ledbetter JA, Press OW. Apoptosis of malignant human B cells by ligation of CD20 with monoclonal antibodies. Blood 1998;91:1644–1652.

21. Shan DM, Ledbetter JA, Press OW. Signaling events involved in anti-CD20-induced apoptosis of malignant human B cells. Cancer Immunol Immunother 2000;48:673–683.

22. Ghetie MA, Bright H, Vitetta ES. Homodimers but not monomers of Rituxan (chimeric anti-CD20) induce apoptosis in human B-lymphoma cells and synergize with a chemotherapeutic agent and an immunotoxin. Blood 2001;97:1392–1398.

23. Alas S, Bonavida B. Rituximab inactivates signal transducer and activation of transcription 3 (STAT3) activity in B-non-Hodgkin's lymphoma through inhibition of the interleukin 10 autocrine/paracrine loop and results in down-regulation of Bcl-2 and sensitization to cytotoxic drugs. Cancer Res 2001;61:5137–5144.

24. Kreitman RJ, Wilson WH, Bergeron K et al. Efficacy of the anti-CD22 recombinant immunotoxin BL22 in chemotherapy-resistant hairy-cell leukemia. N Engl J Med 2001;345:241–247.

25. Dearden CE, Matutes E, Cazin B et al. High remission rate in T-cell prolymphocytic leukemia with CAMPATH-1H. Blood 2001;98:1721–1726.

26. McLaughlin P, Grillo-Lopez AJ, Link BK et al. Rituximab chimeric anti-CD20 monoclonal antibody therapy for relapsed indolent lymphoma: Half of patients respond to a four-dose treatment program. J Clin Oncol 1998;16:2825–2833.

27. Foran JM, Rohatiner AZS, Cunningham D et al. European phase II study of rituximab (chimeric anti-CD20 monoclonal antibody) for patients with newly diagnosed mantle-cell lymphoma and previously treated mantle-cell lymphoma, immunocytoma, and small B-cell lymphocytic lymphoma. J Clin Oncol 2000;18:317–324.

28. Foran JM, Cunningham D, Coiffier B et al. Treatment of mantle-cell lymphoma with Rituximab (chimeric monoclonal anti-CD20 antibody): Analysis of factors associated with response. Ann Oncol 2000;11:117–121.

29. The Non-Hodgkin's Lymphoma Pathologic Classification Project. National Cancer Institute sponsored study of classifications of non-Hodgkin's lymphomas. Summary and description of a Working Formulation for Clinical Usage. Cancer 1982;49:2112–2135.

30. Pan D, Moskowitz C, Zelenetz A et al. Rituximab for aggressive non-Hodgkin's lymphomas relapsing after or refractory to autologous stem cell transplantation. Cancer J 2002;8:371–376.

31. Uppenkamp M, Engert A, Diehl V et al. Monoclonal antibody therapy with CAMPATH-1H in patients with relapsed high- and low-grade non-Hodgkin's lymphomas: a multicenter phase I/II study. Ann Hematol 2002;81:26–32.

32. Keating MJ, Cazin B, Coutre S et al. Campath-1H treatment of T-cell prolymphocytic leukemia in patients for whom at least one prior chemotherapy regimen has failed. J Clin Oncol 2002;20:205–213.

33. Kaminski MS, Zelenetz AD, Press OW et al. Pivotal study of iodine I 131 Tositumomab for chemotherapy-refractory low-grade or transformed low-grade B-cell non-Hodgkin's lymphomas. J Clin Oncol 2001;19:3918–3928.

34. Witzig TE, Flinn IW, Gordon LI et al. Treatment with ibritumomab tiuxetan radioimmunotherapy in patients with rituximab-refractory follicular non-Hodgkin's lymphoma. J Clin Oncol 2002;20:3262–3269.

35. Czuczman MS, Grillo-Lopez AJ, White CA et al. Treatment of patients with low-grade B-cell lymphoma with the combination of chimeric anti-CD20 monoclonal antibody and CHOP chemotherapy. J Clin Oncol 1999;17:268–276.

36. Czuczman MS, Fallon A, Mohr A et al. Rituximab in combination with CHOP or fludarabine in low-grade lymphoma. Semin Oncol 2002;29:36–40.

37. Schulz H, Klein SK, Rehwald U et al. Phase 2 study of a combined immunochemotherapy using rituximab and fludarabine in patients with chronic lymphocytic leukemia. Blood 2002;100: 3115–3120.

38. Howard OM, Gribben JG, Neuberg DS et al. Rituximab and CHOP induction therapy for newly diagnosed mantle-cell lymphoma: Molecular complete responses are not predictive of progression-free survival. J Clin Oncol 2002;20:1288–1294.

39. Romaguera JE, Khouri IF, Kantarjian HM et al. Untreated aggressive mantle cell lymphoma: Results with intensive chemotherapy without stem cell transplant in elderly patients. Leuk Lymph 2000;39:77–85.

40. Vose JM, Link BK, Grossbard ML et al. Phase II study of rituximab in combination with CHOP chemotherapy in patients with previously untreated, aggressive non-Hodgkin's lymphoma. J Clin Oncol 2001;19:389–397.

41. Hainsworth JD, Litchy S, Burris HA et al. Rituximab as first-line and maintenance therapy for patients with indolent non-Hodgkin's lymphoma. J Clin Oncol 2002;20:4261–4267.

42. Joyce RM, Kraser CN, Tetrealt JC et al. Rituximab and ifosfamide, mitoxantrone, etoposide (RIME) with Neupogen (R) support for B-cell non-Hodgkin's lymphoma prior to high-dose chemotherapy with autologous haematopoietic transplant. Eur J Hematol 2001;66:56–62.

43. Wilson WH, Gutierrez M, O'Connor P et al. The role of rituximab and chemotherapy in aggressive B-cell lymphoma: A preliminary report of dose-adjusted EPOCH-R. Semin Oncol 2002;29:41–47.

44. Kewalramani T, Zelenetz A, Bertino J et al. Rituximab significantly increases the complete response rate in patients with relapsed or primary refractory DLBCL receiving ICE as second-line therapy. Blood 2001;98(Suppl 1):346a (abstr 1459).

45. Coiffer B. Treatment of aggressive lymphomas: disseminated cases. In ASCO 2003 Educational Book. 2003:606–611.

46. The International Non-Hodgkin's Lymphoma Prognostic Factors Project. A predictive model for aggressive non-Hodgkin's lymphoma. N Engl J Med 1993;329:987–994.

47. Coiffier B. Diffuse large cell lymphoma. Curr Op Oncol 2001;13:325–334.

48. Hermine O, Haioun C, Lepage E et al. Prognostic significance of bcl-2 protein expression in aggressive non-Hodgkin's lymphoma. Blood 1996;87:265–272.

49. Gascoyne RD, Adomat SA, Krajewski S et al. Prognostic significance of bcl-2 protein expression and bcl-2 gene rearrangement in diffuse aggressive non-Hodgkin's lymphoma. Blood 1997;90:244–251.

50. Mounier N, Briere J, Gisselbrecht C et al. Rituximab plus CHOP (R-CHOP) overcomes bcl-2-associated resistance to chemotherapy in elderly patients with diffuse large B-cell lymphoma (DLBCL). Blood 2003;101:4279–4284.

51. Emmanouilides C, Jazirehi AR, Bonavida B. Rituximab-mediated sensitization of B-non-Hodgkin's lymphoma (NHL) to cytotoxicity induced by paclitaxel, gemcitabine, and vinorelbine. Cancer Biother Radiopharm 2002;17:621–630.

52. Habermann TM, Weller EA, et al. (203). Phase III Trial of Rituximab-CHOP (R-CHOP) vs. CHOP with a Second Randomization to Maintenance Rituximab (MR) or Observation in Patients 60 Years of Age and Older with Diffuse Large B-Cell Lymphoma (DLBCL). Blood 2003; 102 (Suppl. 1):Abst. 8.

53. Pettengell R, Linch D. Position paper on the therapeutic use of rituximab in CD20-positive diffuse large B-cell non-Hodgkin's lymphoma. Br J Haematol 2003;121:44–48.

54. Portlock C. Rituximab and CHOP for elderly patients with diffuse large B-cell lymphoma. Curr Oncol Rep 2003;5:357.

55. Forstpointner R, Hanel A, Repp R et al. Increased response rate with rituximab in relapsed and refractory follicular and mantle cell lymphomas—results of a prospective randomized study of the German Low Grade Lymphoma Study Group. Dtsch Med Wschr 2002;127:2253–2258.

56. Hiddemann W, Dreyling M, Unterhalt M. Rituximab plus chemotherapy in follicular and mantle cell lymphomas. Semin Oncol 2003;30:16–20.

57. Herold M, Dolken G, Fiedler F et al. Randomized phase III study for the treatment of advanced indolent non-Hodgkin's lymphomas (NHL) and mantle cell lymphoma: chemotherapy versus chemotherapy plus rituximab. Ann Hematol 2003;82:77–79.

58. Gianni AM, Magni M, Martelli M et al. Long-term remission in mantle cell lymphoma following high-dose sequential chemotherapy and in vivo rituximab-purged stem cell autografting (R-HDS regimen). Blood 2003;102:749–755.

59. Press OW, Eary JF, Gooley T et al. A phase I/II trial of iodine-131-tositumomab (anti-CD20), etoposide, cyclophosphamide, and autologous stem cell transplantation for relapsed B-cell lymphomas. Blood 2000;96:2934–2942.

60. Press OW, Unger JM, Braziel RM et al. A phase 2 trial of CHOP chemotherapy followed by tositumomab/iodine I 131 tositumomab for previously untreated follicular non-Hodgkin lymphoma: Southwest Oncology Group Protocol S9911. Blood 2003;102:1606–1612.

61. Ghielmini M, Schmite SFH, Cogliatti SB et al. Maintenance treatment with 2-montly rituximab after standard weekly × 4 rituximab induction significantly improves event-free survival in patients with follicular lymphoma [abstract]. Ann Oncol 2002;13 (Suppl 2):38.

62. Horwitz SM, Negrin RS, Blume KG et al. Rituximab as adjuvant to high-dose therapy and autologous hematopoietic cell transplantation for aggressive non-Hodgkin's lymphoma. Blood 2004;103:777–783.

63. Mangel J, Buckstein R, Imrie K et al. Immunotherapy with rituximab following high-dose therapy and autologous stem-cell transplantation for mantle cell lymphoma. Semin Oncol 2002; 29:56–69.

64. Gisselbrecht C, Mounier N. Rituximab: enhancing outcome of autologous stem cell transplantation in non-Hodgkin's lymphoma. Semin Oncol 2003;30:28–33.

65. Gopal AK, Rajendran JG, Petersdorf SH et al. High-dose chemo-radioimmunotherapy with autologous stem cell support for relapsed mantle cell lymphoma. Blood 2002;99:3158–3162.

66. Behr TM, Griesinger F, Riggert J et al. High-dose myeloablative radioimmunotherapy of mantle cell non-Hodgkin lymphoma with the iodine-131-labeled chimeric anti-CD20 antibody C2B8 and autologous stem cell support—results of a pilot study. Cancer 2002;94:1363–1372.

Chapter 11

Novel Schedules of Hormone Therapy for Prostate Cancer

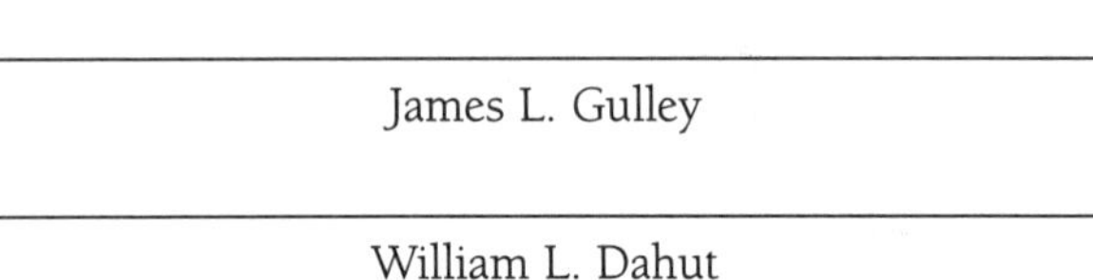
James L. Gulley

William L. Dahut

Prostate cancer is the most common non-cutaneous cancer and second leading cause of cancer death among American men. In 2003, it was estimated that 220,900 new cases would be diagnosed and 28,900 men would die from prostate cancer in the United States.[1] Chemical or surgical castration has become a mainstay for the treatment of metastatic prostate cancer. To understand the rationale behind the use of androgen deprivation therapy (ADT), one must understand the effects of hormones on the prostate gland (Figure 11.1). Normal development of the prostate is dependent on endocrine stimulation, with testosterone being necessary for the prostate to develop into and remain a functional gland. Gonadotropin releasing hormone (GnRH) is made in neurosecretory neurons in the hypothalamus. These neurons terminate in the hypothalamic-hypophysial portal system. This unique vascular bed shuttles the GnRH directly to the anterior lobe of the pituitary (which incidentally gets 90% of its blood from this venous plexus). Luteinizing hormone, produced in the anterior lobe of the pituitary, enters the circulation and subsequently binds to a specific high affinity receptor on the plasma membrane of the testicular interstitial cells of Leydig. The end result of this interaction is an increase in production of testosterone by the testes.

Testosterone then enters the bloodstream. Upon entering the cells of the prostate, it may be converted by 5-alpha reductase into dihydroxytestosterone

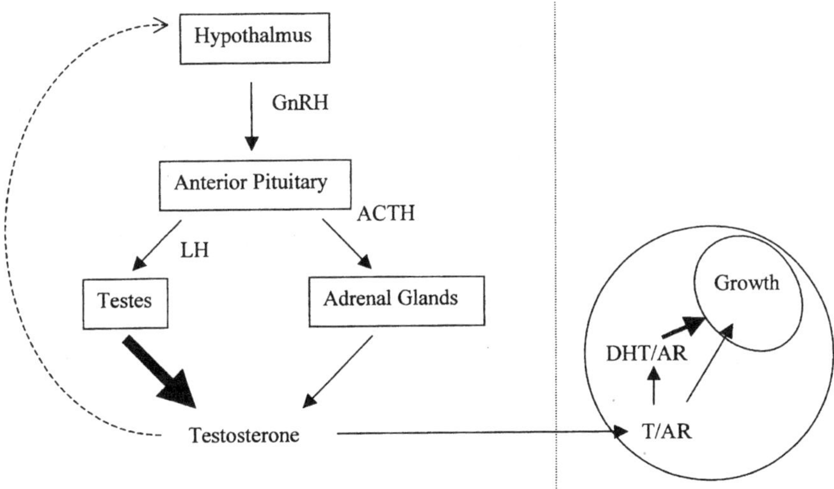

FIGURE 11.1 The hypothalamus/pituitary/testis endocrine loop is shown on the left. Gonadotropin releasing hormone (GnRH) stimulates section of luteinizing hormone (LH) from the anterior pituitary and LH in tern stimulates the production of testosterone. Circulating testosterone (and estrogens) acts in a negative feedback loop to down-regulate the expression of GnRH. Adrenocortocotropic hormone (ACTH), also made by the pituitary stimulates androgens synthesis in the adrenal gland. Testosterone (T) and dihydroxytestosterone (DHT) bind to the androgen receptor (AR) and this causes increased expression of androgen responsive genes leading to cell growth.

(DHT). Either testosterone or DHT can directly bind to the cytoplasmic androgen receptor (the later with increased affinity) and can initiate cell growth. There is a lesser role for prostatatic growth from the 10% to 15% of androgens in the male that come from the adrenal cortex. While all these androgens are important for normal glandular growth, they also serve as strong growth factors for prostate cancer.

In 1941 Huggins and Hodges established the androgen dependence of prostate cancer.[2] In this early human study, they showed that prostate cancer was inhibited by castration or estrogen injections and was activated by androgen injections. This finding led to the use of testosterone suppression as front line therapy for advanced prostate cancer. The first large study looking at the effectiveness of orchiectomy was published in 1967.[3] This study showed that in patients with stage IV disease, orchiectomy was associated with a 73% one-year survival and a 35% five-year survival compared with 66% and 20% for placebo, respectively. In addition, this study showed that DES provided similar efficacy to orchiectomy. In 1971 Schally and colleagues successfully isolated and characterized the decapeptide GnRH.[4] Since GnRH has a half-life of about two to four minutes, further studies were undertaken with single amino acid substitutions to identify compounds with longer half-lives that could be used therapeutically. Substitutions at amino acid position number 6 and 10 led to superagonists which are 50 to 100 times more potent than the native peptide.[5] As one would expect, these GnRH agonists (GnRH-A) initially cause an increase in the level of testosterone; however, within three to four weeks, the levels drop to the castrate range as the physiologic pulsatile release of GnRH is replaced by a continuous low level release, resulting in down-regulation of the pituitary GnRH receptors. GnRH-A have been demonstrated to have similar effectiveness when compared with orchiectomy or estrogens in decreasing levels of testosterone and subsequent clinical benefit to patients with advanced prostate cancer.[6–8] Because of the potential reversibility of testosterone depletion with the GnRH agonists and psychological factors associated with orchiectomy, many patients now choose medical castration (GnRH-A) over surgical castration.

ADJUVANT ADT

While hormonal treatment has clearly been established as an effective therapy for metastatic prostate cancer, there is emerging evidence that hormonal therapy combined with localized disease can provide clinically meaningful improvements in selected patients. While surgery and radiotherapy therapies are generally effective in controlling local disease, those cancer cells that have metastasized will not likely be treated. Thus, the concept of adding effective systemic therapies to local treatment remains appealing.

Probably the most compelling data come from a series of clinical trials combining hormonal therapy with radiation therapy in patients at high risk for recurrent disease (Table 11.1). The first such large trial run by the Radiation Therapy Oncology Group (RTOG 8531) randomized 945 patients with T3 or T1-2 with N1 to radiation therapy (prostate and pelvis) with either adjuvant GnRH-A

TABLE 11.1 Risk Categories for Post-Therapy PSA Failure

Low	Intermediate	High	
Stage	T1c, T2a	T2b	T2c
PSA	< 10	10-20	> 20
Gleason	≤6	7	≥ 8
Qualifier	And	Or	Or
5 year risk of biochemical failure	< 25%	25-50%	> 50%

Source: Reprinted with permission from the American Medical Association. D'Amico AV, Whittington R, Malkowicz et al. Biochemical outcome after radical prostectomy, external beam radiation therapy, or interstitial radiation therapy for clinically localized prostate cancer. JAMA 1998;280:969–974.

therapy for an indefinite period or GnRH-A therapy at the time of relapse.[9,10] The recently presented 10-year overall survival favored the hormone treated group (53% vs. 38%, $P < .0043$).[11]

In addition, the European Organization for Research and Treatment of Cancer (EORTC) performed a trial in 412 patients with poorly differentiated (WHO grade 3) or T3-4 cancers.[12] Patients were randomized to receive radiation with or without concurrent and adjuvant GnRH-A therapy for three years with the first month of GnRH-A therapy given with an antiandrogen. The five-year overall survival was 78% in the hormonal therapy group versus 62% in the radiation alone therapy group ($P = .0002$).[13]

Another trial randomized 91 patients with clinically localized prostate cancer to receive definitive external beam radiotherapy or combined orchiectomy and radiotherapy.[14] All patients underwent surgical lymph node staging and 39 (43%) were found to have lymph node metastasis prior to radiation therapy. After a median follow-up of 9.3 years, clinical progression was seen in 61% of the radiotherapy only group and in 31% of the combined therapy group ($P = .005$). Moreover, the overall mortality was 61% and 38% ($P = .02$) favoring the orchiectomy group. The improvement in median overall survival in the combined treatment arm was seen only in the lymph node positive tumor patients.

A subsequent trial (RTOG 9202) looked at the use of neoadjuvant and concurrent hormonal therapy (GnRH-A with anti-androgen) with or without adjuvant GnRH-A therapy for two years in 1554 patients who had a T stage of at least T2b.[15] This trial demonstrated an overall survival advantage at 5 years (80% vs. 69%, $P = .02$) in the subset of patients who had Gleason 8-10 tumors. Taken together, these trials provide strong evidence that patients at high risk for recurrence who are receiving definitive radiation therapy should be treated with long-term hormonal therapy.

EARLY VERSUS LATE ADT

The Medical Research Council (MRC) reported the results of a trial in which 938 patients with locally advanced or metastatic prostate cancer were randomized to immediate versus delayed hormonal therapy with either a bilateral orchiectomy (>80% of patients) or GnRH-A.[16] The results of this trial consistently favor immediate treatment. Approximately a third of patients in each arm had known metastatic disease. Progression to metastatic disease was significantly decreased and time to painful metastasis was prolonged with immediate treatment. Complications of disease such as pathologic fracture, spinal cord compression, ureteric obstruction, and development of extra-skeletal metastasis were twice as common in the deferred ADT group. In men with locally advanced prostate cancer, 32% of men in the immediate ADT group and 49% of men in the deferred ADT group died from prostate cancer ($P < .001$). It should be noted that of the additional 54 cancer deaths in the deferred treatment group, 29 (54%) did not receive ADT. However, a reanalysis of the data without those 29 patients does not impact the survival data.[17–19]

Additional data are available for patients who have microscopic metastatic disease at time of radical prostatectomy. The Eastern Cooperative Oncology Group (ECOG) performed a trial in which 98 men with microscopic metastatic disease were randomized following radical prostatectomy with lymph node dissection to immediate ADT (GnRH therapy or orchiectomy) versus observation.[20] The difference in overall survival at 10 years was 72.4% versus 49% ($P = .025$) favoring immediate ADT group.[21] Another retrospective study with a larger patient group confirmed these findings. Three hundred and twenty-two patients treated at the Mayo Clinic had lymph node metastasis at the time of radical prostatectomy.[22] Of these, 297 went on to receive adjuvant ADT within 90 days of surgery. Those patients who received ADT had significantly improved five- and ten-year progression-free survivals. Several trials have used a combination of neoadjuvant hormonal therapy and radical prostatectomy, but to date none have shown any survival advantage.[23–25]

The EORTC undertook a Phase III randomized trial comparing early versus late ADT in 234 patients with N+, M0 disease (EORTC protocol 30846) that has been presented in abstract form.[26] The primary endpoint of this trial was overall survival. With a median follow-up of 8.7 years 143 (62%) of the patients have died, 76% from prostate cancer. The hazard ratio for survival with delayed treatment is 1.23; however, this is not statistically significant (95% CI, 0.88–1.71). Another EORTC phase III trial (30891) compares early versus delayed ADT in patients with asymptomatic non-metastatic prostate cancer (T0-4 N0-2 M0).[27] This 900 patient trial in a slightly earlier disease state closed to accrual in January 1999 and results are expected soon.

Thus, although there are data suggesting a survival benefit for immediate ADT for patients with locally advanced disease or microscopic lymph node metastases, there are no definitive survival data available on the timing of ADT in patients with biochemical failure. Some have argued against the use of ADT in patients with biochemical failure following surgery or radiation therapy because of the frequently long interval from first rise of PSA until the development of metastatic disease, and the side effects and economic impact of ADT.[18]

In an effort to decrease the likelihood of recurrence, researchers have added chemotherapy to hormonal therapy as adjuvant for locally advanced prostate cancer that is at high risk for recurrence. A recently published single-arm pilot trial looked at a combination of six courses of vinblastine, doxorubicin and mitomycin with simultaneous radiation and permanent ADT in 25 patients with either clinical evidence of seminal vesicle involvement or lymph node involvement.[28] The 10-year relapse-free survival was 69%. A high priority trial initiated by the South West Oncology Group is looking at the role of adjuvant Gn-RH agonist with anti-androgen alone or with six cycles of mitoxantrone and prednisone in patients with either Gleason 8-10, pT3b-T4, N1, or Gleason 7 and positive margin. The primary endpoint in this 1360 patient trial is to evaluate the difference in overall survival between the two arms.

INTERMITTENT ANDROGEN DEPRIVATION

Based on randomized controlled trials with locally advanced patients as outlined above as well as the MRC data, one could make the argument that immediate ADT is superior to delayed therapy in prolonging survival of patients with advanced prostate cancer. However, with PSA testing, biochemical failure is almost always diagnosed well before clinical failure. There is increasing concern over the significant side effects associated with ADT in this asymptomatic population. In addition, there is potential for restoration of androgen withdrawal-induced apoptosis (i.e., sensitivity) upon androgen replacement in tumors cells that survive ADT (cells that are androgen independent). Preclinical studies have demonstrated that while ADT increases apoptosis of LNCaP cells in a murine model, those cancer cells that escape do not differentiate to become pre-apoptotic again unless there is re-exposure of the cells to testosterone.[29] In addition, ADT is associated with the up-regulation of a number of survival genes that become down-regulated again when testosterone levels return to normal.[30–32] Given these factors, there has been considerable interest in evaluating intermittent scheduling of ADT.

There have been many clinical studies that have explored intermittent ADT. Some of the larger trials are mentioned in Table 11.2. The majority of the trials are phase II studies and to date no definitive clinical results are available comparing intermittent ADT to continuous ADT. Almost all of the studies have utilized GnRH-A with the majority of these studies utilizing an androgen receptor antagonist at least for an initial period of about a month to block any activity caused be the initial surge in testosterone caused by GnRH-A. Current practice trends in the United States were examined for patients who had biochemical failure following external beam radiation therapy and 22% of urologists and an equal proportion of radiation oncologists (both groups from a predominantly private practice setting) recommended intermittent ADT.[42]

There are several factors that have been shown to predict the time off of ADT in patients undergoing intermittent ADT.[38] Patients who achieve an undetectable PSA (<0.05 ng/mg) with one year had a median duration of off ADT (off phase) of 29 months versus 8.5 months for those whose PSA did not become undetectable within one year (P = .00002). In addition, those who had biochemical recurrence without radiographic evidence of disease had a median duration of the off phase twice as long as those patients who had no prior definitive therapy (24 vs. 12 months, P = .028). Seventy-three percent of the latter group had clinically localized disease. Finally, those patients whose testosterone recovered

TABLE 11.2 **Published Reports of Intermittent Androgen Deprivation with at Least 50 Patients**

Author	Year	No. of patients	Treatment	Stage of Disease L/BF/M	Median Time On Therapy (months)	Median Time Off Therapy (months)
Bruchovsky[33]	1998	110	GnRH + AA	0/110/0	9	9
Bracarda[34]	1998	55	GnRH + AA	44/0/11	7	6
Theyer [35]	1998	52	GnRH + AA	15/0/37	6	16
Gleave[36]	1998	70	GnRH + AA	41/0/29	9	9
Crook[37]	1999	54	GnRH + AA	11/4/39	8	9
Strum[38]	2000	52	GnRH + AA	24/19/9	19	24
Grossfeld[39]	2001	61	GnRH + AA	34/27/0	9	6
Prapotnich[40]	2003	233	GnRH + AA	NR[a]	6[b]	13[b]
Tangen[41]	2003	663	GnRH + AA	0/0/663	NR	NR

Abbreviations: L, localized; BF, biochemical failure without radiographic evidence of disease; M, metastatic.
[a]All patients had either biochemical failure, PSA >30 (without local therapy) or metastatic disease.
[b]Median for first cycle. Treatment was stopped when PSA fell below 4 ng/mL and restarted when PSA was >20 ng/mL.

within four months after discontinuing ADT had a shorter median time in the off phase than those whose PSA did not recover within four months (10 vs. 25 months, $P = .0022$).

There are several additional important issues of clinical relevance one should be cognizant of when discussing intermittent hormonal therapy. First, upon discontinuation of a GnRH analogue, testosterone levels remain suppressed for a variable period of time, with variables such as baseline testosterone of the patient, time on testosterone suppression, prior ADT and age likely playing a role in the length of time to normalization of testosterone.[43–46] One study recently presented showed a median of 24.9 weeks to rise of testosterone to above the castrate range after a the second 12 week injection of a –+GnRH analogue with a rise to the normal range in a median of 3.7 weeks after that (about 4 months after the prescribed 6 months of ADT).[43] Second, patients who cycle off hormonal therapy are likely to report improved quality of life.[33,47]

With the previously mentioned rationale for restoring androgen dependence by the addition of androgens after a period of ADT, Dr. Scher at Memorial Sloan Kettering Cancer Center has initiated a trial in which patients with androgen independent metastatic prostate cancer who have been castrate for at least one year are given testosterone replacement.[48] The purpose of this phase I dose escalation study is to determine the safety and maximum tolerated dose of exogenously administered testosterone and to assess the changes in expression of androgen receptor in these patients.

ANTI-ANDROGENS

There are three approved anti-androgens in common use in the United States (Table 11.3). These drugs competitively antagonize the binding of testosterone and DHT to the androgen receptor and thus block the signal for growth caused by androgens. Since about 10% of androgens come from the adrenal gland, there was a push to treat patients with metastatic prostate cancer with combined androgen blockade (CAB) to minimize any effects of these androgens. The clinical benefit of CAB however remains controversial. A trial from the Southwest Oncology Group enrolled men with metastatic prostate cancer and compared treatment with orchiectomy plus placebo (687 patients) to orchiectomy plus flutamide (700 patients).[49] There was no significant difference in overall survival ($P = 0.14$) between the two arms. A recent systematic review and meta-analysis identified 21 trials with a total of 6871 patients who were treated on randomized trials comparing ADT with CAB.[50] The authors found that those trials with survival data out to two years (20 trials) showed no statistical difference in overall

TABLE 11.3 Agents Used in Prostate Cancer Approved by the United States Food and Drug Administration

Generic Name	Trade Name	Manufacturer	Formulation
GnRH Superagonists			
Leuprolide Acetate	Lupron Depot	TAP Pharmaceutical Products (Lake Forest, IL)	IM injection 1 mo: 7.5 mg 3 mo: 22.5 mg 4 mo: 30 mg
Goserelin	Zoladex	AstraZeneca Pharmaceuticals (Wilmington, DE)	SC injection 1 mo: 3.6 mg 3 mo: 10.8 mg
Leuprolide Acetate	Viadur	ALZA Corporation (Mountain View, CA) Dist by Bayer Corporation Pharmaceutical Division (West Haven, CT)	SC implant 12 mo: 65 mg
Androgen Receptor Antagonists			
Flutamide	Eulexin	Schering-Plough (Baulkham Hills, NSW, Australia)	250 mg every 8 hr
Bicalutamide	Casodex	AstraZeneca Pharmaceuticals (Wilmington, DE)	50 mg every day
Nilutamide	Nilandron	Aventis Pharmaceuticals (Kansas City, MO)	300 mg every day for the first 30 days then 150 mg every day

survival; however, in the 10 trials with data out to five years, there was a statistically significant improvement in overall survival of about 3.7 to 7 months. They cautioned that this modest improvement (2.9%) in overall survival must be weighed against the increased risk of adverse events and possible decrease in the patient's quality of life. It is possible that any observed improvement in survival is at least partly due to the anti-androgen blocking the initial surge in testosterone seen when initiating GnRH agonist therapy.

An interesting study reported by Kelly and Scher in 1993 showed that both clinical symptoms and PSA could improve in response to anti-androgen withdrawal.[51] In this study, 21% of patients had a significant PSA decrease after discontinuation of flutamide. Subsequent studies have reproduced this phenomenon with this and other antiandrogens.[52,53] Thus, for patients on an anti-androgen, withdrawal of the anti-androgen should be taken as part of the first therapeutic maneuver upon treatment failure.

MONOTHERAPY

Anti-androgens also have been tested as single agents in patients with prostate cancer. Flutamide has been used as monotherapy for over 20 years, however only two studies have reported survival data.[54,55] Both studies utilized flutamide 250 mg three times daily. One study compared flutamide monotherapy to orchiectomy while the other compared it to CAB. Both reported no significant difference between the arms in terms of time to progression or overall survival. Bicalutamide monotherapy has been studied even more extensively. Trials with 50 mg of bicalutamide daily showed that this dosage was associated with inferior overall survival compared to castration.[56] However, 150 mg daily achieved a PSA response similar to castration and was relatively well-tolerated prompting further evaluation of this dose in large comparative trials.

Survival data on 805 patients with metastatic prostate cancer randomized to receive castration or bicalutamide 150 mg daily were analyzed after a median follow-up of 1.9 years.[57] The bicalutamide arm was not as effective as castration; however, a post-hoc analysis of patients with PSA < 400 showed similar survival outcomes.58 Another study randomized 480 M0 patients to bicalutamide 150 daily or castration and showed no statistically significant difference between the two arms in terms of overall survival and time to progression in this earlier patient population.59 In addition, this trial showed that patients in the bicalutamide arm had statistically significantly better physical capacity and sexual interest.

The largest clinical trial program of prostate cancer treatment to-date analyzed the efficacy and tolerability of bicalutamide 150 mg combined with standard care (radical prostatectomy, radiation therapy or "watchful waiting") in patients with localized or locally advanced disease.[60] Three trials of similar design enrolled 8113 patients randomized to bicalutamide or placebo. After a median follow-up of three years, patients in the bicalutamide arm had 42% less objective disease progression compared with standard care alone ($P < .001$). There were more disease progression events in patients who were treated with "watchful waiting" than the other groups and further follow-up will be require to determine if the decrease progressive disease will continue to hold up for the patients treated with definitive local therapy.

Another trial is evaluating initial anti-androgen monotherapy in comparison with watchful waiting in asymptomatic non-metastatic prostate cancer patients who have not had treatment with curative intent.[61,62] This is a randomized phase III multicenter study (EORTC protocol 30991) in which a target of 1266 patients were enrolled to either treatment with bicalutamide alone followed by the addition of ADT at time of disease progression versus observation followed by bicalutamide with ADT. This trial completed accrual in February 2003 and is designed to compare the overall and cancer-specific survival, the time to first and second clinical progression and the quality of life of patients with prostate cancer treated in the two arms.

KETOCONAZOLE

Ketoconazole is a substituted imidazole that suppresses testicular and adrenal steroidogenesis and is associated with significant PSA declines in patients when used as a second line hormonal agent.[63–65] Indeed, one study that evaluated patients with simultaneous anti-androgen withdrawal and treatment with ketoconazole showed a decline in PSA of at least 50% in 11 of 20 patients (55%) and a median PSA response of 9 months.[66] There can be significant side effects with ketoconazole including nausea, diarrhea, and fatigue.

5-ALPHA REDUCTASE INHIBITORS

Five-alpha-reductase enzymatically converts testosterone into dihydroxytestosterone (DHT), the most active androgen in the prostate. Two FDA approved inhibitors of 5-alpha-reductase are currently available; however, finasteride, a selective inhibitor of the type 2 5-alpha-reductase enzyme, has been more widely tested in prostate cancer than the more recently approved dutasteride. Finasteride decreases levels of DHT by 90%, causing a reduction in gland size by 20% to 30% and improving urinary symptoms for patients with benign prostatic hypertrophy. There have been several reports of patients treated with finasteride in combination with other hormonal therapies. One author reported on 110 consecutive patients treated with a GnRH agonist/anti-androgen/finasteride regimen in patients with clinical stage T1-T3 cancer in lieu of definitive therapy (a so-called triple androgen blockade).[67] All patients were treated for a median of 13 months with the triple androgen blockade before being put on finasteride only as maintenance therapy. At the time of the publication, there was a median follow-up of 36 months with 105 of 110 patients having stable PSA levels.

A Cancer and Leukemia Group B cooperative group trial enrolled 101 patients with rising PSA (between 1 and 10 ng/mL) but no radiographic evidence of disease following local definitive therapy (D0 disease).[68] Of the 69 evaluable patients, 68 had a decline in PSA of at least 80% with the majority (68%) having a PSA <0.2 ng/mL. The median time to PSA nadir was three months. A group from Harvard looked at 20 patients with androgen dependent prostate cancer with 13 having D0 disease, and 7 with overt metastatic disease.[69] At a median follow-up of 88 months, the median castration-free survival was 37 months and the median androgen insensitive prostate cancer survival was 48.6 months. Another phase II study from Harvard evaluated the combination of finasteride and bicalutamide as primary hormonal therapy.[70] Forty-one men were enrolled with 32 of these having biochemical failure following local therapy. The men initially were treated with 150 mg of bicalutamide daily (after prophylactic breast irradiation) until they achieved a PSA nadir, at which time 5 mg of finasteride daily was added. The median PSA nadir following bicalutamide was 3.6% of baseline PSA with the median nadir after starting flutamide at 1.5% of baseline. Toxicities were reportedly mild.

The recently published Prostate Cancer Prevention Trial examined if finasteride could reduce the risk of prostate cancer in men 55 years of age or older who had a normal digital rectal examination and a PSA of 3.0 ng/mL or less.[71] Over 18,000 men were enrolled and placed either on 5 mg/day of finasteride or placebo for seven years. Prostate biopsies were recommended if the PSA (adjusted for the lowering effect of finasteride) exceeded 4.0 ng/mL or if the digital rectal examination became abnormal. In addition, an end of study biopsy was offered to all patients with an impressive 60% of patients either having a biopsy at the end of treatment or to follow-up an abnormal PSA or digital rectal examination. The trial terminated early because the study objectives were met. Thus, 9060 patients were included in the final analysis. A surprisingly large number of patients in both arms developed prostate cancer; however, there was a significant decrease in incidence with the finasteride arm with 24.8% of placebo treated, and 18.4% of finasteride being diagnosed with prostate cancer ($P < .001$).

There were several other differences seen between the arms. Sexual dysfunction was more common in the finasteride treated men, whereas urinary symptoms were more common in those receiving placebo. More worrisome was the increase in Gleason 7–10 tumors identified in the finasteride group, with 6.4% of men in the finasteride group and 5.1% of men in the placebo group having this pathology. One possible explanation is that this is an artificial result of the finasteride treatment as can be seen with androgen deprivation therapy and also has been reported with finasteride.[72]

SIDE EFFECTS OF ADT

Androgen deprivation therapy is associated with both short and long term side effects. Besides the well-described loss of libido, erectile dysfunction and hot flashes, there can be several other side effects (Table 11.4). These have been well

TABLE 11.4 Side Effects of ADT

Sexual Side Effects	
• Decreased Libido	• Erectile dysfunction
Physical Changes	
• Gynecomastia	• Weight gain
• Decreased muscle mass	• Decreased bone mineral density
• Fatigue	• Hair changes
• Decreased size of penis/testis	• Breast pain
Metabolic Changes	
• Lipid changes	• Anemia
Mental Changes	
• Lack of initiative	• Decreased memory
• Emotional lability	• Decreased cognitive function

described in an excellent recent review of the subject.[73] Perhaps the best-known side effect is erectile dysfunction (ED). Loss of libido is seen in many but not all of patients on ADT. For patients who maintain some libido, there are treatments that can reverse ED. Oral sildenafil, and intracavernosal injection or intrauretheral therapy using alprostadil are medical therapeutic strategies to overcome ED. Various devices such as vacuum constriction devices and penile prosthesis may be used also with success. Hot flashes is another common side effect seen in 65% to 80% of men.[74–76] Estrogens, progestins and serotonin reuptake inhibitors such as venlafaxine may be effective in decreasing hot flashes.[73] The incidence of gynecomastia and mastodynia seen with anti-androgen monotherapy may be decreased with either prophylactic breast irradiation or tamoxifen therapy.[77,78]

Other less commonly recognized side effects of ADT include decreases in bone mineral density, decreases in lean muscle and increases in body fat.[79] This is accompanied by increases in insulin total cholesterol, low density lipoprotein (LDL), high density lipoprotein (HDL), and triglycerides.[73] In addition, a normochromic, noromocytic anemia is frequently seen. Loss of body hair and softening of facial hair also may be observed. Finally, there can be significant emotional disturbances with ADT. These can range from emotional lability to irritability to major depression.[80] Thus, it is important to recognize these side effects and recommend a program of diet and exercise, perhaps with adjunctive pharmacologic intervention, intended to decrease or prevent the development of serious consequences caused by long term ADT.

PSA GENE EXPRESSION REGULATED BY ANDROGENS

Standard phase II clinical trials in solid tumors often have objective response with radiographically measurable disease as their primary endpoint. Because only approximately 20% of prostate cancer patients have soft tissue disease, and lesions seen by radioscintigraphy are not measurable, significant interest has been generated in using PSA as a marker for response to experimental agents. PSA is elevated in about 95% of patients with androgen insensitive prostate cancer. Changes in PSA often predate changes seen on radiographic imaging.

The promoter for the PSA gene is under androgen regulation. When the androgen receptor binds to the steroid receptor-binding consensus sequence within the promoter, up-regulation of the PSA gene ensues. Conversely, ADT causes a decrease in expression of PSA.[81,82] Thus, it is possible that PSA may not be an appropriate marker in clinical trials incorporating ADT therapies in hormone naive patients. This could be an explanation for the discrepancy seen in the relative PSA responses and clinical outcomes seen in a recently published trial. In this randomized trial of bilateral orchiectomy with or without flutamide, the combination group had a significantly higher proportion of patients who had a reduction in PSA to less than 4.0 ng/mL compared with the orchiectomy alone group (74% vs. 62%, $P < .001$); however, there was no survival benefit seen.[49] Thus, the anti-androgen may have blocked the binding of the androgen receptor to the PSA promoter and caused down regulation of PSA expression directly.

CONCLUSIONS

ADT remains the standard front-line therapy for metastatic prostate cancer and there are now convincing data for the use of ADT with external-beam radiation therapy for patients at high risk for treatment failure. In addition, hormonal treatment of prostate cancer should be considered for patients who have a high risk of recurrence after local therapy or biochemical recurrence. There is controversy, however, regarding the use of CAB, intermittent androgen blockade, and whether early ADT is superior to delayed therapy. Options for ADT include orchiectomy, GnRH-A, and nonsteroidal anti-androgens. Finally, while hormonal therapy remains a key therapeutic modality for advanced prostate cancer, long-term ADT carries important side effects that need to be carefully weighed against the available evidence of benefit.

ACKNOWLEDGMENT

This chapter was written in a personal capacity and does not represent the opinions of the National Institutes of Health, the Department of Health and Human Services, or the Federal Government

REFERENCES

1. Jemal A, Murray T, Samuels A et al. Cancer statistics, 2003. CA Cancer J Clin 2003;53:5–26.
2. Huggins C, Hodges C. Studies on prostatic cancer: The effect of castration, of estrogen and of

androgen injection on serum phosphatases in metastatic carcinoma of the prostate. Cancer Res 1941;1:293–299.

3. Treatment and survival of patients with cancer of the prostate. The Veterans Administration Cooperative Urological Research Group. Surg Gynecol Obstet 1967;124:1011–1017.
4. Matsuo H, Baba Y, Nair RM et al. Structure of the porcine LH- and FSH-releasing hormone. I. The proposed amino acid sequence. Biochem Biophys Res Commun 1971;43:1334–1339.
5. Schally AV. Luteinizing hormone-releasing hormone analogs: their impact on the control of tumorigenesis. Peptides 1999;20:1247–1262.
6. Soloway MS, Chodak G, Vogelzang NJ et al. Zoladex versus orchiectomy in treatment of advanced prostate-cancer–a randomized trial. Urology 1991;37:46–51.
7. Waymont B, Lynch TH, Dunn JA et al. Phase-Iii randomized study of zoladex versus stilbestrol in the treatment of advanced prostate-cancer. Br J Urol 1992;69:614–620.
8. Seidenfeld J, Samson DJ, Hasselblad V et al. Single-therapy androgen suppression in men with advanced prostate cancer: a systematic review and meta-analysis. Ann Intern Med 2000;132: 566–577.
9. Pilepich MV, Caplan R, Byhardt RW et al. Phase III trial of androgen suppression using goserelin in unfavorable-prognosis carcinoma of the prostate treated with definitive radiotherapy: Report of Radiation Therapy Oncology Group Protocol 85-31. J Clin Oncol 1997;15:1013–1021.
10. Lawton CA, Winter K, Murray K et al. Updated results of the phase III Radiation Therapy Oncology Group (RTOG) trial 85-31 evaluating the potential benefit of androgen suppression following standard radiation therapy for unfavorable prognosis carcinoma of the prostate. Int J Radiat Oncol Biol Phys 2001;49:937–946.
11. Pilepich MV, Winter K, Lawton C et al. Phase III trial of androgen suppression adjuvant to definitive radiotherapy. Long term results of RTOG study 85-31. Proc Am Soc Clin Oncol 2003; 22:A1530a.
12. Bolla M, Gonzalez D, Warde P et al. Improved survival in patients with locally advanced prostate cancer treated with radiotherapy and goserelin. N Engl J Med 1997;337:295–300.
13. Bolla M, Collette L, Blank L et al. Long-term results with immediate androgen suppression and external irradiation in patients with locally advanced prostate cancer (an EORTC study): a phase III randomised trial. Lancet 2002;360:103–108.
14. Granfors T, Modig H, Damber JE, Tomic R. Combined orchiectomy and external radiotherapy versus radiotherapy alone for nonmetastatic prostate cancer with or without pelvic lymph node involvement: A prospective randomized study. J Urol 1998;159:2030–2034.
15. Hanks GE, Lu JD, Machtay M et al. RTOG Protocol 92-02: A Phase III trial of the use of long term androgen suppression following neoadjuvant hormonal cytoreduction and radiotherapy in locally advanced carcinoma of the prostate. Proc Am Soc Clin Oncol 2000;19;A1284.
16. Adib RS, Anderson JB, Ashken MH et al. Immediate versus deferred treatment for advanced prostatic cancer: Initial results of the Medical Research Council trial. Br J Urol 1997;79:235–246.
17. Kirk D. A structured debate: immediate versus deferred androgen suppression in prostate cancer—evidence for deferred treatment. J Urol 2002;167:653.
18. Walsh PC, DeWeese TL, Eisenberger MA. A structured debate: immediate versus deferred androgen suppression in prostate cancer—evidence for deferred treatment. J Urol 2001;166:508–515.
19. Schroder FH. Endocrine treatment of prostate cancer—recent developments and the future. Part 1: maximal androgen blockade, early vs delayed endocrine treatment and side-effects. BJU Int 1999;83:161–170.
20. Messing EM, Manola J, Sarosdy M et al. Immediate hormonal therapy compared with obser-

vation after radical prostatectomy and pelvic lymphadenectomy in men with node-positive prostate cancer. N Engl J Med 1999;341:1781–1788.

21. Messing E, Manola J, Sarosdy M et al. Immediate hormonal therapy compared with observation after radical prostatectomy and pelvic lymphadenectomy in men with node positive prostate cancer: Results at 10 years of EST 3886. J Urol 2003;169:1480a.

22. Cheng L, Zincke H, Blute ML et al. Risk of prostate carcinoma death in patients with lymph node metastasis. Cancer 2001;91:66–73.

23. Gleave ME, Goldenberg L, Chin JL et al. Randomized comparative study of 3 vs 8 months of neoadjuvant hormonal therapy prior to radical prostatectomy: 3 year PSA recurrence rates. J Urol 2003;169:690a.

24. Gleave ME, Goldenberg SL, Chin JL et al. Randomized comparative study of 3 versus 8-month neoadjuvant hormonal therapy before radical prostatectomy: biochemical and pathological effects. J Urol 2001;166:500–506.

25. Aus G, Abrahamsson PA, Ahlgren G et al. Three-month neoadjuvant hormonal therapy before radical prostatectomy: a 7-year follow-up of a randomized controlled trial. BJU Int 2002;90: 561–566.

26. Schroder FH, Kurth KH, Fossa SD et al. Early versus delayed endocrine treatment in PN1-3 MO prostate cancer without local treatment of the primary tumor—results of EORTC 30846 - a phase III study. J Urol 2003;169:1487a.

27. EORTC protocol 30891. Available at: http://www.eortc.be/protoc/details.asp?protocol=30891 . 8-1-1999. 9-26-2003. Accessed December 2003.

28. Bagley CM, Lane RF, Blasko JC et al. Adjuvant chemohormonal therapy of high risk prostate carcinoma—ten year results. Cancer 2002;94:2728–2732.

29. Sato N, Gleave ME, Bruchovsky N et al. Intermittent androgen suppression delays progression to androgen-independent regulation of prostate-specific: antigen gene in the LNCaP prostate tumour model. J Steroid Biochem Mol Biol 1996;58:139–146.

30. Miyake H, Nelson C, Rennie PS, Gleave ME. Testosterone-repressed prostate message-2 is an antiapoptotic gene involved in progression to androgen independence in prostate cancer. Cancer Res 2000;60:170–176.

31. Miyake H, Tolcher A, Gleave ME. Antisense Bcl-2 oligodeoxynucleotides inhibit progression to androgen-independence after castration in the Shionogi tumor model. Cancer Res 1999;59: 4030–4034.

32. Akakura K, Bruchovsky N, Rennie PS et al. Effects of intermittent androgen suppression on the stem cell composition and the expression of the TRPM-2 (clusterin) gene in the Shionogi carcinoma. J Steroid Biochem Mol Biol 1996;59:501–511.

33. Bruchovsky N, Klotz LH, Crook JM et al. A phase II study of intermittent androgen suppression (IAS) in men with a rising serum PSA after radiation for localized prostate cancer [Abstr]. J Urol 1998;159:1287a.

34. Bracarda S, Rosi P, Pizzirusso G et al. Intermittent androgen suppression (IAS) in advanced or inoperable prostate cancer [Abstr]. Ann Oncol 1998;9:2720a.

35. Theyer G, Hamilton G. Current status of intermittent androgen suppression in the treatment of prostate cancer. Urology 1998;52:353–359.

36. Gleave M, Bruchovsky N, Goldenberg SL, Rennie P. Intermittent androgen suppression for prostate cancer: Rationale and clinical experience. Eur Urol 1998;34:37–41.

37. Crook JM, Szumacher E, Malone S et al. Intermittent androgen suppression in the management of prostate cancer. Urology 1999;53:530–534.

38. Strum SB, Scholz MC, McDermed JE. Intermittent androgen deprivation in prostate cancer patients: factors predictive of prolonged time off therapy. Oncologist 2000;5:45–52.

39. Grossfeld GD, Chaudhary UB, Reese DM et al. Intermittent androgen deprivation: update of cycling characteristics in patients without clinically apparent metastatic prostate cancer. Urology 2001;58:240–245.

40. Prapotnich D, Fizazi K, Escudier B et al. A 10-year clinical experience with intermittent hormonal therapy for prostate cancer. Eur Urol 2003;43:233–239.

41. Tangen C, Hussain M, Wilding G et al. Determinants of prostate specific antigen normalization in prostate cancer patients treated with androgen deprivation on Southwest Oncology Group Study 9346 (INT-0162). Proc Am Soc Clin Oncol. 2003;XX:A1591.

42. Sylvester J, Grimm P, Blasko J et al. The role of androgen ablation in patients with biochemical or local failure after definitive radiation therapy: a survey of practice patterns of urologists and radiation oncologists in the United States. Urology 2001;58:65–70.

43. Gulley J, Figg W, Carter J et al. A prospective analysis of the time to normalization of serum testosterone following 6 months of androgen deprivation therapy in patients on a randomized Phase III clinical trial utilizing intermittent hormonal therapy. Proc Am Soc Clin Oncol 2003;22:396, abstr. 1592.

44. Nejat RJ, Rashid HH, Bagiella E et al. A prospective analysis of time to normalization of serum testosterone after withdrawal of androgen deprivation therapy. J Urol 2000;164:1891–1894.

45. Oefelein MG. Serum testosterone-based luteinizing hormone-releasing hormone agonist redosing schedule for chronic androgen ablation: A phase I assessment. Urology 1999;54:694–699.

46. Hall MC, Fritzsch RJ, Sagalowsky AI et al. Prospective determination of the hormonal response after cessation of luteinizing hormone-releasing hormone agonist treatment in patients with prostate cancer. Urology 1999;53:898–902.

47. Higano CS, Ellis W, Russell K, Lange PH. Intermittent androgen suppression with leuprolide and flutamide for prostate cancer: A pilot study. Urology 1996;48:800–804.

48. Scher H. Phase I study of testosterone in patients with progressive androgen-independent prostate cancer. Available at: http://www.cancer.gov/clinicaltrials/view_clinicaltrials.aspx?version=healthprofessional&cdrid=68060&protocolsearchid=537893 . 5-1-2002. Accessed December 2003.

49. Eisenberger MA, Blumenstein BA, Crawford ED et al. Bilateral orchiectomy with or without flutamide for metastatic prostate cancer. N Engl J Med 1998;339:1036–1042.

50. Samson DJ, Seidenfeld J, Schmitt B et al. Systematic review and meta-analysis of monotherapy compared with combined androgen blockade for patients with advanced prostate carcinoma. Cancer 2002;95:361–376.

51. Kelly WK, Scher HI. Prostate specific antigen decline after antiandrogen withdrawal—the flutamide withdrawal syndrome. J Urol 1993;149:607–609.

52. Schellhammer PF, Venner P, Haas GP et al. Prostate specific antigen decreases after withdrawal of antiandrogen therapy with bicalutamide or flutamide in patients receiving combined androgen blockade. J Urol 1997;157:1731–1735.

53. Herrada J, Dieringer P, Logothetis CJ. Characterization of patients with androgen-independent prostatic carcinoma whose serum prostate specific antigen decreased following flutamide withdrawal. J Urol 1996;155:620–623.

54. BocconGibod L, Fournier G, Bottet P et al. Flutamide versus orchidectomy in the treatment of metastatic prostate carcinoma. Eur Urol 1997;32:391–395.

55. Pavone-Macaluso M. Flutamide monotherapy versus combined androgen blockade in advanced prostate cancer. Interim report of an Italian multicenter randomized study. SIU 23rd Congress. 1994;abstract 354.

56. Kolvenbag GJCM, Nash A. Bicalutamide dosages used in the treatment of prostate cancer. Prostate 1999;39:47–53.

57. Tyrrell CJ, Kaisary AV, Iversen P et al. Randomised comparison of 'Casodex'(TM) (bicalutamide) 150 mg monotherapy versus castration in the treatment of metastatic and locally advanced prostate cancer. Eur Urol 1998;33:447–456.

58. Kaisary AV, Iversen P, Tyrrell CJ et al. Is there a role for antiandrogen monotherapy in patients with metastatic prostate cancer? Prostate Cancer Prostatic Dis 2001;4:196–203.

59. Iversen P, Tyrrell CJ, Kaisary AV et al. Bicalutamide monotherapy compared with castration in patients with nonmetastatic locally advanced prostate cancer: 6.3 years of followup. J Urol 2000;164:1579–1582.

60. See WA, Wirth MP, McLeod DG et al. Bicalutamide as immediate therapy either alone or as adjuvant to standard care of patients with localized or locally advanced prostate cancer: First analysis of the early prostate cancer program (abstr #2558). J Urol 2002;168:429a.

61. EORTC protocol 30991. Available at: http://www.eortc.be/protoc/Details.asp?Protocol=30991 . 2-28-2003. 9-25-2003. Accessed December 2003.

62. Mickisch G. Phase III randomized study of initial bicalutamide versus observation followed by bicalutamide with either goserelin or bilateral orchiectomy in patients with prostate cancer. Available at: http://www.cancer.gov/clinicaltrials/view_clinicaltrials.aspx?version=health professional&cdrid=68560 . 4-17-2003. 9-25-2003. Accessed December 2003.

63. Trachtenberg J, Halpern N, Pont A. Ketoconazole—a novel and rapid treatment for advanced prostatic-cancer. J Urol 1983;130:152–153.

64. Trachtenberg J. High-dose ketoconazole in the treatment of metastatic prostatic-cancer [Abstr]. Prostate 1985;6:455a.

65. Harris KA, Weinberg V, Bok RA et al. Low dose ketoconazole with replacement doses of hydrocortisone in patients with progressive androgen independent prostate cancer. J Urol 2002; 168:542–545.

66. Small EJ, Baron A, Bok R. Simultaneous antiandrogen withdrawal and treatment with ketoconazole and hydrocortisone in patients with advanced prostate carcinoma. Cancer 1997;80: 1755–1759.

67. Leibowitz RL, Tucker SJ. Treatment of localized prostate cancer with intermittent triple androgen blockade: Preliminary results in 110 consecutive patients. Oncologist 2001;6:177–182.

68. Picus J, Halabi S, Hussain A et al. Efficacy of peripheral androgen blockade on prostate cancer: initial results of CALGB 9782. Proc Am Soc Clin Oncol 2002;21:182a.

69. Oh W, Manola J, Bittman L et al. Finasteride and flutamide therapy in patients with advanced prostate cancer: long-term follow-up and response to subsequent castration. Proc Am Soc Clin Oncol 2003;22:412a.

70. Leibowitz S, Kaufman D, Oh W et al. Primary hormonal therapy with finasteride and bicalutamide in advanced prostate cancer (CaP). Proc Am Soc Clin Oncol 2003;22:402a.

71. Thompson IM, Goodman PJ, Tangen CM et al. The influence of finasteride on the development of prostate cancer. N Engl J Med 2003;349:215–224.

72. Civantos F, Soloway MS, Pinto JE. Histopathological effects of androgen deprivation in prostatic cancer. Semin Urol Oncol 1996;14[suppl 2]:22–31.

73. Higano CS. Side effects of androgen deprivation therapy: monitoring and minimizing toxicity. Urology 2003;61:32–38.

74. Karling P, Hammar M, Varenhorst E. Prevalence and duration of hot flushes after surgical or medical castration in men with prostatic-carcinoma. J Urol 1994;152:1170–1173.

75. Spetz AC, Hammar M, Lindberg B et al. Prospective evaluation of hot flashes during treatment with parenteral estrogen or complete androgen ablation for metastatic carcinoma of the prostate. J Urol 2001;166:517–520.

76. Schow DA, Renfer LG, Rozanski TA, Thompson IM. Prevalence of hot flushes during and after neoadjuvant hormonal therapy for localized prostate cancer. South Med J 1998; 91:855–857.

77. Widmark A, Fossa SD, Lundmo P et al. Does prophylactic breast irradiation prevent antiandrogen- induced gynecomastia? Evaluation of 253 patients in the randomized Scandinavian trial SPCG-7/SFUO-3. Urology 2003;61:145–151.

78. Staiman VR, Lowe FC. Tamoxifen for flutamide/finasteride-induced gynecomastia. Urology 1997;50:929–933.

79. Smith JC, Bennett S, Evans LM et al. The effects of induced hypogonadism on arterial stiffness, body composition, and metabolic parameters in males with prostate cancer. J Clin Endocrinol Metabol 2001;86:4261–4267.

80. Pirl WF, Siegel GI, Goode MJ, Smith MR. Depression in men receiving androgen deprivation therapy for prostate cancer: A pilot study. Psycho-Oncology 2002;11:518–523.

81. Wolf DA, Schulz P, Fittler F. Transcriptional regulation of prostate kallikrein-like genes by androgen. Mol Endocrinol 1992;6:753–762.

82. Riegman PHJ, Vlietstra RJ, Vanderkorput JAGM et al. The promoter of the prostate-specific antigen gene contains a functional androgen responsive element. Mol Endocrinol 1991;5: 1921–1930.

Chapter 12

The Immunotherapy of Patients with Metastatic Melanoma by Inducing Clonal Repopulation with Antitumor Lymphocytes

Steven A. Rosenberg

Mark E. Dudley

Cancer immunotherapies can be divided into approaches that involve active immunization (also referred to as cancer vaccines) or passive immunization (also referred to as adoptive or cell transfer immunotherapy). T lymphocytes are the major immune effector cells involved in tissue destruction, and both active and passive immunotherapies are aimed at inducing specific antitumor T-cells that can traffic to and destroy cancer deposits.

Active immunization approaches involve exposing the cancer-bearing host to antigens aimed at generating cellular immune responses against determinants expressed by the growing cancer. The discovery over the last decade of a wide variety of human cancer antigens has stimulated interest in the development of this approach to cancer treatment.[1] Most human cancer antigens are either differentiation antigens expressed on the tumor and the cell of origin of the malignancy, cancer-testis antigens expressed on selected epithelial cancers as well as germ cells, or mutated proteins exclusively expressed on the cancer and not on normal tissues. Attempts to immunize cancer patients have utilized recombinant viruses or DNA plasmids encoding the cancer antigen, irradiated tumor cells, tumor lysates, purified protein antigens, peptides derived from those proteins, or antigens that are pulsed onto professional antigen presenting cells such as dendritic cells. Although these approaches can generate immune T-cells capable of recognizing peptides on the surface of tumor cells, the regression of growing cancers in patients utilizing this approach has been sporadic and rare.[2] Thus, the generation of antitumor T-cells in the tumor-bearing host may be necessary, but certainly is not sufficient to mediate the regression of clinically significant cancers.

Extensive studies have attempted to understand the mechanisms used by tumors to escape immune destruction.[3] Several of these tumor escape mechanisms are listed in Table 12.1. In contrast to active immunization approaches, cell transfer therapies have unique qualities that enable them to overcome many of these tumor escape mechanisms.

TABLE 12.1 Possible Mechanisms of Tumor Escape from Immune Destruction

Lymphocyte Factors
Lack of T-cell help
Insufficient number of antitumor T-cells
Insufficient avidity of T-cells for tumor
T-cells are "tolerized"
Downregulation of T-cell receptor signal transduction
Apoptosis of T-cells when encountering tumor
Inadequate T-cell function (cytokines, lysis)
T-cells cannot enter tumor stroma
Inhibition by "suppressor" T-cells
Tumor Factors
Tumor cannot activate quiescent precursors
Insufficient tumor antigen expression
Loss of HLA expression by tumor
Tumor produces local immunosuppressive factors
Tumor lacks sufficient apoptotic or other cell destruction pathways

ADVANTAGES OF CELL TRANSFER THERAPY

Cell transfer therapies involve the administration of lymphocytes with antitumor activity and have a variety of advantages compared to active immunization approaches. In contrast to the relatively small numbers of antitumor T-cells that are generated by active immunization, cell transfer therapies can involve the administration of very large numbers of antitumor lymphocytes.

Most cell transfer therapies used to treat cancer patients utilize tumor infiltrating lymphocytes (TIL) from resected tumor specimens that are expanded in vitro in interleukin-2 (IL-2).[4,5] Lymphocytes can be grown from tumor cell fragments, from enzymatic digests, or from mechanical disruption of tumor fragments. We recently reported an analysis of 860 attempted TIL cultures from 90 sequential melanoma biopsy specimens from 62 HLA-A2$^+$ patients (Table 12.2).[6] Tumor-specific activity was detected from 81% of patients that were screened for tumor reactivity. Multiple independent TIL cultures derived from a single tumor often exhibited substantial functional and phenotypic variation, and the characteristics of TIL obtained from different lesions from the same patient exhibited variability as well. These lymphocytes can grow with a doubling time of two to three days, and thus it is possible to generate up to 10^{11} lymphocytes in one to two months after initiating the cultures.

The ability to grow autologous antitumor lymphocytes in vitro also provides an opportunity to test individual cultures to identify cells with a very high affinity for tumor antigen recognition. There is substantial redundancy in the phenotype and function of tumor reactive lymphocytes in any individual patient. The ability to grow cells ex vivo and test them for function prior to cell transfer potentially enables the identification of the exact cell subpopulations and effector functions that are required to mediate cancer regression in vivo.

Because tumor cells do not express costimulatory molecules such as B7-1, tumor cells may not be able to adequately activate lymphocytes generated by active immunization. An advantage of cell transfer therapy is the ability to administer cells activated ex vivo to exhibit an antitumor effector function. Further, lymphocytes with antitumor activity may be "ignorant" or "tolerized" in the local environment of the tumor, and the ability to expand and activate lymphocyte subpopulations ex vivo has the potential to overcome these mechanisms and to substantially improve their effectiveness.

Perhaps the greatest advantage of cell transfer therapies is the ability to manipulate the host prior to cell transfer to provide an altered environment for the transferred cells. In early clinical trials of cell transfer therapies, cells were administered to the intact host and thus competed with endogenous lymphocytes for the homeostatic cytokines that provide the stimulus for maintenance and growth of host lymphocytes.[4,5] By treating patients with a nonmyeloablative chemotherapy and administering in vitro grown lymphocytes at a time when natural lymphocytes are at a low level, the administered lymphocytes have increased

TABLE 12.2 Melanoma Excisional Biopsies Processed to Established TIL for Potential Adoptive Cell Transfer Therapy

				Active TIL[a]		
	Total Initiated	"+" growth[b]	Cryo-preserved[c]	Allogeneic HLA-A2$^+$ (not screened)	Autologous (not screened)	REPed for treatment[d]
Fragments						
Patients	62	59	23	23 (36)	21 (27)	6
Tumors	90	83	33	34 (50)	34 (44)	7
Cultures	710	496	194	87 (302)	151 (247)	9
Digests						
Patients	33	32	11	3 (21)	10 (17)	3
Tumors	42	41	16	3 (25)	11 (21)	3
Cultures	119	112	44	16 (68)	26 (54)	4
Medimachine						
Patients	17	14	5	4 (9)	3 (8)	0
Tumors	26	20	8	7 (12)	5 (11)	0
Cultures	31	28	5	9 (23)	13 (21)	0

[a]At least one TIL culture demonstrated a specific IFN-γ release when stimulated with indicated tumor cells (defined as an IFN-γ release greater than 100 pg/mL and at least twice the value of any A2$^-$ cell lines).

[b]At least one culture expanded sufficiently for screening or cryopreservation (more than approximately 5×10^6 cells).

[c]No TIL were screened, but at least one culture was cryopreserved at sufficient cell numbers for screening.

[d]Eight of the 62 patients included in this data set were treated with the REPed cultures included in this table.

Eight additional patients had an initial biopsy that led to cultures included in this data set, but were ultimately treated with cells derived from later biopsies or other sources.[6]

"space" and preferential exposure to these homeostatic cytokines. Perhaps of greater importance is the ability of immunosuppressive chemotherapy to eliminate regulatory T-cells that can compromise the function of the transferred antitumor T-cells.

CLINICAL TRIALS OF CELL TRANSFER THERAPY FOLLOWING NONMYELOABLATIVE CHEMOTHERAPY

Although earlier trials of cell transfer therapy using TIL from patients with metastatic melanoma could mediate cancer regression in some patients, these responses were very often short lived. In these earlier studies there was a correlation between TIL reactivity against autologous tumor and cancer regression, although many administered TIL populations did not have antitumor reactivity.[7,8]

The development of techniques to clone lymphocytes from TIL and peripheral blood lymphocytes (PBL) enabled the in vitro generation of large numbers of cloned lymphocyte populations with antitumor activity.[9] These techniques utilized limiting dilution followed by multiple rounds of expansion with antiOKT3 antibody in conjunction with IL-2.[10] A phase I trial was performed in fifteen patients with metastatic melanoma who received these cloned cells following nonmyeloablative chemotherapy.[11] Examples of the reactivity of these cells are shown in Table 12.3. All but one of these cells (patient 11) had reactivity against either the gp100 209-217 epitope or the MART-1:27-35 epitope. In all cases melanoma cell lines were recognized by the cloned lymphocyte populations. Because cell transfer had not been performed previously in patients treated with a nonmyeloablative chemotherapy, a phase I trial was performed in which patients received increasing doses of cyclophosphamide and fludarabine along with increasing doses of IL-2. A final regimen was established in which patients received 60 mg/kg of cyclophosphamide for two days followed by five days of fludarabine at 25 mg/m^2. On the day after the last fludarabine dose, when absolute lymphocyte and neutrophil counts were near zero, lymphocytes were administered along with IL-2 at a dose of 720,000 IU/kg every eight hours to tolerance. No objective cancer responses were seen in these patients.

Two limitations of this clinical approach were suggested. Cloned cell populations that began from single starting cells and were then expanded to greater than 10^{10} lymphocytes may have exhausted much of their proliferative potential. This may have accounted for the inability to detect a persistence of these cells for more than several days following administration. In addition, the cloned cells were CD8$^+$ and studies in both animals and humans have emphasized the importance of CD4 helper cells to sustain the survival and activity of effector CD8$^+$ lymphocytes.

The clinical protocol thus was modified to administer the nonmyeloablative chemotherapy at the highest doses achieved in the phase I study, followed by the administration of heterogeneous TIL populations often containing both CD4 and CD8$^+$ cells that had been grown for much shorter periods of time (Table 12.2 and growth techniques described in reference[6]). Because TIL populations were grown from tumors and not cloned, it was often possible to administer the cells after just a single expansion with anti-CD3 antibody and IL-2. The characteristics of the first thirteen patients treated in this trial are shown in Table 12.4 and the reactivity of cells administered are shown in Table 12.5.[12] All thirteen patients previously had been refractory to treatment with high-dose IL-2 and eight were refractory to aggressive chemotherapy. Six patients showed an objective cancer response and four additional patients showed mixed responses. Three of the responding patients previously had received the identical nonmyeloablative

TABLE 12.3 Specificity and Activity of T-Cell Clones

	T2 + peptide[a]									
			g209[d]			$A2^-$ Tumor line		$A2^+$ Tumor line		
Patient	m27[b] 1.0	g280[c] 1.0	1.0	0.01	0.0001	888mel	938mel	526mel	624mel	Auto[e]
1		131	19770	11050	>1000	143	179	2195	996	
2		4	55150	43100	512	0	0	3335	2815	
3		85	71000	59400	9300	90	87	5245	2130	
4		20	30750	6400	70	25	24	825	567	
5	1235		10			8	11	>29700	8270	
6		90	45400	31450	537	47	52	5810	3980	
7		30	>128000	65400	299	36	11	>12000	5350	
8		17	58900	35750	373	13	15	>14900	4625	
9		27	15850	5160	248	18	24	4450	3690	
10	47050		657			419	418	27150	>9665	
11	1	1	1			2		2		19900
12		17	18515	3874	265	12	12	778	56	
13		32	21750	19750	2950	28	39	2385	2710	
14	9		25900	8720	151	10	8	1840	3120	
15	24		52150	34950	>16360	20	15	>11180	7995	

[a]Interferon-gamma secretion (pg/mL) by cloned T cells when stimulated with T2 cells pulsed with the indicated peptide concentration (micromolar) or with melanoma cell lines.
[b]MART-1:27-35 peptide
[c]gp100:280-288 peptide
[d]gp100:209-217 peptide
[e]Autologous tumor-cell line[11]

TABLE 12.4 Patient Demographics, Treatments Received, and Clinical Outcomes

			Treatment[a]					
Patient	Auto-immunity	Age/sex	Cells infused[b] ($\times 10^{-10}$)	CD8/CD4 Phenotype[c] (%)	Antigen Specificity[d]	IL-2 (Doses)	Sites of Evaluable Metastases	Response Duration[e] (months)
1	None	18/M	2.3	11/39	Other	9	Lymph nodes (axillary, mesen-teric, pelvic)	PR (24+)[f]
2	Vitiligo	30/F	3.5	83/15	MART-1, gp100	8	Cutaneous, subcutaneous	PR (8)
3	None	43/F	4.0	44/58	gp100	5	Brain, cutaneous, liver, lung	NR
4	None	57/F	3.4	56/52	gp100	9	Cutaneous, subcutaneous	PR (2)
5	None	53/M	3.0	16/85	Other	7	Brain, lung, lymph nodes	NR-mixed
6	None	37/F	9.2	65/35	Other	6	Lung, intraperi-toneal, subcuta-neous	PR (15+)
7	Vitiligo	44/M	12.3	61/41	MART-1	7	Lymph nodes, subcutaneous	NR-mixed
8	None	48/M	9.5	48/52	gp100	12	Subcutaneous	NR
9	Viltilgo	57/M	9.6	84/13	MART-1	10	Cutaneous, subcutaneous	PR (10+)
10	Uveitis	55/M	10.7	96/2	MART-1	12	Lymph nodes, cutaneous, subcutaneous	PR (9+)
11	Vitiligo	29/M	13.0	96/3	MART-1	12	Liver, pericardial subcutaneous	NR-mixed

12	None	37/M	13.7	72/24	MART-1	11	Liver, lung, gallbladder, lymph nodes	NR-mixed
13	None	41/F	7.7	92/8	MART-1	11	Subcutaneous	NR

[a]Each patient was treated with chemotherapy starting 7 days before cell administration, consisting of 2 days of cyclophosphamide at 60 mg per kg of body weight, followed by 5 days of fludarabine at 25mg/m^2. On the day after the final dose of fludarabine, when circulating lymphocyte and neutrophil counts had dropped to less than 20/mm^3, each patient received an intravenous infusion of autologous lymphocytes over approximately 30 to 60 min. After cell infusion, patients received high-dose IL-2 therapy consisting of 720,000 IU/kg bolus intravenous infusion every 8 hours to tolerance. Some patients with mixed or responding lesions received an additional course of cell transfer therapy.

[b]T cell cultures for infusion were derived from TILs by minor modifications of established techniques. Multiple cultures were started from each resected melanoma specimen and were screened independently by cytokine secretion assay for recognition of autologous tumor cells (if available) and HLA-A2$^+$ tumor cell lines.[11] TIL cultures that exhibited specific tumor cell recognition were expanded for treatment using one or two cycles of a rapid expansion protocol with irradiated allogeneic feeder cells, OKT3 (anti-CD3) antibody, and 6000 IU per ml of IL-2.

[c]Percent of lymphocyte gated cells from the infusion sample that stained with each antibody. Values do not add to 100% if a significant fraction of infused cells was negative or double positive for CD4 and CD8 antigen expression.

[d]Antigen specificity was determined by cytokine release assay. Other: recognition of autologous tumor cells, but no HLA-A2-restricted epitope derived from MART-1, tyrosinase, tyrosinase related protein 1(TRP1), TRP2, NY-ESO-1, gp100, MAGE1, or MAGE3.

[e]Abbreviations: NR, no response; PR, partial response.

[f]Microscopic residual focus of disease resected; patient remains free of disease. Patient 1 had a 6-mm brain density that increased to 8 mm at 8 months. After localized stereotactic radiotherapy, the density disappeared.

TABLE 12.5 Activity and Specificity of Infused Lymphocyte Cultures (IFN-γ pg/ml)

	Stimulation by Tumor Lines (HLA-A2)[b]				Stimulation by 293-A2 Gene Transfectants[c]								
Patient[a]	None	938 (–)	526 (+)	Autol. (+)	GFP	MART-1	TRP1	TRP2	TYR	NY-ESO-1	gp100	MAGE1	MAGE3
1	204	143	155	**5140**	155	151	123	137	126	128	110	133	151
2	9	7	**9850**	**7020**	0	**6850**	53	0	0	65	**950**	0	0
3	1	3	**20420**	**615**	0	0	0	0	2	0	**7100**	0	0
4	0	4	**9090**	nd	0	0	75	0	0	0	**4390**	0	0
5	0	2	19	**3535**	0	0	0	0	2	0	0	0	0
6	0	9	**798**	**2620**	68	121	94	87	121	104	118	96	104
7	0	279	**5170**	**5230**	0	**3790**	0	0	0	0	28	23	83
8	0	849	**4990**	nd	0	0	0	2	0	0	**458**	0	0
9	11	43	**2528**	nd	12	**>1361**	17	13	17	30	17	14	19
10	0	0	**15150**	nd	0	**13360**	13	0	0	0	20	0	33
11	0	0	**9025**	nd	0	**12110**	10	0	7	65	**287**	0	70
12	11	72	**1200**	**1006**	126	**1970**	120	80	96	60	145	88	209
13	0	234	**3545**	**703**	75	**1730**	0	0	0	0	19	0	0

All samples for infusion demonstrated significant cytokine release when stimulated with autologous or HLA-A2$^+$ tumor cell lines. Six infusion samples recognized MART-1, five recognized gp100, and three recognized unidentified antigens expressed by the autologous tumor cell line. There was no correlation between the antigen specificity of the infused cells and objective response, the onset of autoimmunity, or treatment toxicity.

[a]The results in this table are combined from three different experiments. Values indicated pg/ml of IFN-γ. Significant T-cell reactivity was defined by value that are at least two times all controls and greater than 100 pg/ml (bold typeface and underlined).

[b]Melanoma cell lines were derived from tumor specimens obtained at the Surgery Branch, NCI. If a patient had no autologous melanoma cell line available at the time of the assay, the value is listed as "nd" (not done).

[c]The human embroyonic kidney cell line 293 was first stably transfected with an expression construct for HLA-A2, then transiently transfected with a panel of plasmids encoding shared melanoma antigens. Efficient transfection was confirmed in each experiment by visual assessment of green florescent protein (GFP) expression in GFP transfected cells and in some assays by the stimulation of T-cell clones by the appropriate transfectants including MART-1, tyrosinase-related protein (TRP)2, tyrosinase (TYR), NY-ESO-1, and gp100.

chemotherapy but with cloned CD8+ cells plus IL-2, and they had not responded. Thus, it appeared that the combination of the nonmyeloablative chemotherapy with the more heterogeneous TIL cultured for shorter periods was responsible for the substantial objective response rate in these patients with metastatic melanoma.

Responses were seen at a variety of sites including skin, subcutaneous tissue, liver and lung. Examples of these antitumor responses are shown in Figures 12.1 through 12.7.

Of significance was the ability of the transferred cells to survive and grow in the patient for many months following the adoptive cell transfer, the first time we had seen this in any of our cell transfer studies. Examples of two such patients are shown in Figure 12.8. In these two patients almost 80% of all circulating CD8+ lymphocytes were the transferred lymphocytes with antitumor activity.[12]

The antitumor cells continued to expand following intravenous injection, which thus magnified their antitumor activity. In this way, cell transfer therapies differ substantially from chemotherapeutic approaches whose effector functions are eliminated shortly after chemotherapy administration.

FUTURE DIRECTIONS FOR STUDY OF CELL TRANSFER THERAPIES FOR PATIENTS WITH METASTATIC CANCER

Although the development of cell transfer therapies is still in early stages, a variety of possibilities exist for modifying and possibly improving upon these efforts. Although current studies have been performed in patients with melanoma, tumor antigens have been identified in a variety of common

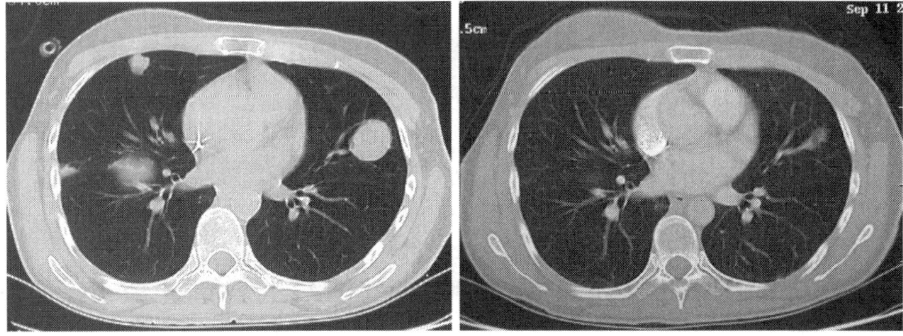

FIGURE 12.1 Regression of the lung metastasis in a patient receiving cell transfer therapy following nonmyeloablative chemotherapy. Pretreatment (left); post-treatment (right).

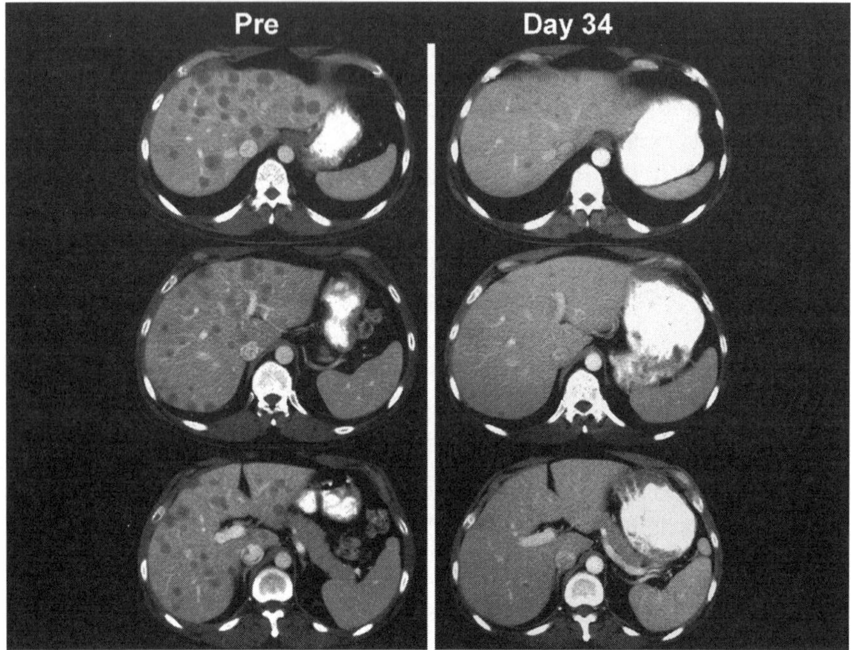

FIGURE 12.2 Regression of the liver metastases in a patient receiving cell transfer therapy following nonmyeloablative chemotherapy. Pretreatment (left); post-treatment (right).

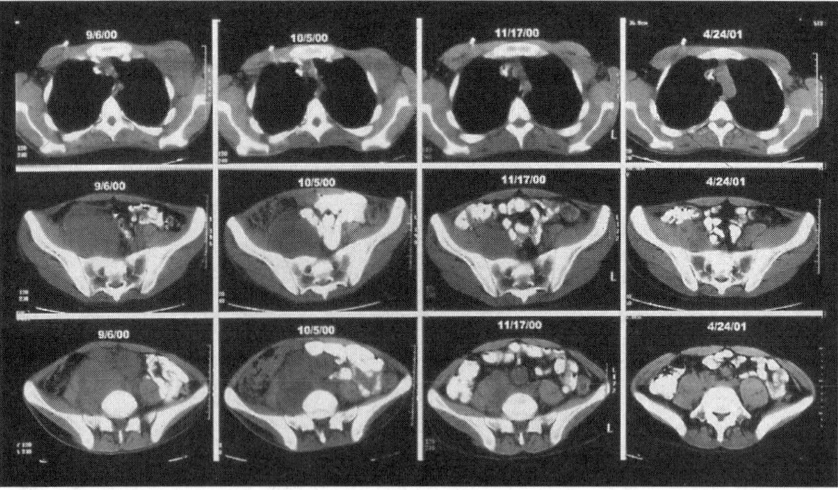

FIGURE 12.3 Regression of large axillary (upper), pelvic (middle), and intra-abdominal (lower) metastases in a patient receiving cell transfer therapy following nonmyeloablative chemotherapy. Sequential shrinkage of these lesions is seen (right to left).

Pre-therapy: 11/04/02 | **Post-therapy: 01/16/03**

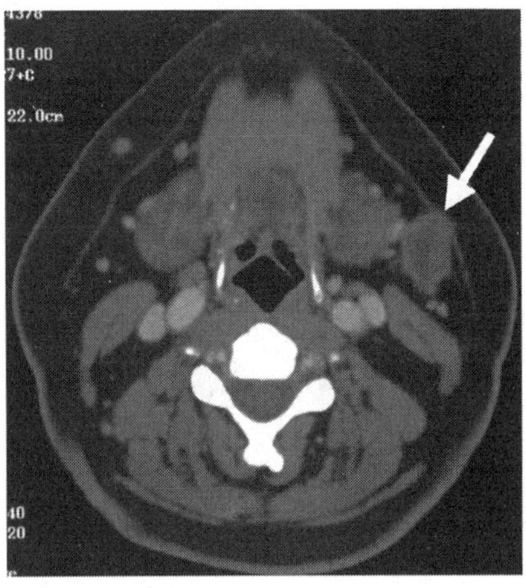

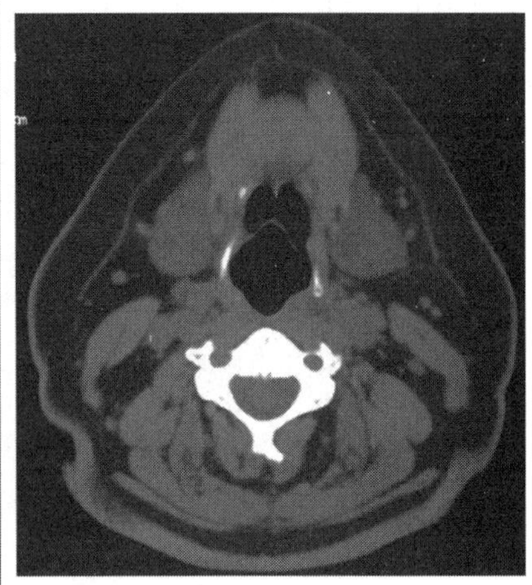

FIGURE 12.4 Regression of lymph node metastasis in the neck in a patient receiving cell transfer therapy following nonmyeloablative chemotherapy. Pretreatment (left); post-treatment (right).

Pre-therapy: 11/04/02

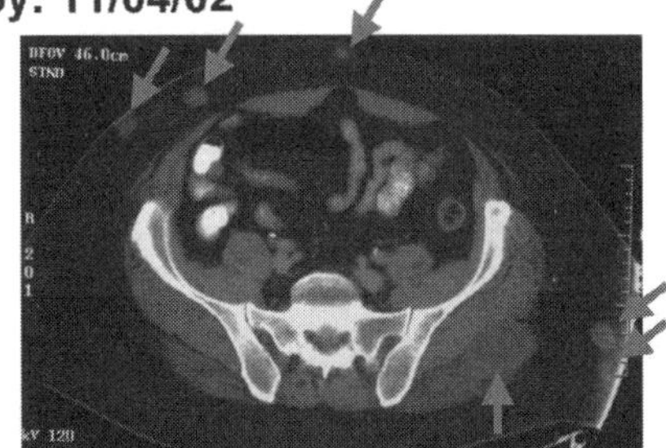

Post-therapy: 01/15/03

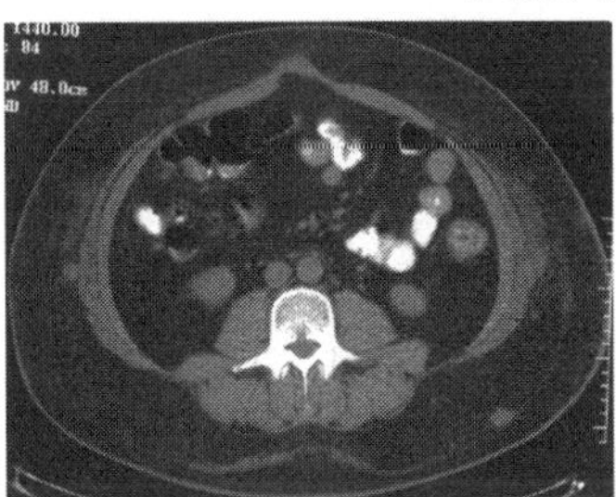

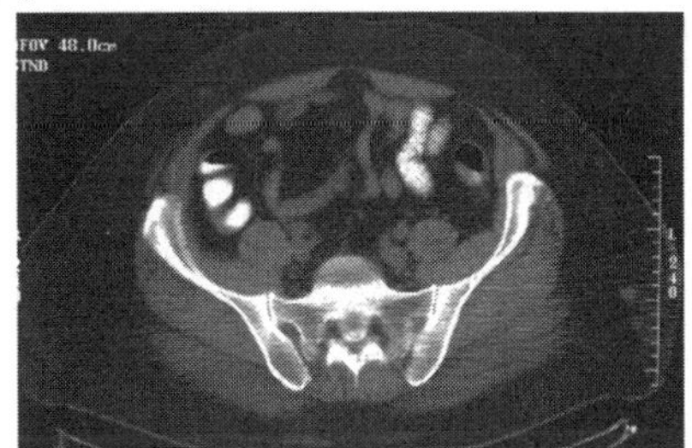

FIGURE 12.5 Regression of multiple subcutaneous metastases in a patient receiving cell transfer therapy following nonmyeloablative chemotherapy. Pretreatment (upper); post-treatment (lower).

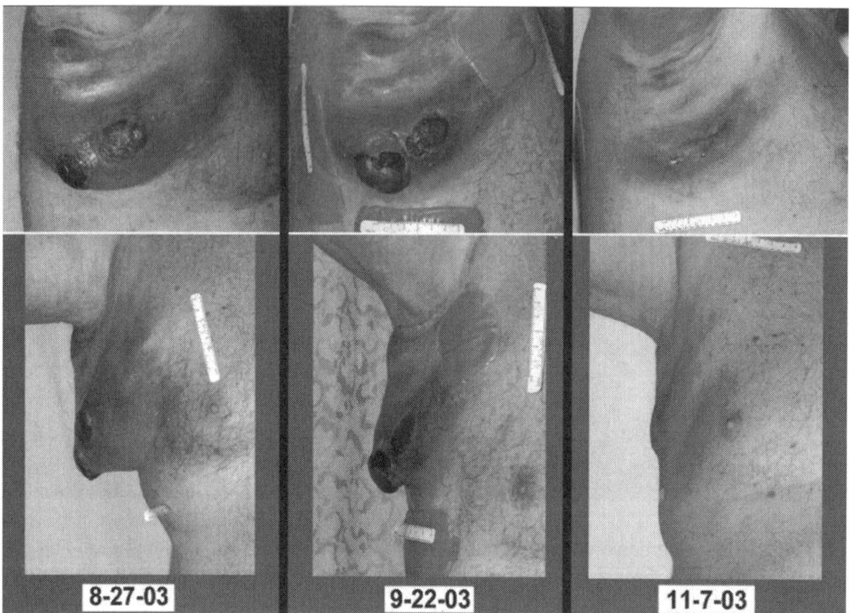

FIGURE 12.6 Regression of a large axillary mass in a patient undergoing cell transfer therapy following nonmyeloablative chemotherapy. Pretreatment (left); post-treatment (middle and right).

epithelial tumors that can serve as the target of cell transfer approaches.[1] Preliminary studies in patients have indicated that the administration of antitumor lymphocytes directly into the arterial supply of tumors may be more effective than the intravenous injection of these cells.[13] Patients tolerated only about three days of high-dose IL-2 and perhaps lower doses of IL-2 administered for prolonged periods of time may be more effective. In addition, perhaps cytokines other than IL-2, such as IL-7 or IL-15, may be more effective in sustaining the survival and growth of the transferred cells. Animal models have suggested that immunization of patients utilizing the antigen recognized by the administered cells can improve tumor regression and clinical protocols to attempt this in humans are planned.[14] The cyclophosphamide-flurdarabine preparative regimen mentioned above is only one possible conditioning regimen and the exploration of others is warranted. Genetic modification of transferred lymphocytes with genes encoding antitumor T-cell receptors or genes encoding cytokines such as IL-2 or IL-15 are being explored.[15-17]

Cell transfer immunotherapy can mediate tumor regression in patients with metastatic melanoma refractory to other treatments. The further application and improvement of this approach is under vigorous investigation.

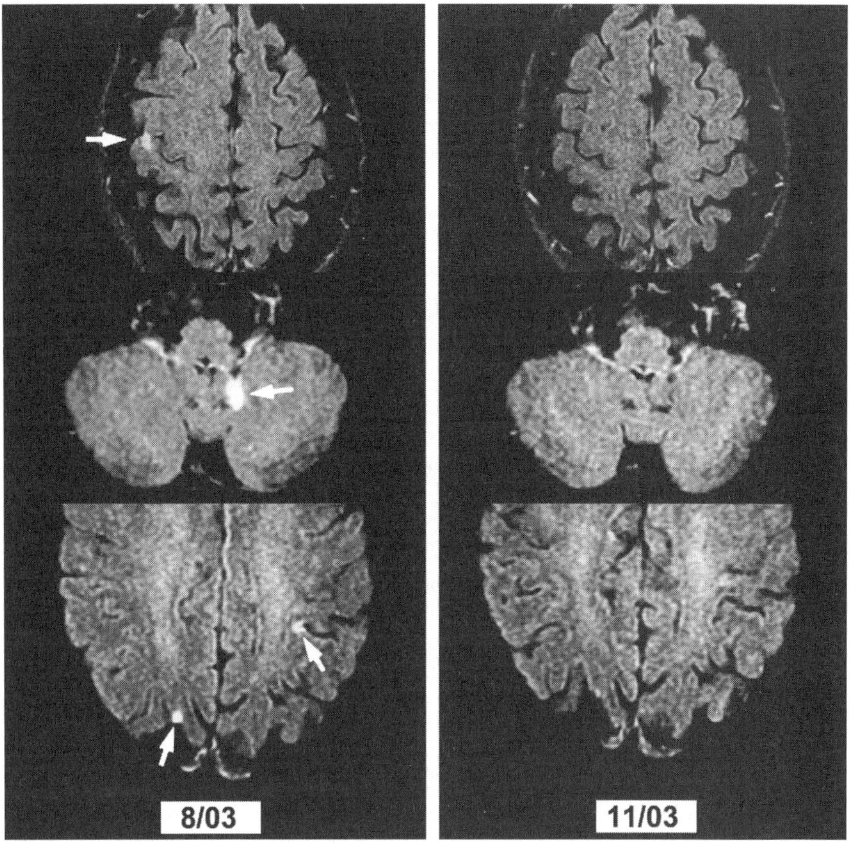

FIGURE 12.7 Regression of multiple brain metastases in a patient undergoing cell transfer therapy following nonmyeloablative chemotherapy. Pretreatment (left); post-treatment (right).

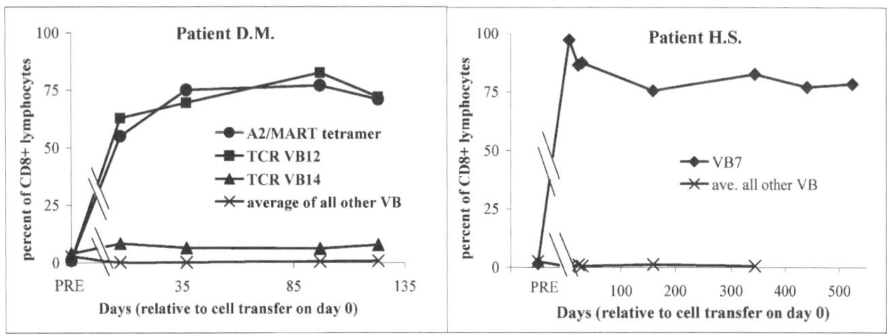

FIGURE 12.8 Tumor reactive clones persist as the predominant lymphocyte population in the PBL of some treated patients. PBL from patients DM (left) or HS (right) at the indicated days after cell transfer were analyzed by FACS using antibodies specific for the indicated T cell receptor (TCR) V-beta families or HLA-A2/MART-1: 26–35 (27L) tetrameric complexes.

REFERENCES

1. Rosenberg SA. Progress in human tumour immunology and immunotherapy. Nature 2002;411:380–384.
2. Rosenberg SA, Yang JC, Schwartzentruber DJ, et al. Immunologic and therapeutic evaluation of a synthetic peptide vaccine for the treatment of patients with metastatic melanoma. Nat Med 1998;4:321–327,.
3. Khong HT, Restifo NP. Natural selection of tumor variants in the generation of "tumor escape" phenotypes. Nat Immunol 2002;3:999–1005.
4. Rosenberg SA, Packard BS, Aebersold PM, et al. Use of tumor infiltrating lymphocytes and interleukin-2 in the immunotherapy of patients with metastatic melanoma. Preliminary report. N Engl J Med 1988;319:1676–1680.
5. Rosenberg SA, Yannelli JR, Yang JC, et al. Treatment of patients with metastatic melanoma using autologous tumor-infiltrating lymphocytes and interleukin-2. J Natl Cancer Inst 1994;86:1159–1166.
6. Dudley ME, Wunderlich JR, Shelton TE, et al. Generation of tumor-infiltrating lymphocyte cultures for use in adoptive transfer therapy for melanoma patients. J Immunother 2003;26:332–342.
7. Rosenberg SA. Interleukin-2 and the development of immunotherapy for the treatment of patients with cancer. Cancer J 2000;6(suppl):S2–S7.
8. Schwartzentruber DJ, Hom SS, Dadmarz R, et al. In vitro predictors of therapeutic response in melanoma patients receiving tumor infiltrating lymphocytes and interleukin-2. J Clin Oncol 1994;12:1475–1483.
9. Dudley ME, Ngo LT, Westwood J, et al. T cell clones from melanoma patients immunized against an anchor-modified gp100 peptide display discordant effector phenotypes. Cancer J 2000;6:69–77.
10. Riddell SR, Greenberg PD. The use of anti-CD3 and anti-CD28 monoclonal antibodies to clone and expand human antigen-specific T cells. J Immunol Meth 1990;128:189–201.
11. Dudley M, Wunderlich J, Yang JC, et al. A Phase I study of non-myeloablative chemotherapy and adoptive transfer of autologous tumor antigen-specific T lymphocytes in patients with metastatic melanoma. J Immunother 2002;25:243–251.
12. Dudley ME, Wunderlich JR, Robbins PF, et al. Cancer regression and autoimmunity in patients following clonal repopulation with anti-tumor lymphocytes. Science 2002;298:850–854.
13. Rosenberg SA, Yang JC, Robbins PF, et al. Cell transfer therapy for cancer: lessons from sequential treatments of a patient with metastatic melanoma. J Immunother 2003;26:385–393.
14. Overwijk WW, Theoret MR, Finkelstein SE, et al. Tumor regression and autoimmunity after reversal of a functionally tolerant state of self-reactive CD8+ T cells. J Exp Med 2003; 198:569–580.
15. Cole DJ, Weil DP, Shilyansky J, et al. Characterization of the functional specificity of a cloned T-cell receptor heterodimer recognizing the MART-1 melanoma antigen. Cancer Res 1995;55:748–752.
16. Morgan RA, Dudley ME, Yu Y, et al. High efficiency TCR gene transfer into primary human lymphocytes affords avid recognition of melanoma tumor antigen glycoprotein 100 and does not alter the recognition of autologous melanoma antigens. J Immunol 2003;171:3287–3295.
17. Liu K, Rosenberg SA. Transduction of an interleukin-2 gene into human melanoma-reactive lymphocytes results in their continued growth in the absence of exogenous IL-2 and maintenance of specific antitumor activity. J Immunol 2001;167:6356–6365.

Chapter 13

Focused Ultrasound for the Treatment of Patients with Cancer

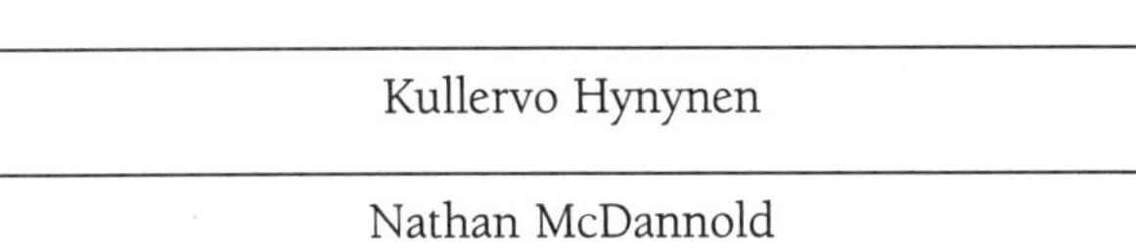

Kullervo Hynynen

Nathan McDannold

Ultrasound is used extensively in medicine to obtain diagnostic information of anatomy and blood flow. It is considered to be perhaps the safest form of noninvasive imaging, as indicated by its common use in prenatal care. However, ultrasound also has several characteristics that make it well suited for localized energy deposition for targeted tumor treatments. These include the feasibility of constructing applicators of practically any shape and size, and the good penetration of the ultrasound beam at frequencies where the wavelengths are on the order of millimeters. Such small wavelengths allow the beams to be focused and the energy deposition controlled. The major disadvantages of ultrasound are its high absorption in bone and its reflection from gas interfaces, both of which make certain organs difficult to target.

PROPAGATION THROUGH TISSUE

Ultrasound is a high frequency sound wave above the audible frequency range (over 20,000 vibrations/second), or in other words, it is as a form of vibrational energy that is propagated as mechanical wave by the motion of molecules within the medium. The characteristics of the wave are a function of both the original disturbance that generates the motion and the acoustic properties of the medium through which it travels. For therapeutic purposes, the ultrasound frequency is typically between 0.5 and 10 MHz. The speed of the propagating wave is independent of the frequency and is about 1500 m/s in soft tissues and water. The distance between the molecules in the same phase of motion (for example, the distance between two compressions) is the wavelength, which is inversely proportional to the frequency. For example, the wavelength in soft tissues at 1 MHz is about 1.5 mm, and at 3 MHz it is about 0.5 mm.

As the ultrasound energy passes through tissue, it is attenuated according to an exponential law (Figure 13.1). The rate of energy flow through a unit area normal to the direction of the wave propagation is called the acoustic intensity. At 1 MHz the ultrasound wave is attenuated approximately 50% after propagating through 7 cm of tissue. At 2 MHz, the wave is reduced to approximately 25% of its initial value by the same tissue. The attenuated energy is translated to temperature elevation in the tissue (for a review of the theory and references, see[1]).

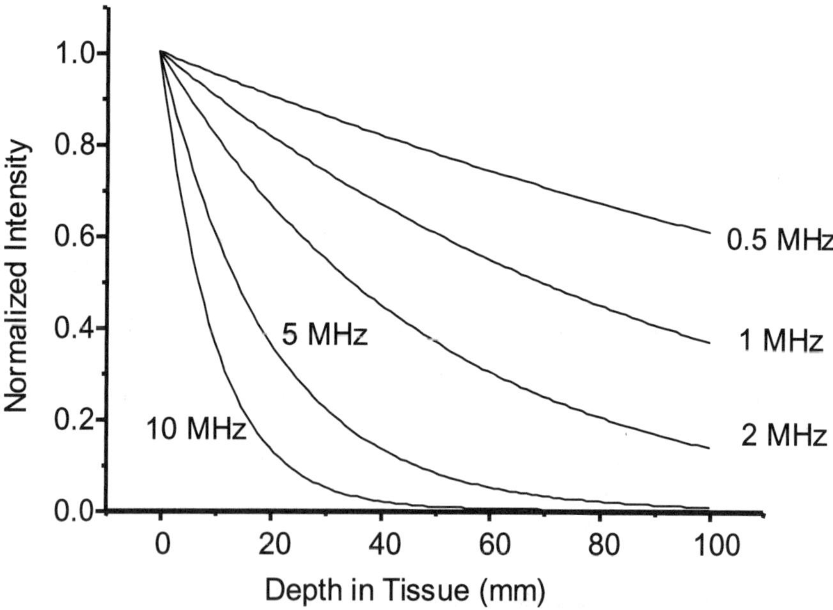

FIGURE 13.1 Theoretical ultrasound intensity versus depth in tissue graphs for different frequencies. The beam is assumed to be a collimated plane wave, and the tissue attenuation is assumed to be 5 Np/m/MHz.

By focusing the ultrasound beam, the attenuation losses can be compensated for and more energy can be delivered at a deep region than at the surface (Figure 13.2). Similar to optics, ultrasonic beams can be focused by using focused radiators, lenses, or reflectors. Focusing also can be achieved by using transducer arrays that are driven with individual signals that have phase differences such that the resulting beams possess a common focal point. Phased arrays with a large number of elements allow the location of the focal spot and the shape of the field to be controlled electronically, and they can even induce multiple focal points simultaneously (Figure 13.3).

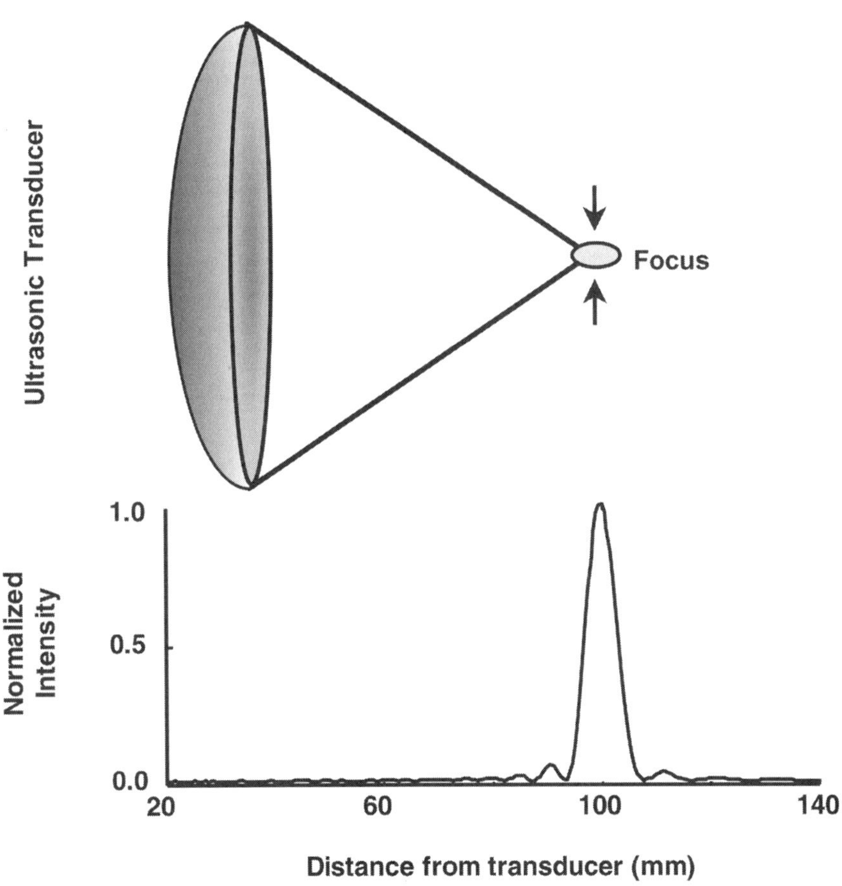

FIGURE 13.2 A plot showing the ultrasound intensity distribution from a spherically curved focused transducer calculated in tissue.

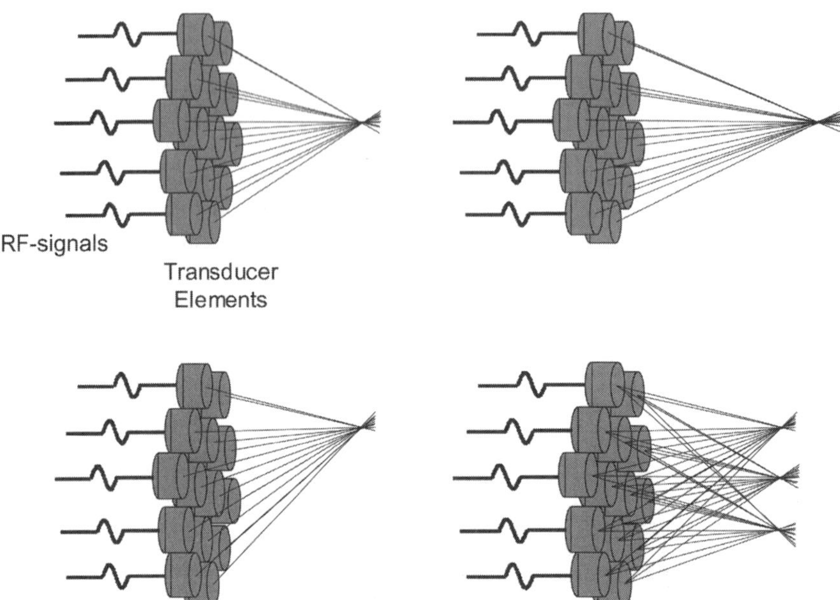

FIGURE 13.3 An ultrasound phased array applicator. The focal spot location can be steered electronically, and even multiple foci can be created simultaneously.

The size of the focal region is limited by the wavelength. A focal diameter of 1 mm can be achieved in practice at 1.5 MHz with a sharply focused transducer. The length of the focus is typically 5 to 20 times larger than the diameter (Figure 13.2). Large tissue volumes can be exposed by multiple exposures,[2] scanning the focus during the sonication,[3] or by generating optimized energy deposition patterns with multiple focal spots using phased arrays.[4]

Since the ultrasound beam is transmitted from an applicator that is several cm in diameter, the ultrasound intensity at the millimeter sized focal spot can be several hundred times higher than in the over overlying tissues. Similarly, the ultrasound exposure drops off rapidly across the focus, thus, limiting the high ultrasound exposure to the focus (Figure 13.2). This gain is reduced when the focal spot size is increased, with a practical limit that is dependent on the applicator size and the depth of the target.[5]

Ultrasound is effectively transmitted from one soft tissue layer to another with a small amount (a few percent) of wave reflected back. At soft tissue-bone interfaces, about 1/3 of the incident energy is reflected back at normal incidence. In addition, the amplitude attenuation coefficient of ultrasound is about 10 to 20 times higher in bone than in soft tissues. This causes the transmitted beam to be absorbed rapidly and results in a hot spot at the bone surface.[6] At a soft tissue-gas interface, all of the energy is reflected back.

TISSUE EFFECTS

The ultrasound beam can interact with tissue by elevating the temperature due to energy absorption from the wave. The temperature elevation during short (a few seconds) sonications follows closely the ultrasound field distribution. At longer exposures, thermal conduction and perfusion smooth the temperature distribution, resulting in less sharp gradients and a more variable temperature elevation. The variability in the temperature elevation is induced by the increased influence of blood flow and perfusion, which is highly location and tissue-dependent. In addition, tissue close to large blood vessels will be cooled by the flow if the energy delivery is slow. Short exposures can coagulate tissues next to the large blood vessels, as has been shown by theoretical models and in vivo animal experiments.[7,8] Therefore, exposures of 10 to 20 s or less should be used to reduce the variability caused by blood flow and perfusion, unless three-dimensional temperature monitoring can be used.

The effect of elevated temperature on cells and tissues has been found to be a nonlinear function of both time and temperature.[9] For exposures of a few seconds, temperatures of above approximately 60°C are needed to cause irreversible tissue damage. The elevated temperature can block the microvasculature[10] and even large blood vessels,[11] stopping blood perfusion in the coagulated tissue volume. When the temperatures reach 100°C, the tissue water boils and results in gas formation. The gas blocks the propagation of the ultrasound beam and significantly modifies the energy deposition pattern.

While ultrasound surgery has mainly exploited thermal effects so far, ultrasound also can induce mechanical tissue destruction when pressure amplitudes are used that are high enough to induce gas bubbles.[12] The large amplitude pressure wave causes these bubbles to expand and then collapse. The collapse of the bubbles causes shock waves with high pressures and shear forces that can cause direct mechanical damage to the tissue. This phenomenon is called transient or inertial cavitation. The ultrasound exposures that induce cavitation can increase the ultrasound absorption also, thereby increasing the tissue temperature elevation. This phenomenon can be used to enhance the thermal effects.[13]

By using short bursts at high pressure amplitudes, these thermal effects can be minimized or eliminated, and the non-thermal effects of cavitation can be mostly isolated. Various mechanical effects have been observed with such exposures. Histological studies have shown that cavitation can disrupt the blood brain barrier, cause selective vascular damage, generate tissue necrosis, and produce complete tissue disintegration.[14] In addition, animal tumor studies have shown that focused ultrasound-induced cavitation can activate certain chemicals.[15] An increase in blood vessel permeability has been demonstrated in muscle tissue in vivo after ultrasound exposures.[16] The cavitation effects can be further amplified by injecting preformed microbubbles into the vasculature. These bubbles were developed for imaging, but have been shown to reduce the power required for inducing tissue effects by at least two orders of magnitude.[17,18] The utilization of these mechanical effects may offer new therapeutic options.

HISTORY OF ULTRASOUND FOR CANCER THERAPY

In the 1930s, ultrasound was proposed for use in cancer treatments in a manner similar to x-rays: by using the intensity and the exposure time as the measures of the ultrasound exposure and assuming that the propagating wave had some direct and selective effect on the cancer cells. The first report of using ultrasound for cancer therapy did not show any effect on the tumor growth.[19] The next report[20] demonstrated stimulation of tumor growth in a mouse model by a 60 s ultrasound exposure at 0.5 MHz and at an intensity of 2 W/cm^2. Later papers demonstrated that longer exposures would be required to inhibit tumor growth. The first clinical study by Hovarth[21] induced significant enthusiasm, and a number of clinical studies with variable ultrasound exposures followed. When the results of these studies were reviewed in the Ultrasound in Medicine conference held in Erlangen, Germany in 1949, it was concluded that ultrasound was not suitable for cancer therapy and that its clinical use should be discontinued. This statement known as the "Erlangen Resolution" stopped the clinical use of ultrasound in cancer therapy. This early history is reviewed in detail by Kremkau.[22]

During the 1950s and 1960s, a few studies investigated the combined effects of ultrasound and radiation. It was observed that good therapeutic effects could be obtained if the ultrasound exposures were delivered such that they induced a temperature elevation in tissue.[23] In the early 1970s, there was a significant increase in interest in using temperature in the range of 41°C to 45°C for 30 to 60 min (hyperthermia) to enhance radiation and chemotherapy with promising clinical studies.[24] Mechanically-scanned focused ultrasound beams were demonstrated to be a good method for controlling the temperature distributions at locations where bone or air did not prevent the propagation of the beam.[25] Although single institutional phase II and III studies (using ultrasound and other heating modalities) showed a potentially significant increase in tumor control when compared with radiation alone,[26,27] the treatments were labor-intensive and compromised by the need to place invasive temperature sensors to monitor and control the treatments. Finally, the failure of multi-institutional randomized phase III clinical trials in the U.S. to show an increased tumor response[28,29] collapsed the clinical interest for hyperthermia treatments. It has been argued that this failure was due to the inadequate heating equipment used in the trials (for example, scanned focused ultrasound systems were not used in these treatments) and not because hyperthermia itself was ineffective.[28] The clinical temperature data, the device characteristics, and the success in small, superficial tumors that could be well heated in this trial support this argument. However, technologically it could be argued that in order to properly deliver desired hyperthermia treatments, noninvasive temperature monitoring methods are required, and therefore the trials were premature.

During the same period there was a parallel effort aimed in using the ability to focus ultrasound energy through soft tissues so that focal tissue volumes could be noninvasively destroyed. This method aimed to replace conventional invasive surgery and was first studied for functional brain surgery. Such noninvasive surgery using focused, high-intensity ultrasound beams was first proposed by Lynn et al.[30] This technique was later modified and used in destruction of small tissue volumes in the central nervous system in animals and in humans.[31] It has been used also in spinal commissurotomy[32] and for the treatment of glaucoma.[33]

First, as related to cancer therapy, Burov[34] used high-intensity pulsed ultrasound and produced resorption of rabbit carcinomas and also of human malignant melanomas. Later, this high intensity approach was tested in the treatment of human breast[35] and brain tumors.[35] Although the tumor responses achieved were promising, the above phase I clinical feasibility studies were not conclusive. However, systematic studies with experimental animal tumor models have clearly indicated that ultrasound surgery has significant potential. For example, good responses were obtained in murine gliomas implanted in abdominal walls.[36]

Finally, during the 1990s several commercial companies started to develop clinical focused ultrasound surgery devices that are currently in clinical trials or on early stages of clinical practice.

IMAGING GUIDANCE AND TREATMENT MONITORING

Accurate anatomical information is needed online to take advantage of the precise nature of the energy deposition possible with ultrasound systems. In addition, the energy deposition must be localized and the exposure quantified to assure desired therapeutic effect. This can be accomplished by combining the sonication system with modern imaging methods. Three imaging techniques—ultrasound, computed tomography (CT), and magnetic resonance imaging (MRI)—have been used for guiding ultrasound beams. Each may detect the induced temperature elevation, though so far only MRI has been shown to work accurately in vivo. Since only ultrasound and MRI have been used to guide clinical focused ultrasound treatments, they will be reviewed here.

Ultrasound

It has long been known that thermally induced lesions are visible in the diagnostic ultrasound images under certain experimental conditions.[37] The first commercial clinical devices have utilized diagnostic ultrasound to aim the therapeutic beam to the target volume and attempted to utilize the ultrasound imaging also to detect the induced tissue coagulation. Although bright echoes often appear at the focal location during sonication, it has not been possible to correlate the coagulated tissue volume with the B-scan images. Therefore, all of the clinical experience is based on aiming the beam under ultrasound guidance without exposure feedback.

Ultrasound guided focused ultrasound surgery may be improved in future. Recent studies have demonstrated that diagnostic ultrasound can be combined either with ultrasound contrast agent imaging[38] or ultrasound elastography[39] in a clinical setting to determine the coagulated tissue volume after the sonications. Similarly, ultrasound may be used to detect the increase in the attenuation coefficient induced by the coagulation.[40] Finally, there is a considerable effort in developing ultrasound methods for temperature imaging,[41,42] but reliable temperature monitoring method has not yet been demonstrated in vivo.

MRI

Since MRI generally has the best soft tissue contrast of the imaging modalities, several groups[43–45] have tested the feasibility of using MRI to guide and monitor the focused ultrasound exposures. These studies have demonstrated that temperature-sensitive MRI sequences can be used to detect the temperature elevations at levels that do not induce any histologic or physiologic tissue damage.[46] Thus, the location of the focus can be detected at low powers to verify that the targeting is accurate. Temperature sensitive sequences allow an estimation to be made on the achieved focal temperature and thus on the thermal exposure produced. This can be useful in assuring that the target volume is adequately covered.

Noninvasive MRI thermometry utilizes the temperature dependence of a physical property from which the spatial distribution can be visualized. Three tissue properties have been used for this purpose: spin-lattice decay time (T1),[47] molecular diffusion of water molecules,[48] and proton resonance frequency.[49] Increased interest in MRI thermometry has been evident over the past few years and several research groups have published reports on this topic (for references, see[50]). Much of this research confirms that in many cases, the proton resonance frequency (PRF) shift is the most useful for thermal surgery monitoring. The changes in the PRF induced by the temperature elevation are related to variations in the molecular screening constant of the water molecules. This constant is linearly dependent on temperature at a rate of about -0.01×10^{-6} $(^{o}C)^{-1}$ in water[49] and in most soft tissues.[51] The exception is fat, which has a much smaller coefficient.[52] In addition, the local magnetic flux density also varies because of the temperature dependent susceptibility constant. To obtain the temperature information, the frequency shifts can be measured from the phase images of gradient-echo sequences.[53] The mean phase shift in a voxel built up during the echo time is proportional to the frequency shift. This linear temperature dependency of the PRF shift continues with temperatures that are above the threshold for tissue coagulation.[54]

Although several issues have been reported that contribute to small uncertainty in the method,[55] a growing number of animal studies have demonstrated the usefulness of MRI-derived thermometry using the PRF method in detecting the threshold for tissue damage,[56,57] accurately mapping the areas that reached lethal thermal dosages,[58] and for guiding thermal tumor treatments.[58,59] The method also has been demonstrated in clinical thermal tumor treatments. The ability to measure the temperature distribution noninvasively during the sonication may provide a method that allows closed-loop computer controlled energy delivery and control.[60,61]

Finally, the tissue changes induced by the sonications can be detected using MRI. The signal intensities in T1- and T2-weighted images are affected by thermal tissue damage. Similarly, the tissue volume with coagulated capillaries can be detected by utilizing contrast agent uptake.[10]

CLINICAL DEVICES

Extracorporeal Focused Ultrasound Systems

Ultrasound Guided Systems Diagnostic ultrasound has been used to guide the focused ultrasound beams in most clinical treatments to date. Three extracorporeal approaches with diagnostic ultrasound guidance have been extensively tested clinically.

The first type of devices are functionally similar to a focused ultrasound system that was used for clinical tests of hyperthermia,[62] which included a transducer gantry immersed in a water bath on top of which the patient was positioned (Figure 13.4). In such devices, the diagnostic transducer is located in the middle of the gantry and surrounded by the therapy transducer(s). The whole gantry can be moved with motors so that the therapy beam can be aimed at the desired location. Before the treatment sonications, a series of diagnostic ultrasound images are obtained to localize the tumor. Then the treatment is planned and the beams are aimed to target locations. The target volume is covered by multiple sonications. The power values are based on animal and clinical experience. Although the aim is to thermally coagulate the tissue, the intensity levels are in the range that most likely will induce generation of gas bubbles resulting in increased energy absorption and higher temperatures.[69] The first device, which was developed by EDAP (France)[64] had an array of focused transducers that operated at a frequency of approximately 1 MHz and delivered short (0.125–1 s) sonications at intensities above 10,000 W/cm². A system with similar functionality was developed in China[65] and operates at frequencies between 0.8 and 1.6 MHz and peak intensities up to 20,000 W/cm².

The second type of device is similar to an early focused ultrasound hyperthemia device[25] that used an open water bag hanging on top of the patient to provide acoustic coupling (Figure 13.4A). In the surgery system, the diagnostic

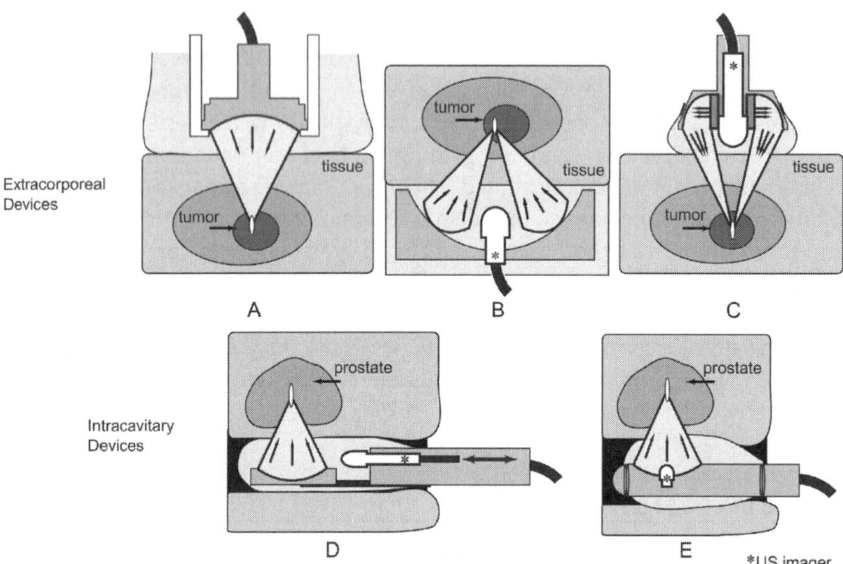

FIGURE 13.4 A diagram of the clinical ultrasound-guided focused ultrasound surgery systems that have been employed. Extracorporeal systems are in panels A[63], B[64,65], C[66] and transrectal systems are illustrated in panels D[67] and E[68]. The ultrasound imager is operated online during the treatments for the systems shown in B, C, and E, and each is indicated in the diagrams. In the systems in A and D, the imager is introduced only when the sonications are not being performed.

ultrasound transducer is first placed in the holder in the water bag to locate the tumors, and then the therapy transducer is placed in the holder in a way that it is registered with the imaging transducer coordinates and the sonications performed.[63] The system uses a single focused transducer with a diameter of 10 cm, a radius of curvature of 15 cm, and a frequency of 1.7 MHz. This system used lower intensities that the above systems, between 1000 and 4660 W/cm^2 (measured in water), so it most likely operates in the range below the cavitation threshold and induces purely thermal effects.

The third type of device combines a cylindrical ultrasound source with a parabolic reflector to focus the therapy beam. The treatment is guided by a diagnostic ultrasound transducer that is place in the middle of the applicator through a hole in the cylindrical source (Figure 13.4C). This device is positioned manually on patient's skin and aimed free-hand with the aid of the diagnostic ultrasound imaging.[66] The treatment parameters used are: frequency 1 MHz, diameter of the aperture and focal length 100 mm, and an ultrasound intensity of approximately 5400 W/cm^2.

MRI Guided Systems The first prototype MR-guided ultrasound device was manufactured for breast tumor surgery by General Electric Medical System and Center of Research and Development in collaboration with the personnel from the Brigham and Women's Hospital. The ultrasound fields were generated by a single, focused, transducer (frequency 1.5 MHz, diameter 10 cm, focal length 8 or 10 cm, maximum focal intensity 3000 to 4000 W/cm^2) that was mounted in a standard MRI table. The transducer could be moved by a computer controlled positioning device.[70] A functionally similar device (with different mechanical transducer positioning) also was developed by Siemens[45] for breast cancer treatments.

The second-generation system was developed by InSightec Inc. (Haifa, Israel) in collaboration with the Boston team, and was based on the clinical experience and developments in ultrasound phased array technology. A focused ultrasound phased array transducer with over 200 elements and a 120-mm diameter, 160-mm radius of curvature generates the ultrasound beam at a variable frequency approximately between 0.9 and 1.3 MHz.[71] Each of the transducer elements are driven with an independent radiofrequency (RF) signal with a computer controlled phase and amplitude. The electronic control allows the focus to be moved along the axial direction between 5 cm (skin depth) and 200 cm. Thus, the depth of the focus can be controlled electronically without the need of mechanically moving the transducer. The transducer array is mounted in a plastic chamber filled with degassed deionized water and covered with a plastic membrane that is secured on top of the container (Figure 13.5). The chamber is mounted in a standard MR imaging table. The transducer can be moved in a plane and be tilted

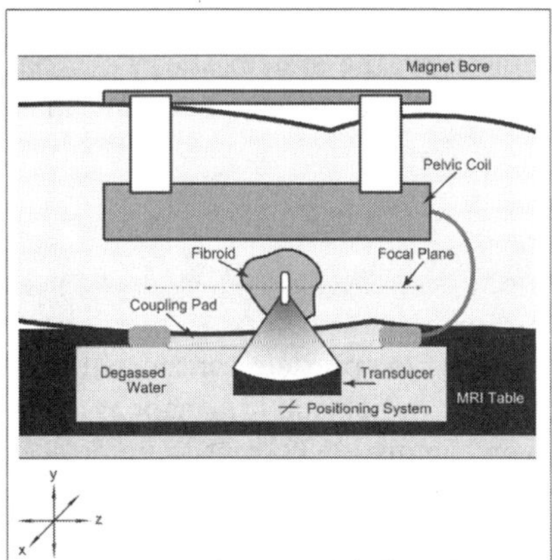

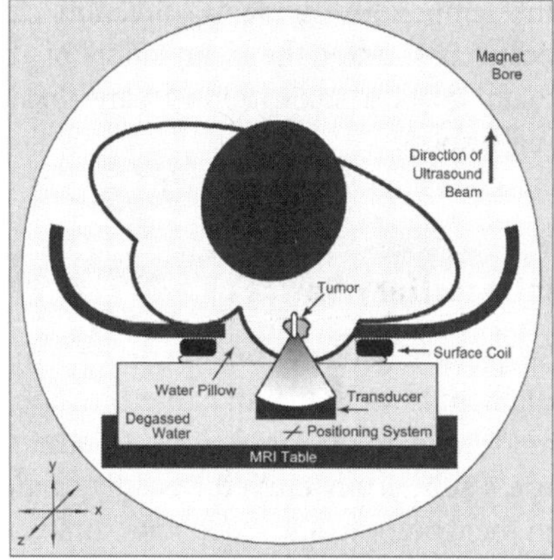

FIGURE 13.5 Diagrams of the clinical MRI guided focused ultrasound system for the treatment of pelvic and breast tumors.[72,73].

approximately 20 degrees in both x and z directions with a computer-controlled mechanical positioning device. The central element of the transducer array is used as a hydrophone to receive the acoustic emissions from the focal spots. This allows online monitoring of cavitation and ensures that the exposures are kept below the inertial cavitation threshold.

Treatment Execution After the treatment planning, a low energy test pulse with the beam aimed in a single location in the target volume is delivered. The MRI-derived temperature imaging is performed across the beam direction at the focal depth. The power is increased until the temperature elevation at the focus is visible on the temperature sensitive image. The user then corrects any mismatch between the location of the temperature elevation and the planned target, a correction generally of a few millimeters. After this targeting correction is verified with another sonication, the same alignment procedure is repeated while performing the temperature imaging along the axis of the beam. With the use of thermal imaging, the accuracy of the targeting is ensured to be within the resolution of the MR images, which is typically about 1 mm.

When the test pulse is located in the planned position, the complete target volume is sonicated with a series of high power pulses. Additional targeting adjustments can be made after any of the sonications. The pulse duration is under operator control, and in most cases is 10 to 20 seconds. The sonication power, duration and focal spot size are predicted by the system software. The operator can adjust the sonication power based on the measured temperature and thermal dose values so that predetermined volume of tissue coagulation can be achieved with each sonication. During the volume sonications, the temperature imaging direction can be selected either along or across the beam axis. After the completion of the sonication, the system allows the operator to add sonications to any location that did not receive adequate thermal exposure.

Intracavitary Devices

Several trials have used single transducer devices for prostate cancer with two different devices manufactured by Focus Surgery (Sonoblate, Indianapolis, Indiana)[68] and EDAP TMS S.A. (Ablatherm; Lyon, France).[67] Both of these devices use a spherically curved transducer mounted in an applicator that is positioned in the rectum to allow accurate sonications of the prostate tissue through the rectal wall. The applicators also include a diagnostic ultrasound transducer that is used to map the prostate and to guide the therapy beam (Figure 13.4 C and D). A water-filled latex condom is used to ensure acoustic coupling to the rectal wall.

CLINICAL STUDIES

Prostate Cancer Treatments

The first study conducted by Madersbacher et al[74] demonstrated the feasibility of the procedure in 10 patients. In a second study reported by Gelet et al,[75] 50 patients were treated with an average of 24 months follow-up time. These patients also received radiation therapy. Among these patients, 56% were cancer free (Biopsy and PSA) at the follow-up. The treatment had 50% complication rate with the first device and a 17% rate with a second-generation system that had safety features added. In a later study, only 5% of the patients had complications, while the 83% of the patients had negative biopsy in a group where the aim was to ablate the whole gland.[76] A similar high success rate (60%–100%) has been observed in a number of clinical studies[77–81] with devices from both manufacturers that are currently in clinical studies. In a later study, the post-treatment quality of life (for example catheter time, urinary infections, and incontinence) was significantly improved by combining the focused ultrasound treatment with transurethral resection of the prostate (TURP).[82]

Liver and Kidney Treatments

The first focused ultrasound liver and kidney treatments were performed by Vallancien et al,[64] who treated two liver patients and five renal cancer patients using an ultrasound guided system with post-treatment surgical removal of the tumor. The results demonstrated tissue necrosis at the focal zone.

The most significant experience in treating liver tumors comes from China. In a report where 68 patients were treated,[83] 30 of the treated tumors were surgically removed posttreatment, and histology verified that the tumors were completely coagulated in all cases. More patients have been treated in multiple institutions in China, but the results have not yet been published in the peer-reviewed literature.

In a recent study, ter Haar used a single focused transducer guided by ultrasound to coagulate small segments of tumors prior to their surgical removal.[84] This treatment has been performed in six liver, two kidney and five prostate tumors, and it demonstrated the ability of focused to coagulate tumor tissue safely through the skin and body wall. Similar feasibility was demonstrated with the handheld device in a study that treated three kidney tumors in one patient.[66]

Breast Cancer

The feasibility of using ultrasound surgery in treating breast tumors was demonstrated by ablating fibroadenoma tumors in the breast MRI guided single transducer first generation system.[85] A breast cancer trial in another institution followed and 24 patients treated with the same device in combination with tamoxifen.[86] The needle biopsies performed at six months after the treatments showed that 58 % of the patients did not have residual tumor, whereas the remaining ten patients had various amounts of viable tumor. After a second treatment, the tumor free patient population increased to 19 (79%). Only one second-degree burn was observed in these treatments.

The second generation MRI-guided phased array system was used to treat breast cancer.[72] In this trial, the tumors (8 patients) were sonicated under MRI guidance, and the tumor was surgically removed within two weeks for histology evaluation to determine the completeness of the tumor necrosis. The results demonstrated that MRI provided excellent targeting with 95.6 (± 8.5% of the tumor volume was in the treated volume. Complete tumor necrosis was induced in two patients, with an average over all patients of 88 ± 14% tumor volume necrosed. There were only two minor skin burns, and no other complications. The study also demonstrated that the proton resonance frequency shift did not provide temperature information in fat. Thus, in areas outside the tumor, the focal heating could not be quantified. The measured temperatures that could be performed within the bulk tumor were used to guide the treatment.

An ultrasound-guided system also has been used to treat 106 breast cancer patients in China.[65] The paper reports good results, but little detail or the long-term effects are not currently available from the study.

Uterine Leiomyomas

A multi-institutional feasibility study has been performed for the treatment of uterine leiomyomas (55 patients).[73,87] In this study, only part of this benign tumor was treated. The long-term goals are to eventually treat larger volumes to reduce the tumor volume and thus the symptoms. In this study, the patients returned for follow up imaging approximately 72 hours after the treatment, and then a hysterectomy was performed within one month. The thermally-coagulated tissue volume was then histologically evaluated. The histology and the posttreatment MRI revealed that 75% of tumors had a coagulated volume. In the cases that the coagulation failed, the MRI thermometry (Fig. 13.6) showed inadequate thermal exposures. The reason for the failure in those cases was poor acoustic coupling in the first patients and a lack of an ultrasound window due to bowel between the abdominal wall and the fibroid in others. The complication rate was small, with two first-degree skin burns that spontaneously healed. The histologically documented tissue necrosis was three times larger than the targeted treatment volume. In one patient the thermal damage extended into the normal surrounding myometrium. This was caused by motion of the target tissue due to filling of the bladder. There were two first-degree skin burns. These treatments demonstrate that deep pelvic tumors can be safely treated with MRI guided focused ultrasound.

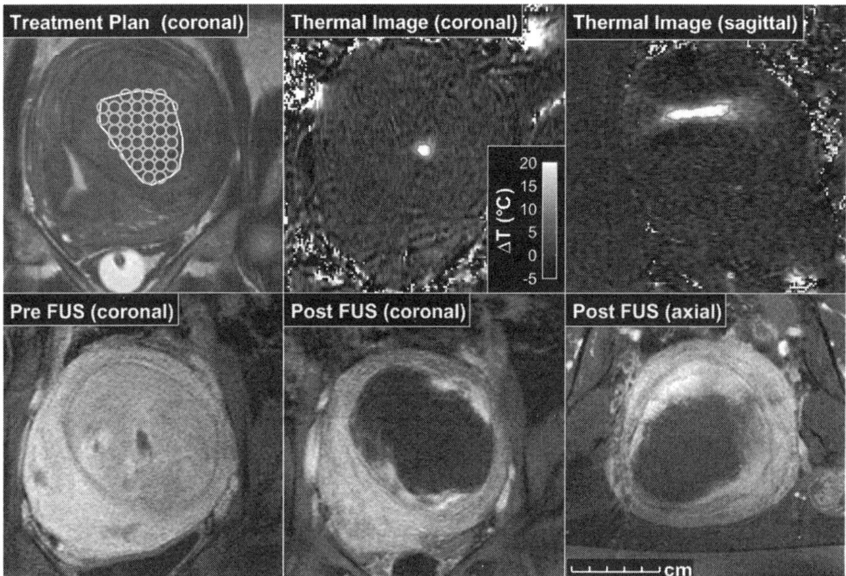

FIGURE 13.6 Magnetic resonance images of a focused ultrasound treatment of uterine leiomyomas. Top: T2-weighted image showing the treatment plan, and temperature maps showing the heating induced during two sonications. Thermal dose[88] contours of 240 equivalent min at 43°C are shown and were used to guide the exposures. Bottom: Contrast enhanced T1-weighted images acquired before and after treatment shows the non-enhancing volume that was induced by the procedure.

Brain Tumors

Finally, a more advanced ultrasound phased array system that may be able to ablate deep tumors in the brain through an intact skull has been developed.[89,90] This procedure will require more sophisticated treatment planning and an advanced sonication system.[91,92] A clinical prototype with these capabilities has been constructed, and it is currently under preclinical testing (Fig. 13.7).

Other Applications

Blood vessel occlusion may be useful for treating tumors with an identifiable blood supply. Such occlusion can be induced noninvasively with focused ultrasound and has been demonstrated in animal experiments.[11,93] Similarly, there is experimental evidence that MRI guided and monitored focused ultrasound can modify the permeability of blood vessels and cell membranes.[16,18] Ultimately, focused ultrasound may thus become a key tool in targeted drug delivery and gene therapy.[94–96] The localized and controlled temperature elevations

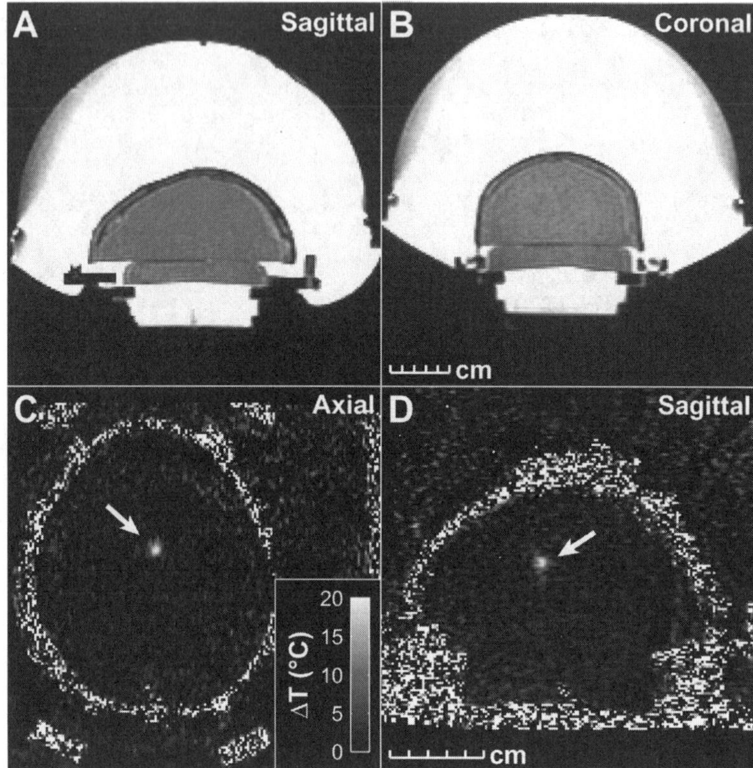

FIGURE 13.7 Magnetic resonance images of tests of an experimental 500 element hemispherical ultrasound phased array system for the treatment of brain tumors. Top: T2-weighted images showing a human skull mounted inside the array and filled with MRI/ultrasound phantom material. Bottom: Temperature-sensitive images acquired during two sonications showing focal heating achieved while sonicating through the skull.

that can be produced with focused ultrasound also may prove useful in localizing gene therapy.[97]

SUMMARY

Focused high-power ultrasound beams are well suited for noninvasively concentrating thermal or mechanical energy into precisely targeted locations deep in soft tissues. The feasibility of guiding and monitoring the thermal energy deposition using MRI and the implementation of large scale phased array transducers have been shown in clinical settings and shows great promise for tumor coagulation. With these developments, this technology has a good chance of advancing to widespread use in the clinic.

The main disadvantages of focused ultrasound are its need for an acoustic window and its small focal size. First, the strong attenuation in bones and reflection from gas interfaces limits the use of ultrasound to sites that offer a soft tissue window for the beam propagation. Second, ultrasound propagation through the overlying tissues limits the amount of energy transfer to deep tissues and increases the treatment time for large tumors.

REFERENCES

1. Wells PNT. Biomedical Ultrasound. Boston, MA: Academic Press, 1977.
2. Fry WJ, Fry FJ. Fundamental neurological research and human neurosurgery using intense ultrasound. IRE Trans Med Electron 1960;ME-7:166–181.
3. Palussiere J, Salomir R, Le Bail B, et al. Feasibility of MR-guided focused ultrasound with real-time temperature mapping and continuous sonication for ablation of VX2 carcinoma in rabbit thigh. Magn Reson Med 2003;49:89–98.
4. Ebbini ES, Cain CA. Multiple-focus ultrasound phased-array pattern synthesis: optimal driving-signal distributions for hyperthermia. IEEE Trans Ultrason Ferroelectr Freq Control 1989;36:540–548.
5. Daum DR, Hynynen K. Theoretical design of a spherically sectioned phased array for ultrasound surgery of the liver. Eur J Ultrasound 1999;9:61–69.
6. Hynynen K, DeYoung D. Temperature elevation at muscle-bone interface during scanned, focussed ultrasound hyperthermia. Int J Hypertherm 1988;4:267–279.
7. Dorr LN, Hynynen K. The effect of tissue heterogeneities and large blood vessels on the thermal exposure induced by short high power ultrasound pulses. Int J Hypertherm 1992; 8:45–59.
8. Kolios MC, Sherar MD, Hunt JW. Blood flow cooling and ultrasonic lesion formation. Med Phys 1996;23:1287–1298.
9. Dewhirst MW, Viglianti BL, Lora-Michiels M et al. Basic principles of thermal dosimetry and thermal thresholds for tissue damage from hyperthermia. Int J Hypertherm 2003;19:267–294.
10. Hynynen K, Darkazanli A, Damianou C et al. The usefulness of contrast agent and GRASS imaging sequence for MRI guided noninvasive ultrasound surgery. Invest Radiol 1994;29:897–903.
11. Hynynen K, Colucci V, Chung A, Jolesz FA. Noninvasive artery occlusion using MRI guided focused ultrasound. Ultrasound Med Biol 1996;22:1071–1077.
12. Coakley A. Acoustical detection of single cavitation events in a focussed field in water at 1 MHz. J Acoust Soc Am 1971;49:792–801.
13. Chavrier F, Chapelon JY, Gelet A, Cathignol D. Modeling of high-intensity focused ultrasound-induced lesions in the presence of cavitation bubbles. J Acoust Soc Am 2000;108:432–440.
14. Vykhodtseva NI, Hynynen K, Damianou C. Histologic effects of high intensity pulsed ultrasound exposure with subharmonic emission in rabbit brain in vivo. Ultrasound Med Biol 1995;21:969–979.
15. Umemura S-I, Kawabata K-I, Sasaki K. In vitro and in vivo enhancement of sonodynamically active cavitation by second-harmonic superimposition. J Acoust Soc Am 1997;101:569–577.
16. Bednarski MD, Lee JW, Callstrom MR, King CP. In vivo target-specific delivery of macromolecular agents with MR-guided focused ultrasound. Radiology 1997;204:263–268.
17. Miller DL, Gies RA. The influence of ultrasound frequency and gas-body composition on the contrast agent-mediated enhancement of vascular bioeffects in mouse intestine. Ultrasound Med Biol 2000;26:307–313.

18. Hynynen K, McDannold N, Vykhodtseva N, Jolesz F. A. noninvasive MR imaging-guided focal opening of the blood-brain barrier in rabbits. Radiology 2001;220:640–646.

19. Szent-Gorgyi A. Chemical and biological effects of ultrasonic radiation. Nature 1933;131:278.

20. Nakahara W, Kabayashi R. Biological effects of ultrasound: mechanisms and clinical application. Jpn J Exp Med 1934;12:137.

21. Horvath J. Ultraschallwirkung Beim Menshlichen Sarkom. Strahlentherapie 1944;75:119.

22. Kremkau FW. Cancer therapy with ultrasound: a historical review. J Clin Ultrasound 1979;7:287–300.

23. Clarke PR, Hill CR. Synergism between ultrasound and x-rays in tumor therapy. Br J Radiol 1970;43:97–99.

24. Overgaard J. The current and potential role of hyperthermia in radiotherapy. Int J Radiat Oncol Biol Phys 1989;16:535–549.

25. Lele PP, Parker KJ. Temperature distributions in tissues during local hyperthermia by stationary or steered beams of unfocussed or focussed ultrasound. Br J Cancer 1982;45:108–121.

26. Overgaard J, Gonzalez Gonzalez D, Hulshof MCCM. et al. Randomized trial of hyperthermia as adjuvant to radiotherapy for recurrent or metastatic malignant melanoma. Lancet 1995;345:540–543.

27. Scott R, Gillespie B, Perez CA et al. Hyperthermia in combination with definitive radiation therapy: results of a phase I/II RTOG study. Int J Radiat Oncol Biol Phys 1988;15:711–716.

28. Perez CA, Pajak T, Emami B et al. Randomized phase III study comparing irradiation and hyperthermia with irradiation alone in superficial measurable tumors. Final report by the Radiation Therapy Oncology Group. Am J Clin Oncol 1991;14:133–141.

29. Emami B, Scott C, Perez CA et al. Phase III study of interstitial thermoradiotherapy compared with interstitial radiotherapy alone in the treatment of recurrent or persistent human tumors. A prospectively controlled randomized study by the Radiation Therapy Group. Int J Radiat Oncol Biol Phys 1996;34:1097–1104.

30. Lynn JG, Zwemer RL, Chick AJ, Miller AE. A new method for the generation and use of focused ultrasound in experimental biology. J Gen Physiol 1942;26:179–193.

31. Fry WJ, Barnard JW, Fry FJ. Ultrasonically produced localized selective lesions in the central nervous system. Am J Phys Med 1955;34:413–423.

32. Richards ED, Tyner CF, Shealy CN. Focused ultrasonic spinal commissurotomy: experimental evaluation. J Neurosurg 1966;24:701–707.

33. Coleman DJ, Lizzi FL, Driller J et al. Therapeutic ultrasound in the treatment of glaucoma. Ophthalmology 1985;92:339–246.

34. Burov AK. High intensity ultrasonic oscillations for the treatment of malignant tumors in animal and man. Dokl Akad Nauk SSSR 1956;106:239–241.

35. Oka M. Surgical application of high-intensity focused ultrasound. Clin All Round (Jpn) 1960;13:1514.

36. Kishi M, Mishima T, Itakura T et al. Experimental studies of effects of intense ultrasound on implantable murine glioma. Proceedings of the 2nd European Congress on Ultrasonics in Medicine. Amsterdam, The Netherlands: Exerpta Medica, 1975.

37. Fry FJ. Intense focused ultrasound: its production, effects and utilization. In Fry FJ. Ultrasound: Its Applications in Medicine and Biology. New York, New York: Elsevier, 1978: 689–736.

38. Sedelaar JP, Aarnink RG, Van Leenders GJ et al. The application of three-dimensional contrast-enhanced ultrasound to measure volume of affected tissue after HIFU treatment for localized prostate cancer. Eur Urol 2000;37:559–568.

39. Souchon R, Rouviere O, Gelet A et al. Visualisation of HIFU lesions using elastography of the human prostate in vivo: preliminary results. Ultrasound Med Biol 2003;29: 1007–1015.

40. Damianou CA, Sanghvi NT, Fry FJ, Maas-Moreno R. Dependence of ultrasonic attenuation and absorption in dog soft tissues on temperature and thermal dose. J Acoust Soc Am 1997;102:628–634.

41. Maas-Moreno R, Damianou CA, Sanghvi NT. Noninvasive temperature estimation in tissue via ultrasound echo-shifts. Part II. In vitro study. J Acoust Soc Am 1996;100:2522–2530.

42. Simon C, VanBaren P, Ebbini ES. Two-dimensional temperature estimation using diagnostic ultrasound. IEEE Trans Ultrason Ferroelectr Freq Control 1998;45:1088–1099.

43. Hynynen K, Darkazanli A, Unger E, Schenck JF. MRI-guided noninvasive ultrasound surgery. Med Phys 1993;20:107–115.

44. Suzuki T, Fujimoto K, Aida S et al. MRI monitoring during high-intensity focused ultrasound treatment. Proc SMR 3rd Meeting, ISSN 1065-9889 1995;2:1177.

45. Huber PE, Jenne JW, Rastert R et al. A new noninvasive approach in breast cancer therapy using magnetic resonance imaging-guided focused ultrasound surgery. Cancer Res 2001;61:8441–8447.

46. Hynynen K, Vykhodtseva NI, Chung A et al. Thermal effects of focused ultrasound on the brain: determination with MR imaging. Radiology 1997;204:247–253.

47. Parker DL. Applications on NMR imaging in hyperthermia: an evaluation of the potential for localized tissue heating and noninvasive temperature monitoring. IEEE Trans Biomed Eng 1984;31:161–167.

48. Delannoy J, Chen CN, Turner R et al. Noninvasive temperature imaging using diffusion MRI. Magn Reson Med 1991;19:333–339.

49. Hindman JC. Proton resonance shift of water in the gas and liquid states. J Chem Phys 1966; 44:4582–4592.

50. Wlodarczyk W, Hentschel M, Wust P et al. Comparison of four magnetic resonance methods for mapping small temperature changes. Phys Med Biol 1999;44:607–624.

51. Kuroda K, Abe K, Tsutsumi S et al. Water proton magnetic resonance spectroscopic imaging. Biomed Thermol 1995;13:43–62.

52. Kuroda K, Oshio K, Chung A et al. Temperature mapping using water proton chemical shift: chemical shift selective phase mapping method. Magn Reson Med 1997;38:845–851.

53. Ishihara Y, Calderon A, Watanabe H et al. Precise and fast temperature mapping using water proton chemical shift. Magn Reson Med 1995;34:814–823.

54. Kuroda K, Chung A, Hynynen K, Jolesz FA. Calibration of water proton chemical shift with temperature for noninvasive temperature imaging during focused ultrasound surgery. J Magn Res Imaging 1998;8:175–181.

55. De Poorter J. Noninvasive MRI thermometry with the proton resonance frequency method: study of susceptibility effects. Magn Reson Med 1995;34:359–367.

56. Graham SJ, Chen L, Leitch M et al. Quantifying tissue damage due to focused ultrasound heating observed by MRI. Magn Reson Med 1999;41:321–328.

57. McDannold NJ, King RL, Jolesz FA, Hynynen KH. Usefulness of MR imaging-derived thermometry and dosimetry in determining the threshold for tissue damage induced by thermal surgery in rabbits. Radiology 2000;216:517–523.

58. Hazle JD, Stafford RJ, Price RE. Magnetic resonance imaging-guided focused ultrasound thermal therapy in experimental animal models: correlation of ablation volumes with pathology in rabbit muscle and VX2 tumors. J.Magn Reson Imaging 2002;15:185–194.

59. McDannold N, Hynynen K, Wolf D, Wolf G, Jolesz F. MRI evaluation of thermal ablation of tumors with focused ultrasound. J Magn Reson Imaging 1998;8:91–100.

60. Hutchinson EB, Dahleh MA, Hynynen K. The feasibility of MRI feedback control for phased array hyperthermia treatments. Int J Hypertherm 1998;14:39–56.

61. Salomir R, Vimeux FC, De Zwart JA, Grenier N, Moonen CTW. Hyperthermia by MR-guided focused ultrasound: accurate temperature control based on fast MRI and a physical model of local energy deposition and heat conduction. Magn Reson Med 2000;43:342–347.

62. Hynynen K, Roemer R, Anhalt D et al. A scanned focussed multiple transducer ultrasonic system for localized hyperthermia treatments. Int J Hypertherm 1987;3:21–35.

63. Visioli AG, Rivens IH, ter Haar GR et al. Preliminary results of a phase I dose escalation clinical trial using focused ultrasound in the treatment of localised tumours. Eur J Ultrasound 1999;9:11–18.

64. Vallancien G, Harouni M, Veillon B et al. Focused extracorporeal pyrotherapy: feasibility study in man. J Endourol 1992;6:173–180.

65. Wu F, Chen WZ, Bai J et al. Pathological changes in human malignant carcinoma treated with high-intensity focused ultrasound. Ultrasound Med Biol 2001;27:1099–1106.

66. Kohrmann KU, Michel MS, Gaa J et al. High intensity focused ultrasound as noninvasive therapy for multilocal renal cell carcinoma: case study and review of the literature. J Urol 2002;167:2397–2403.

67. Chapelon JY, Ribault M, Vernier F et al. Treatment of localised prostate cancer with transrectal high intensity focused ultrasound. Eur J Ultrasound 1999;9:31–38.

68. Sanghvi NT, Hawes RH. High-intensity focused ultrasound. Gastrointest Endosc Clin N Am 1994;4:383–395.

69. Hynynen K. The threshold for thermally significant cavitation in dog's thigh muscle in vivo. Ultrasound Med Biol 1991;17:157–169.

70. Cline HE, Hynynen K, Watkins RD et al. A focused ultrasound system for MRI guided ablation. Radiology 1995;194:731–737.

71. Daum DR, Hynynen K. A 256 element ultrasonic phased array system for treatment of large volumes of deep seated tissue. IEEE Trans Ultrason Ferroelect Freq Control 1999; 46:1254–1268.

72. Gianfelice D, Khiat A, Amara M et al. MR imaging-guided focused US ablation of breast cancer: histopathologic assessment of effectiveness—initial experience. Radiology 2003; 227:849–855.

73. Tempany CM, Stewart EA, McDannold N et al. MR imaging-guided focused ultrasound surgery of uterine leiomyomas: a feasibility study. Radiology 2003;226:897–905.

74. Madersbacher S, Kratzik C, Susani M et al. Transcutaneous high-intensity focused ultrasound and irradiation: an organ-preserving treatment of cancer in a solitary tesis. Eur Urol 1998;33:195–201.

75. Gelet A, Chapelon JY, Bouvier R et al. Local control of prostate cancer by transrectal high intensity focused ultrasound therapy: preliminary results. J Urol 1999;161:156–162.

76. Chaussy C, Thuroff S. High-intensity focused ultrasound in prostate cancer: results after 3 years. Mol Urol 2000;4:179–182.

77. Beerlage HP, Thuroff S, Debruyne FM et al. Transrectal high-intensity focused ultrasound using the ablatherm device in the treatment of localized prostate carcinoma. Urology 1999;54:273–277.

78. Gelet A, Chapelon JY, Bouvier R, et al. Transrectal high-intensity focused ultrasound: minimally invasive therapy of localized prostate cancer. J Endourol 2000;14:519–528.

79. Gelet A, Chapelon JY, Bouvier R, et al. Transrectal high intensity focused ultrasound for the treatment of localized prostate cancer: factors influencing the outcome. Eur Urol 2001;40:124–119.

80. Kiel HJ, Wieland WF, Rossler W. Local control of prostate cancer by transrectal HIFU-therapy. Arch Ital Urol Androl 2000;72:313–319.

81. Uchida T, Sanghvi NT, Gardner TA et al. Transrectal high-intensity focused ultrasound for treatment of patients with stage T1b-2n0m0 localized prostate cancer: a preliminary report. Urology 2002;59:394–398.

82. Chaussy C, Thuroff S. The status of high-intensity focused ultrasound in the treatment of localized prostate cancer and the impact of a combined resection. Curr Urol Rep 2003;4:248–252.

83. Wu F, Chen WZ, Bai J et al. Pathological changes in human malignant carcinoma treated with high-intensity focused ultrasound. Ultrasound Med Biol 2001;27:1099–1106.

84. ter Haar GR. High intensity focused ultrasound for the treatment of tumors. Echocardiography 2001;18:317–322.

85. Hynynen K, Pomeroy O, Smith DN et al. MR imaging-guided focused ultrasound surgery of fibroadenomas in the breast: a feasibility study. Radiology 2001;219:176–185.

86. Gianfelice D, Khiat A, Boulanger Y et al. Feasibility of magnetic resonance imaging-guided focused ultrasound surgery as an adjunct to tamoxifen therapy in high-risk surgical patients with breast carcinoma. J Vasc Interv Radiol 2003;14:1275–1282.

87. Stewart EA, Gedroyc WM, Tempany CM et al. Focused ultrasound treatment of uterine fibroid tumors: safety and feasibility of a noninvasive thermoablative technique. Am J Obstetr Gynecol 2003;189:48–54.

88. Sapareto SA, Dewey WC. Thermal dose determination in cancer therapy. Int J Radiat Oncol Biol Phys 1984;10:787–800.

89. Hynynen K, Jolesz F. Demonstration of potential noninvasive ultrasound brain therapy through intact skull. Ultrasound Med Biol 1998;24:275–283.

90. Clement GT, White J, Hynynen K. Investigation of a large-area phased array for focused ultrasound surgery through the skull. Phys Med Biol 2000;45:1071–1083.

91. Clement GT, Hynynen K. A non-invasive method for focusing ultrasound through the human skull. Phys Med Biol 2002;47:1219–1236.

92. Thomas J-L, Fink MA. Ultrasonic beam focusing through tissue inhomogeneities with a time reversal mirror: application to transskull therapy. IEEE Trans Ultrason Ferroelectr Freq Control 1996;43:1122–1129.

93. Vaezy S, Martin R, Crum L. High intensity focused ultrasound: a method of hemostasis. Echocardiography 2001;18:309–315.

94. Greenleaf WJ, Bolander ME, Sarkar G et al. Artificial cavitation nuclei significantly enhance acoustically induced cell transfection. Ultrasound Med Biol 1998;24:587–595.

95. Huber PE, Pfisterer P. In vitro and in vivo transfection of plasmid DNA in the Dunning prostate tumor R3327-AT1 is enhanced by focused ultrasound. Gene Ther 2000;7:1516–1525.

96. Ng KY, Liu Y. Therapeutic ultrasound: its application in drug delivery. Med Res Rev 2002;22:204–223.

97. Moonen C, Madio D, de Zwart J et al. MRI-guided focused ultrasound as a potential tool for control of gene therapy. Eur Radiol 1997;7:1165.

Chapter 14

The Concept of Dose Density and Its Application to the Adjuvant Chemotherapy of Node-Positive Primary Breast Cancer

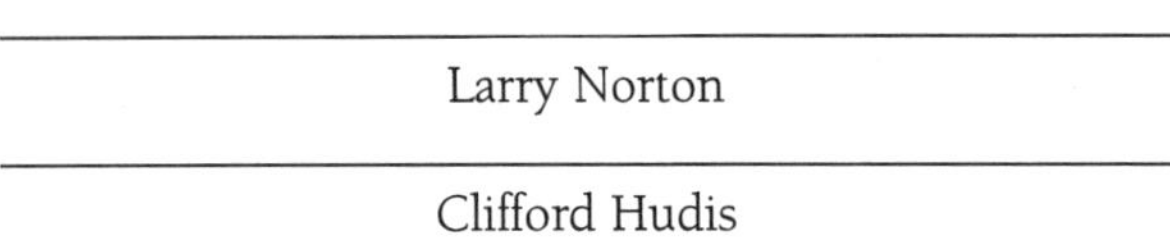

Larry Norton

Clifford Hudis

Modern medical oncology has two foundations, both of which have been evolving continuously since the mid-twentieth century. The first is the discovery of agents that adversely affect the growth and viability of cancer cells. The second is a set of principles that guide their successful application.[1] The analogy to antibiotic therapy is apt: Having drugs that kill bacteria is useless without knowledge of appropriate choice of drug or combination of drugs, proper dose levels and routes of administration, optimal intervals between doses and necessary duration of therapy. Yet for several reasons it is even more important to have well-developed principles for the chemotherapy of cancer than for the chemotherapy of infections: Few anticancer drugs are as effective as modern antibiotics in their respective tasks, the toxicity of chemotherapy is usually greater, and, unlike many bacterial infections, few cancers are uniformly sensitive to any one drug.

These considerations have motivated the development and refinement of sophisticated concepts of drug administration, which have largely stood the test of time.[1] Examples are the use of combinations of drugs at meaningful doses, chosen so as to have non-overlapping toxicities and in an effort to minimize cross-resistance, and applied beyond the achievement of clinical complete remission. The application of these principles has resulted in cures for many cases of several different types of cancer. These currently curable cancers have the common property of being particularly sensitive to anticancer drugs. However, the principles informing the development of curative regimens could be as important in the treatment of less-sensitive tumor types. This chapter will attempt to develop these principles further by considering their application in the more common settings of reduced, partial, or mutable drug sensitivity. In particular, we will discuss two ideas, sequential therapy and dose density, which have proven effective in recent clinical trials in early breast cancer.

It is essential for both historical and practical reasons to note that all of the principles mentioned above, including the sequential therapy and dose density, are products of the phenomenological, mathematical modeling of tumor growth kinetics. As demonstrated by their value in planning successful drug therapy, phenomenological models are important in themselves. Yet in this era of vastly improved molecular biology, phenomenological models certainly will serve another purpose, that of guiding the search for the biochemical and biophysical etiologies of cancerous and normal growth. A translational connection between models and quantitative observations is in fact a frequent requirement in the advance of science. In mechanics, fluidics, optics, electronics, and all other areas of quantitative science, the mathematical definition of a phenomenon is a prerequisite for its elucidation and eventual control. Ideally, refinements in the mathematical models follow their testing against observations so that in the end the model is improved. Should oncologic science follow this paradigm, improvement may and should be seen in cancer prevention, diagnosis, and prognostication in addition to therapy.

THE SKIPPER-SCHABEL MODEL AND ITS IMPLICATIONS

The founders of medical oncology made a historic decision in their early emphasis on in vivo rather than just in vitro experimental models of cancer growth-and-response.[2] Unlike the antibiotic chemotherapy of bacteria, in which the killing of cells in vitro is an excellent predictor of clinical benefit, cancer therapeutics involves more intricate phenomena. This may well be because any clinical cancer represents a heterogeneous mix of neoplastic cells that are often polyclonal in origin plus host reactive cells, including elements of the immune system, supporting stroma, including blood vessels, non-cellular structural elements, and anatomic derangements that are only just now beginning to be explicated for individual patients and tumors.[3] Furthermore, our reliance on classifications based solely on histologic appearance may obscure potentially more important biological underpinnings for neoplastic transformation and growth. These molecular bases for phenotypic behavior are likely to explain some of the heterogeneity among tumors of the same histologic type in different patients.[4–6]

Because our theoretical and computational knowledge is still inadequate to handle such complexity, it has proven advantageous to study in vivo experimental models that are biologically realistic and hence predictive of clinical events.

One of the earliest, conceptually and practically most important—and hence influential—of these models is the murine leukemia L1210. Howard Skipper, Frank Schabel, and colleagues pioneered this model with U.S. National Cancer Institute support, and it soon became the premier focus of experimental oncology.[7] The model now has been supplanted by more useful models, by virtue of their defined genetic background, in the dissection of molecular events in carcinogenesis, and the regulation of growth and apoptosis.[8,9]

The value of L1210, in contrast, was in its reproducible growth characteristics, predictable impact on mouse survival, and sensitivity to drugs that affect human cancer. Among other features, L1210 is notable for its ability to spontaneously generate drug-resistant cells, mimicking the heterogeneity in drug sensitivity typical of most clinical neoplasms. Its importance has been closely linked to the invention of mathematical means of summarizing and predicting experimental observations, a quintessential phenomenological model. The coupling of experimental and mathematical models is critical since many questions simply cannot be answered without a quantitative approach. For example, given a drug with both dose-response (regarding the killing of cancer cells) and dose-toxicity relationships, should that drug be given less frequently at a higher dose level or more frequently at a lower dose level? There is no qualitative way to address this question productively. The question implicates the magnitude of cell-kill as a function of dose level, the rate of cancer regrowth between drug administrations, and complicated considerations of drug toxicity and rate of host recovery. These are all quantitative issues that may be constant in direction even as they vary in magnitude among hosts and tumors.

What Skipper and colleagues discovered is that L1210 grows almost perfectly exponentially from the cell number at the time of implantation until the achievement of a cell number incompatible with host survival (Fig. 14.1). In exponential growth, the time for a population to double is constant, independent of population size. Hence, if it takes x days for 10^4 L1210 cells to grow to 10^5 cells, it will take x days for 10^5 to become 10^6, x days for 10^6 to become 10^7, and so on. Moreover, once the population reaches a certain level (usually in the range of 10^4 (10^5 cells) homogeneous sensitivity to a given drug evolves by spontaneous mutation into heterogeneity by virtue of the emergence of relatively or totally resistant strains. (This process, first quantified in the early 1940s by Delbrück and

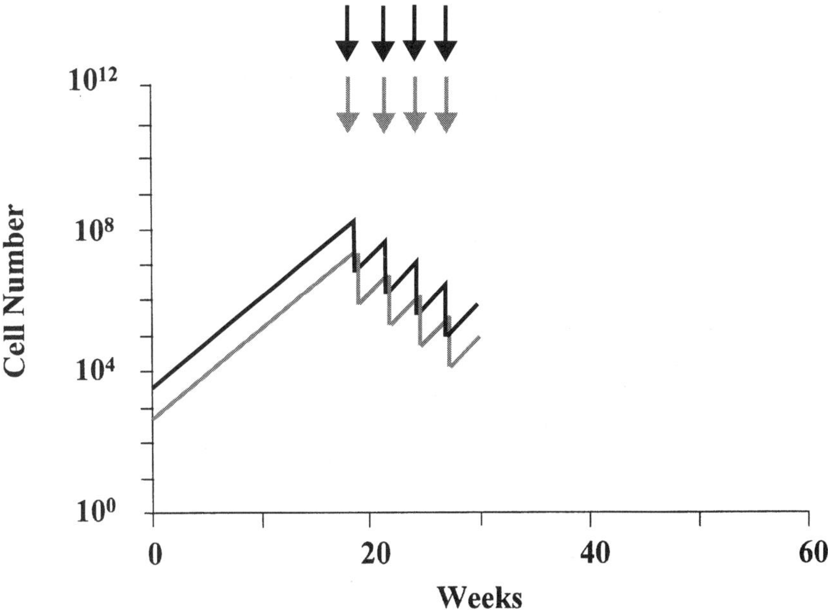

FIGURE 14.1 The Skipper-Schabel model. An example of an exponentially-growing cancer (like murine L1210) comprised of two cellular subpopulations is symbolized by the blue and the green lines. Exponential growth results in straight lines on this semi-logarithmic plot, which has as a vertical axis the logarithm to the base ten of cell number and as a horizontal axis an arithmetic scale of weeks. Each subpopulation is sensitive only to the treatments symbolized by the same-colored arrows. Each blue treatment, given at a constant dose level, causes a constant fractional (or *log*) kill of the blue-sensitive cells, as does each green treatment of the green-sensitive cells.

Luria using a bacteriophage-bacteria model, within a decade had been applied to the treatment of cancer with drugs by Law.[10,11]) Hence, any hope of causing a volume regression of all but the smallest cancers required the use of multiple anticancer agents. Furthermore, it was discovered that if one dose of a drug improved survival by a certain interval, that the number z additional doses would delay death by another z times that interval. Both theoretical arguments and empirical measurements established that this was because a given dose of a given agent against a given homogeneously-sensitive sub-line always killed a constant fraction of the cells present regardless of their number at the time of treatment. Expressing this fractional cell kill in logarithms means that if a drug at a given dose can reduce 10^6 cells to 10^4, a *log-kill* of two, the same drug at the same dose against the same tumor if it was 10^5 cells in size would reduce those 10^5 cells to 10^3, 10^4 to 10^2, and so on. In this model, any number of cancer cells under 10^2 could be cured by a single dose of that drug at that dose, since the resulting cell number would be less than one! This pattern of tumor regression in response to cytotoxic chemotherapy has been termed the *log-kill hypothesis* and this has been critical in the development of effective treatments.[2]

The discovery of this phenomenon and its mathematical expression was important for many reasons. It allowed the quantification of cell-kill using survival data, greatly simplifying experimental analysis. It also hinted at how anticancer drugs do their work, not by a gross cytotoxicity, which would result in a given number of cells dying per dose rather than a given fraction, but by an interaction with the cellular biochemistry of cell division and cell death. From a practical point of view, the log-kill hypothesis justified an approach to the design of treatment regimens that was already emerging from empirical studies of leukemia, malignant lymphoma, and breast cancer. These principles—historically termed the *MOPP principles* because of their elegant and well-documented application to the curative chemotherapy of Hodgkin's disease—included the simultaneous use of multiple agents, each at their maximum tolerated dose *within that combination*, in equally-spaced cycles of equal intensity administered beyond the achievement of clinical complete remission. Subsequent analysis of clinical data by Vincent DeVita, Emil Frei, III, George Canellos, and others underscored the importance of each of the components of MOPP principles, especially the critical nature of adequate dose level.[12,13]

Without question, the MOPP principles have dominated investigative and practical medical oncology, and for good reason. The curative chemotherapies of pediatric acute lymphoblastic leukemia, Hodgkin and other lymphomas, testicular carcinoma in adults, and several pediatric non-hematologic cancers are direct consequences of the application of these principles. In the field of breast cancer management, circumstantial evidence would seem to point in a similar direction. That is, combinations of drugs are more active in terms of response rates than single agents, adjuvant chemotherapy regimens need to be administered for longer than two months to be effective, and lower dose levels of drugs within a given combination are often inferior to higher dose levels.[14–16] A huge commitment of investigative clinical oncology, in all diseases, not just breast cancer, concerns defining the combinations of agents already shown to be active as single agents.

Yet clinical experience, while sometimes, even often, consistent with the predictions of the Skipper-Schabel model, also has raised some provocative questions in this regard. For example, while simultaneous combination chemotherapy improves response rates in the treatment of metastatic breast cancer, sequential single agents have been shown to yield identical survival statistics and actually improve total duration of disease control.[17] For two of the most active agents against breast cancer—doxorubicin and paclitaxel—dose levels have been documented that are more effective than lower dose levels and not inferior to higher dose levels.[18–20] In the post-operative adjuvant combination chemotherapy of breast cancer, dose levels of doxorubicin higher than 60 mg/m^2 and of cyclophosphamide higher than 600 mg/m^2 are not superior and, in fact, the concurrent application of these drugs at standard doses is no better than their sequential application as single agents.[21–23] In the management of stage IV breast cancer with paclitaxel, the dose level of 175 mg/m^2 is as active as a higher level.[20] Hence, these examples illustrate that in terms of log-kill the dose-response relationships for these agents are not only non-linear, but are not strictly rising. Thus, there should be no facile assumption regarding dose and cell kill for any agent in the treatment of breast cancer. (It remains to be determined if this statement applies to the chemotherapy of other malignant diseases.) In addition, there seems to be no advantage to durations of adjuvant breast cancer chemotherapy longer than four to six months.[24–26] How can we reconcile these observations—that higher doses and larger number of treatment applications are not necessarily more effective—with the principles derived from the study of L1210?

GOMPERTZIAN GROWTH AND THE NORTON-SIMON HYPOTHESIS

To approach a resolution of this enigma let us examine the relevance of exponential growth kinetics—the basis for the log-kill hypothesis—in human cancer. In the early nineteenth century, the British actuary Benjamin Gompertz formulated a mathematical equation that over the next century and a half was shown to apply to many growth phenomena in biology.[27,28] In particular, Anna Laird and colleagues demonstrated the relevance of Gompertzian kinetics to malignant growth.[29] As shown in Figure 14.2, on a semilogarithmic plot of logarithm of cell number versus an arithmetic time scale, the same plot that makes exponential growth look like a straight line (Fig. 14.1), the Gompertzian curve bends continuously away from linearity. If allowed to grow unimpeded, the Gompertzian curve eventually approaches a *plateau phase* of very slow growth, operationally equivalent to stable population size. For an individual tumor, the rate of deviation from the exponential pattern has been shown to be quite consistent, so consistent in fact that a few measurements early in the growth history of a cancer can be used to accurately predict later tumor size.[28] At the same time, it is important to note that the plateau phase may not occur in many or nearly all metastatic tumors until after the attainment of a lethal volume (Fig. 14.2).[30]

Although Gompertzian growth is an observed fact, its existence not dependent on theory, it is tempting to recognize that during the initial phase of growth, when the relative rate of growth is fastest, cell production by mitosis must be much greater than cell loss by apoptosis or other mechanism. This may be because of a greater fraction of mitotic than apoptotic cells, a shorter cell-cycle duration than the length of cell longevity, or (most likely) a combination of factors. As the population approaches its plateau size the rates of cell production and loss must approach equivalence. How rates of mitosis and apoptosis relative to population size are regulated remains unknown, although a link to fractal geometry

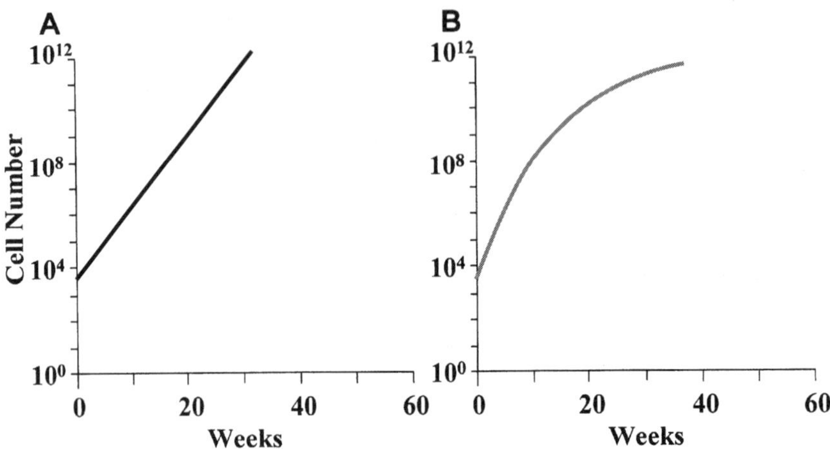

FIGURE 14.2 The contrast between exponential (A) and Gompertzian (B) growth. While exponential growth appears as a straight line on a semi-logarithmic plot, Gompertzian growth appears as a line of constantly decreasing slope. In any example of exponential growth the relative growth rate—the increment in population size as a proportion of cell number—is constant, although that constant may vary among different exponential tumors. The relative growth rate in the Gompertzian case, in contrast, is always decreasing. While the growth rate asymptotically approaches zero (no further growth), the cancer may achieve a lethal size while considerably below its asymptotic limit.

has been considered.[31] Yet differences between mitotic cell production and apoptotic loss form a plausible biological basis for both unperturbed Gompertzian growth and the observation of Norton and Simon regarding the response of Gompertzian cancers to chemotherapy.[32] Informed by a growing understanding of the biological impact of chemotherapy agents on the balance of apoptosis and mitosis, one therapeutic goal might be to alter the magnitude of or the timing of achievement of the plateau phase so that a lethal tumor volume is never reached within the natural life span of the patient.

From clinical and laboratory observations, Norton and Simon hypothesized that log-kill was not constant, but rather proportional to relative growth rate.[33] That is, the rate of tumor volume regression or cell number reduction in response to therapy is faster when the growth rate is faster, and slower when the growth rate is slower. (If chemotherapy impedes mitosis and augments apoptosis, the difference between the rates of mitosis and apoptosis that is present immediately pre-chemotherapy could account for this effect, although this mechanism remains as yet uninvestigated.)

Why wasn't the proportionality of the rates of regression and growth observed by Skipper and colleagues? In fact, it was, but it was not noticed because in the exponential case one cannot distinguish between log-kill that is proportional to growth rate and a constant log-kill! L1210's growth rate, being exponential, is always proportional in absolute terms to cell number. That is, a change from 10^4 to 10^5 cells in x days is a rate of 9×10^4 cells divided by x days. The number 10^5 is one log greater than 10^4, and a change from 10^5 to 10^6 cells in x days is a rate of 9×10^5 cells divided by x days, also one log greater. It is important to emphasize that in absolute or arithmetic terms, the rate of growth increases as the tumor size increases, but the relative growth rate—the increase in size as a proportion of the cell mass—is constant in logarithmic terms. Per Norton and Simon this relationship would be true in reverse if treatment was applied. For example, if a given dose of a given therapy reduces 10^5 L1210 cells over x days to 10^4, this is a rate of regression of 9×10^4 cells divided by x days. The log-kill hypothesis would state that the same dose of the same drug would reduce 10^4 L-1210 cells over x days to 10^3. This is a rate of 9×10^3 cells divided by x days, which is one log smaller. In other words, a rate of regression proportional to the rate of growth would explain the log-kill hypothesis in the case of exponential growth. Yet, the assumption of exponential growth and log-kill usually would predict greater efficacy for proven effective chemotherapy than is commonly observed in the clinic. The Gompertzian model can explain this divergence of predicted and actual impact.

For Gompertzian growth, a rate of regression proportional to the rate of growth would not produce a constant log-kill. As illustrated in Figure 14.3, since a cancer is growing relatively more quickly when it is smaller, the log-kill will be greater than it would if it is treated at a larger size. This, however, does not necessarily mean that clinical results will always be superior when therapy is initiated against a small cancer. As shown in Figure 14.3, if the tumor nadir achieved is not small enough to preclude regrowth, the cancer will grow back relatively more rapidly when it is small than when it is large. The magnitude of the regrowth from a small size would be just rapid enough to exactly compensate for the increased log kill, so that the eventual growth curve would be the same in both treatment situations. This may account for the common observation that improving response rates in the clinic are not always accompanied by improvements in survival.[33–36] It also can specifically explain why a complete clinical response may be a necessary but not a sufficient condition for the cure of clinically apparent disease.

Rapidly-growing types of cancer—many leukemias and lymphomas, testicular carcinoma, gestational choriocarcinoma—may be thought of as low enough on their Gompertzian curves that they behave like exponential tumors. That is, although they may in fact be growing in a Gompertzian fashion, their predicted plateau phase would be well above the lethal tumor volume. Hence, in the clinic only an early, pseudo-exponential growth phase is ever witnessed.[30] When these pseudo-exponential cancers are also very sensitive to available drugs, they seem to behave as if they were exponential in terms of the log-kill hypothesis. In addition, the rapid growth rates of subpopulations, that are likely to be present by

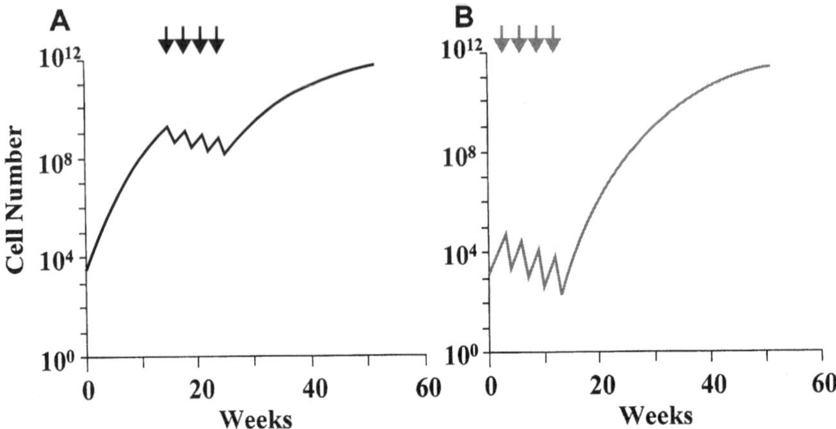

FIGURE 14.3 The Norton-Simon model. Two identical Gompertzian tumors (A and B) are treated with identical therapies of the "Skipper-Schabel" type: Equally-spaced cycles of equal dose level. The only difference between the two examples is that A is treated at a larger size than example B. At the time of initiation of therapy the relative growth rate of tumor B is greater than that of tumor A. Hence, the log-kill (i.e., cells killed as a proportion of cell number) is greater in example B than in example A. However, because the cells in example B are not eradicated or otherwise prevented from re-growing, the relative re-growth rate is also greater in example B than in example A, so that the eventual outcome is the same.

virtue of genetic lability, with differing specific drug sensitivities would make concurrent application of two or more drugs essential for cure. This is because the delayed use of a critical agent might allow a drug-sensitive subpopulation to mutate toward drug resistance or even reach a lethal tumor volume.

However, many cancer types—including most breast adenocarcinomas—have plateau phases closer to their lethal size and hence a slower growing phase within the clinically-apparent range. When these cancers are not very sensitive to drug therapy also, their optimal treatment may require a different approach. It was the search for new therapeutic rules applicable to less sensitive Gompertzian tumors that led to the hypothesis that sequential chemotherapy, rather than strict adherence to simultaneous combination, is sometimes preferable, for reasons of minimizing toxicity and, under certain conditions, maximizing efficacy.[37] Furthermore, this work led to the hypothesis that dose density, rather than dose escalation, could have significant advantages in some clearly-defined clinical settings.

SEQUENTIAL CHEMOTHERAPY

Let us consider a case in which a Gompertzian cancer is comprised of two subpopulations, one sensitive to drug A and the other sensitive to drug B. (All of the arguments below could be generalized to cases of multiple sub-lines, but the two sub-line example is chosen for ease of exposition.) As shown in Figure 14.4A, which simulates the Norton-Simon model in the Gompertzian case, if both drugs can be given at full dose levels then a certain tumor cell nadir can be achieved. If that nadir is small enough to impair or preclude regrowth, a good clinical result would ensue. Hence, full dose simultaneous chemotherapy is the optimal way of combining agents in the treatment of a cancer heterogeneous in drug sensitivity. It is similarly optimal were all the cells sensitive to A alone or to B alone. However, in many or even most cases simultaneous combinations cannot be given at full doses. Instead, reductions in dose levels are required for considerations of toxicity. Even when simultaneous combinations are feasible, lesser toxicity may ensue when the same agents are given sequentially. A good example is the TAC regimen for the adjuvant chemotherapy of operable breast cancer. In TAC the full dose of docetaxel (T) of 100 mg/m^2 is reduced to 75 mg/m^2, doxorubicin (A) of 60 mg/m^2 reduced to 50 mg/m^2, and cyclophosphamide (C) of 600 mg/m^2 reduced to 500 mg/mg^2.[38] Despite these modifications, six three-week cycles of this regimen caused febrile neutropenia in 24% of patients and other severe toxicity. In a randomized trial the regimen was superior to six cycles of FAC, with 5-fluorouracil substituting for docetaxel, in terms of disease-free survival. The usual course of FAC is eight cycles, not six.[39] Nevertheless, the TAC trial accomplished its planned goal, clearly demonstrating the activity of adjuvant docetaxel.[38] But would the results have been better had it been possible to give full dose levels and number of cycles of docetaxel, doxorubicin and cyclophosphamide? This specific question will be addressed in an ongoing NSABP trial (B-30) in which the sequence of standard AC (four cycles of 60 and 600 mg/m^2, respectively) followed by four courses of full dose docetaxel (100 mg/m^2) will be compared to four cycles of a concurrent TAC regimen requiring dose reductions to 75, 50, and 500 mg/m^2, respectively. A third arm of this trial eliminates the cyclophosphamide completely, but maintains concurrent application of the AT combination at these dose levels.

The computer simulation of Figure 14.4B illustrates that dose modifications that result in inferior log-kills do not achieve the desirable nadir. If full-dose simultaneous combination chemotherapy (Fig. 14.4A) is impossible and reduced dose treatment (Fig. 14.4B) is insufficient, are there other options? In fact, two other options have been proposed, and both merit careful consideration.

In the mid-1980s Drs. Goldie and Coldman presented a mathematical argument that a strict alternation of agents would be the best way to reduce tumor volume while minimizing the odds of sensitive cells mutating toward drug resistance.[40,41] (This model is critiqued.[42]) However, as first proposed shortly thereafter, and as illustrated by the simulation in Figure 14.4C, alternating chemotherapy at full dose levels would not provide optimal log-kill. While full-dose therapy A is being administered the cells sensitive only to B would be growing, and while full-dose therapy B is being given the A-sensitive cells would be left unperturbed. As a consequence both subpopulations would be under-treated.

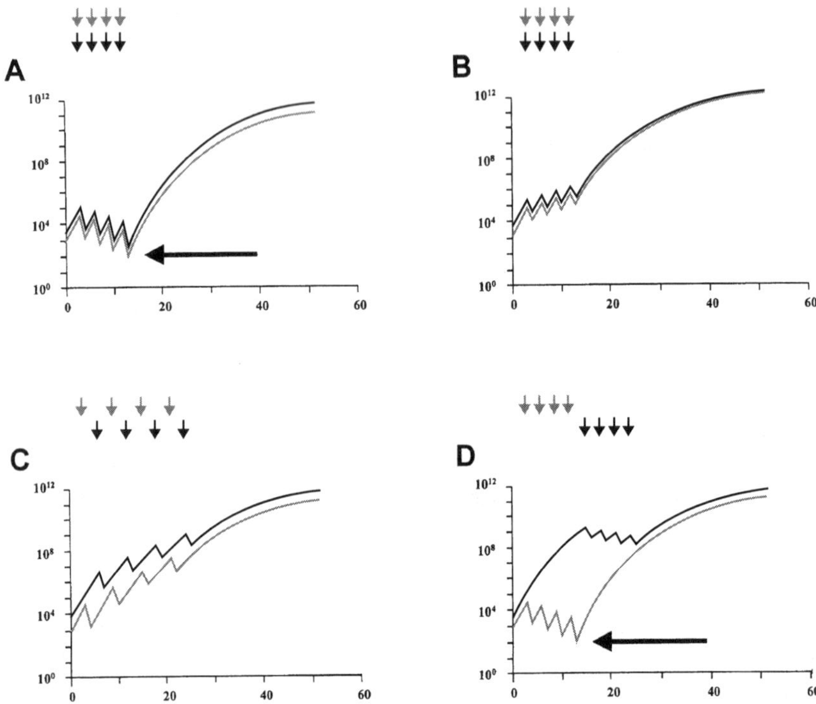

FIGURE 14.4 Simulation of four patterns of therapy against Gompertzian tumors that are heterogeneous in drug sensitivity. (A) Simulation of simultaneous therapy using full dose levels of two (black and gray) treatments against two (blue and green) cellular subpopulations sensitive only to their respective therapies. This results in maximum tumor cell nadirs (large black arrow). If it was possible to deliver full dose levels (defined in the text) of both treatments simultaneously, this would be the best pattern. (B) However, this panel illustrates the most common case: Both treatments must be delivered at reduced dose levels to avoid unacceptable toxicity. The result is a markedly reduced anti-cancer effect. (C) The two treatments are given at full dose levels in an alternating fashion. Because the black subpopulation is allowed to grow during the application of the gray therapy, and the gray subpopulation grows during black treatment, neither subpopulation is adequately treated. (D) Sequential full-dose therapy. Because the dose rate of each treatment type is preserved, the cytoreduction is preserved as well, with the dominate subpopulation achieving the same nadir as in panel A (large black arrow). Hence, if the treatment pattern in panel A is impossible to deliver, the pattern in panel D is preferable to that of panels B and C.

Full-dose sequential therapy (simulation in Fig. 14.4D), however, does achieve the same nadir as full dose simultaneous chemotherapy for one subpopulation, and is not inferior to the full dose regimen in eventual outcome for the other population. The reason is recalled by reference to Figure 14.3. Hence, when full dose chemotherapy cannot be given simultaneously, it has been suggested that the drugs should be given at full dose, but sequentially.[37,43,44] To test the validity of the above analysis, in 1985 Gianni Bonadonna and colleagues at the Istituto Nazionale Tumoi in Milan initiated a direct comparison of full-dose alternating chemotherapy and full-dose sequential chemotherapy.[45] The alternating schedule used two three-week cycles of CMF (cyclophosphamide, methotrexate, 5-fluorouracil) followed by one dose of doxorubicin (A), repeated four times for a total of eight cycles of CMF and four of doxorubicin (CMF-CMF-A-CMF-CMF-A-CMF-CMF-A-CMF-CMF-A). The sequential treatment gave four three-week cycles of doxorubicin followed by eight of CMF (A-A-A-A-CMF-CMF-CMF-CMF-CMF-CMF-CMF-CMF). Drugs, dose levels, cycle length, number of cycles and total duration of therapy were identical. At five and ten years of follow-up the sequential therapy was statistically superior to the alternating in both disease-free and overall patient survival.[46]

One question that was left unanswered by the above study was the role of the anthracycline: Did doxorubicin contribute at all to the efficacy of CMF, then the international standard? To address this point two large prospective randomized trials in the United Kingdom were conducted and analyzed jointly.[47] Both compared variants of CMF alone or in the sequence of the anthracycline epirubicin at full dose for four cycles followed by CMF. As presented in 2003, sequential epirubicin clearly added to both disease-free and overall survival. Hence, the sequential inclusion of an anthracycline clearly improves outcomes, lending support to the previous conclusion that sequential use is superior to an alternating approach.[46]

One of the major advantages of sequential therapy, as illustrated by the case of anthracycline, is the ease with which new agents can be integrated into established regimens. Another example is the integration of paclitaxel with the AC (doxorubicin plus cyclophosphamide) combination. In 1993 the U.S. Breast Intergroup conducted a clinical trial, chaired by Craig Henderson of the Cancer and Leukemia Group B (C9344), which asked two questions: Are dose levels of doxorubicin higher than 60 mg/m^2 more effective? Does paclitaxel, given for four three-week cycles at 175 mg/m^2 sequentially after four three-week cycles of AC, add to disease-free and overall survival?[21] A previous CALGB-coordinated Intergroup trial (C8541) had already demonstrated that 60 mg/m^2 of doxorubicin was superior to the reduced dose level of 30 mg/m^2.[18,19] Trial C9344, previously presented and recently published, provides convincing evidence that AC with doses of doxorubicin of 75 mg/m^2 and even 90 mg/m^2 (requiring amelioration of granulocytopenia with filgrastim) conveyed no superiority.[21] Consistent with this theme, the National Surgical Adjuvant Breast and Bowel Project (NSABP) also showed in clinical trials B22 and B25 that AC with dose levels of cyclophosphamide greater than 600 mg/m^2 produced no better clinical results.[22,23] Regarding the second question asked in C9344, the addition of paclitaxel, given sequentially after AC was of benefit, and this benefit was not offset by severe toxicity. A recent overview of CALGB trials including C8541 and C9344 has shown that the benefits of the proper dose level of doxorubicin in the first trial and of the addition of paclitaxel in the second extended to older patients as well as younger ones.[48]

In confirmation of the C9344 results, the NSABP recently presented the first statistically-valid results of a trial (B28) comparing AC (four three-week cycles at 60 mg/m^2 of doxorubicin plus 600 mg/m^2 of cyclophosphamide) followed or not by paclitaxel at 225 mg/m^2 for four three-week cycles.[49] (A prior presentation of study B28, mandated for completeness at a National Cancer Institute Consensus Conference and triggered by a predefined interim analysis, included immature data, admittedly inadmissible for drawing conclusions.[50]) The most recent presentation confirmed a significant impact of the paclitaxel in improving disease-free survival. While no survival benefit was observed by the time of this analysis, the curves could yet diverge, and indeed are expected to diverge based on the well-documented and logical phenomenon that survival benefit always lags behind improvement in disease-free survival. NSABP's B28 may be maturing more slowly than C9344 because of differences in prognostic factors in their respective patient populations. The patients on the NSABP trial were older, had fewer involved ipsilateral axillary lymph nodes, more frequently had hormone receptor positive tumors, and were more likely to receive adjuvant tamoxifen compared to those enrolled on the CALGB/Intergroup trial. It is especially notable that in a subset analysis the positive effects of paclitaxel on disease-free survival as defined prospectively in B28 were largely in the patients with potentially hormone responsive disease (those with estrogen receptor-positive cancers). This is of interest because in the CALGB/Intergroup experiment, the patients with estrogen receptor-negative tumors benefited more than the others from the addition of paclitaxel. An exploratory analysis of the NSABP study limited only to relapse-free survival events demonstrated no significant interaction between hormone receptor status and benefits from tamoxifen. These observations illustrate the folly of relying on unplanned subset analyses for making clinical decisions. The history of B28 and C9344 highlights the importance of using such analyses only for their intended purpose, the generation of hypotheses for future study. At present there is no reason to believe that the use of a taxane would not benefit any patient with involved axillary lymph nodes regardless of the hormone receptor status of their primary cancer.

Critics have correctly cited a flaw in the above experimental designs as regards their "proof" of the value of sequential therapy. The flaw is that the sequential regimens in these studies were longer in duration than the control treatments. Could the advantages of sequential therapy be entirely due to this duration difference? The duration question is a legitimate topic for further clinical research, and is indeed the focus of ongoing studies. However, it already appears unlikely that duration alone could account for all of the therapeutic benefits described above. The two arms of the NCI-Milan trial of alternative *vs.* sequential doxorubicin and CMF were of equal duration, yet sequential therapy was superior.[46] Other evidence is provided by a clinical trial in node-positive primary breast cancer conducted by the CALGB starting in 1980 (C8082).[51] This study, chaired by Marjorie Perloff, used two minor scheduling variations of CMF (with vincristine and prednisone, termed CMFVP) chosen to compare their ability to deliver close to full dose treatment for eight to thirteen months. The two schedules were found to deliver equivalent dose levels and yield equivalent therapeutic results; hence, their data were pooled for analysis. The experimental arms gave CMFVP for eight months, then sequentially six three-week cycles of a doxorubicin combination at very modest doses of doxorubicin: 15 mg/m^2 for two cycles, 30 mg/m^2 for two cycles, then 45 mg/m^2 for the last two cycles. The dose level of doxorubicin, therefore, never reached the optimal dose level as discussed above. Also biasing the trial away from a positive result in favor of the experimental treatment was the decision to have the CMFVP-alone arms deliver a total duration of therapy longer than the sequential experimental arms. Yet despite these impediments, the sequential therapies that crossed over from CMFVP to the doxorubicin combination gave results that statistically were significantly superior in disease-free survival and better in overall survival as well. (The *P* value for the difference in survival duration is .06, but the magnitude of the difference is consistent with the magnitude of the disease-free survival benefit at $P = .0037$, and is based on a clearly inadequate sample size of less than 700 patients. This study was conducted before the era of very large Intergroup-style trials.) This trial, therefore, confirmed the activity of doxorubicin delivered in a sequential fashion, and provided evidence that longer treatment duration alone is not necessarily beneficial. As a third example, a trial at the M. D. Anderson Hospital, compared eight three-week cycles of adjuvant FAC with four three-week cycles of paclitaxel followed by four of FAC in patients with node-positive breast cancer.[39] The results were in the same direction and of the same magnitude as C9344 and B28. While they failed to reach statistical significance, this is likely due to the small size of the trial (524 patients). Consistent with this observation, a neo-adjuvant therapy trial in which docetaxel replaced continued doxorubicin-based combination therapy demonstrated an increase in tumor response and improved disease-free and overall survival despite the delivery of the same number of cycles and duration of therapy on both arms.[52]

Several studies now underway or with completed accrual do control for number of cycles and duration of therapy. Hence, we anticipate more data concerning this issue in the coming years. Currently, however, all available evidence supports the conclusion that the sequential use of full doses of different, effective agents is the key to improved therapeutic results, and that this benefit is not due entirely to longer duration of therapy.

Dose Level

The term *full dose* is used frequently in the above examples. The concept of full dose clearly is critical, as shown by a comparison of Figures 14.4 A and B, but the existence of the concept begs the question of what is meant by the term *full*. Clinical research described above clearly demonstrates that the dose-response curves for several main agents, doxorubicin and cyclophosphamide, in the adjuvant setting, and paclitaxel in the treatment of stage IV disease, are not strictly rising in dose-ranges relevant to out-patient use. The dose-response curve must rise steeply from a dose level of zero to a dose level that gives a maximum log-kill, but it is clear that once the maximum log-kill is achieved further increases in dose level for these agents do not increase log-kill (which is implicit in the use of the term *maximum*). Furthermore, the dose levels of doxorubicin, cyclophoshamide, and paclitaxel that cause their respective maximum log-kills are well below their maximally tolerable dose levels. However, what about other drugs and extremely high dose levels, especially of alkylating agents? Here we are considering dose levels so high that autologous bone marrow reinfusion plus granulocyte colony-stimulating factor support are necessary to avoid potentially fatal bone marrow suppression or ablation. Could such high escalation of dose levels of various drugs be associated with a second step up in the dose-response relationship? If so, could a single application of such high-dose therapy have profoundly beneficial anticancer effects? As discussed below, data from randomized clinical trials do not as yet support this hypothesis.[33,53–57] Multiple applications of high dose level therapy, when feasible and tolerable, might improve efficacy to some degree, but this approach is more difficult to interpret in that it implicates dose density (defined below) as well as dose escalation.[58,59]

If the dose-response relationship is not strictly rising, then it is not surprising that single applications of drugs at ultra-high dose levels do not produce the clinical benefits that we would expect to result from greater, or substantially greater, cancer cell killing. However, there may be another problem with the high-dose approach that has more to do with Gompertzian growth kinetics than with dose-response relationships. Figure 14.5 presents a computer simulation using the Norton-Simon Model. In it the residual tumor size after induction chemotherapy is well above the small size necessary to preclude regrowth. The log-kill from high-dose therapy is assumed to be significantly increased (which, of course, may not be realistic). Yet even if the single application of high-dose therapy was more effective in terms of log-kill, this would not produce major therapeutic benefits in terms of disease-free or overall survival. In Figure 14.5 the time to diagnosable recurrence (at about 10^{10} to 10^{11} cells) is improved slightly, but any small survival benefit (tumor lethality being expected in the range of 10^{12} cells) readily could be erased by increased fatal toxicities from the high-dose treatment. Among the many studies that have addressed the effects of ultra-high dose level therapy in early breast cancer, the two Intergroup trials that were well controlled, audited, multi-institutional and monitored by independent data and safety committees, produced results consistent with this hypothesis.[55,60]

Dose Density

A comparison of Figure 14.4 panels C and D reveals that the expected difference in efficacy between the two treatment plans (alternating and sequential), a dif-

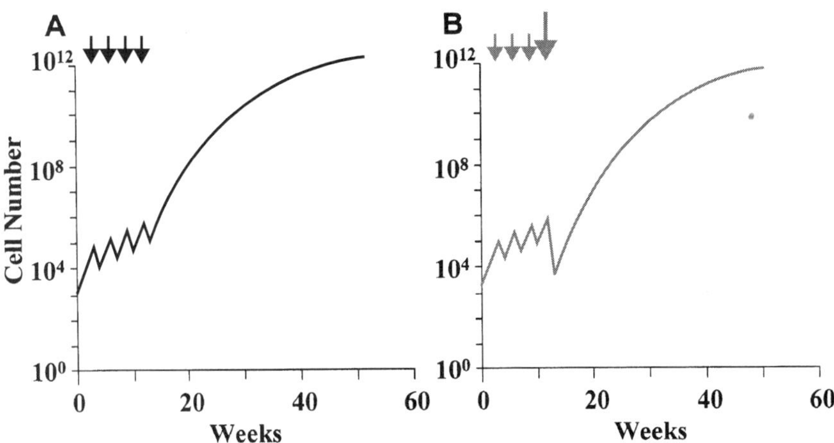

FIGURE 14.5 Simulation of the induction followed by single administration of high-dose chemotherapy. (A) The effects of a classical chemotherapy regimen with equally spaced cycles of equal dose level. (B) The effect of substituting for the last cycle a single administration of a high dose level of chemotherapy. For the sake of this example, the induction chemotherapy leaves a significant number of cancer cells and the high dose level treatment is assumed to result in increased log-kill (which, as discussed in the text, is not always true). Even if the log-kill was increased by the application of an increased dose level, as shown here, the number of cancer cells residual after such treatment is large enough to permit tumor regrowth. In addition, the increased log-kill is balanced by rapid Gompertzian regrowth. As a result the eventual tumor growth is only slightly inproved compared with the simulation in panel A, which does not include the final high-dose treatment.

ference confirmed by clinical trial, is due to the *density* of the treatment. That is, in Figure 14.4C both treatments A and B are delivered in dose-sparse six-week cycle lengths, allowing for the significant growth of cancer cells between drug administrations. The treatment simulated in Figure 14.4D, in contrast, gives the same treatments over more dose-dense three-week cycles, resulting in an improved tumor nadir for one subpopulation of cancer cells. This raises the theoretical question: What would happen if the treatments were given in an even denser schedule, say in two-week cycles? Figure 14.6 uses the Norton-Simon Model to simulate this schedule, to obvious good effect.

This simulation shows that the ability of dose dense chemotherapy to eradicate a population of cancer cells is due to several factors. The first is that the full dose level of the chemotherapy is preserved, avoiding the reduced log-kill that could well accompany dose reductions (as in Fig. 14.4B). The second is that the time of regrowth between cycles of chemotherapy is reduced, meaning that when the second and subsequent doses are administered they are being applied to a smaller number of cancer cells. The third is that because of the Gompertzian growth pattern, the smaller number of cells that are left following the more lim-

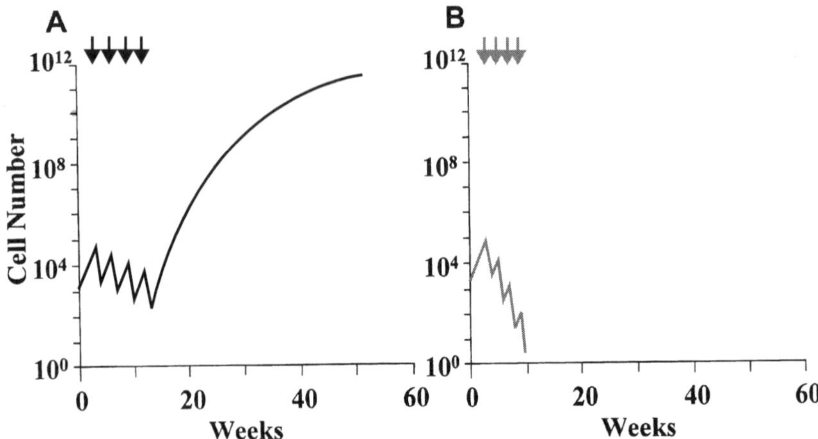

FIGURE 14.6 (A) Dose density or increased rate of drug administration (increased dose rate). (B) The effect of giving the same therapy as in panel A, but with less time between cycles. Because of the shorter re-growth time the number of cancer cells at the time of treatment is reduced in all cycles after the first. Because of Gompertzian kinetics the log-kill is increased and because the starting tumor size is small, the tumor in panel B is eradicated.

ited regrowth time are growing relatively faster, so that—by the Norton-Simon Hypothesis—the log-kill resulting from the next application of treatment, at an optimal dose level, is greater. Lastly, because the number of cancer cells at the time of initiation of therapy is small enough, the *cure limit*—the number of cancer cells small enough that the tumor cannot regrow—can be achieved by this treatment plan.

Testing of Sequential Therapy and Dose Density

In 1990, in preparation for a definitive test of these concepts, investigators at the Memorial Sloan-Kettering Cancer Center initiated a series of clinical trials culminating in a regimen called ATC.[61,62] This treatment was designed to test the feasibility of maximizing dose level and dose density simultaneously in a purely sequential regimen. In the final study in this pilot series, doxorubcin was given at 80 mg/m^2 for three two-week cycles, then paclitaxel at 200 mg/m^2 over 24 hours for three two-week cycles, and then cyclophosphamide at 3,000 mg/m^2 for the final three two-week cycles.[63] The two-week cycle length was made possible by the use of filgrastim, as previously shown in the treatment of bladder cancer.[64] Dose levels in the context of this multi-cycle treatment plan were intentionally high for several reasons. The first was that the results of the clinical trials of dose-response described above were not yet available to challenge the hypothesis prevailing at that time was that higher dose levels would be more effective. Also, it was reasoned that if it were feasible to deliver sequential dose-dense chemotherapy at elevated dose levels, it would certainly be feasible to do so at dose levels below that tested. ATC was found to be tolerable. In addition, its noncomparative efficacy when used to treat patients with node-positive disease was encouraging.[63] (A randomized comparison of ATC with a regimen applying induction chemotherapy followed by an ultra-high dose level chemotherapy against high-risk node positive disease was initiated by the Breast Intergroup, coordinated by Scott Bearman of the Southwest Oncology Group (personal communication), but was discontinued because of poor accrual that followed the release of negative clinical trial data regarding the ultra-high dose approach.)

In 1997, building on the results of many prior clinical trials, a major study was designed and initiated by the Breast Intergroup, coordinated by the CALGB and chaired by Marc Citron.[65] C9741 was a two-by-two factorial comparison with one axis being dose density and the other sequential therapy (Fig. 14.7). Volunteer patients with successfully operated breast cancer that had involved axillary lymph nodes but who had no other evidence of disease were enrolled. The four postoperative treatments were as follows: AC followed by paclitaxel exactly as was given in C9344 (four three-week cycles of each); the same regimen but with two-week cycle lengths (using the pilot data from ATC); a regimen using the

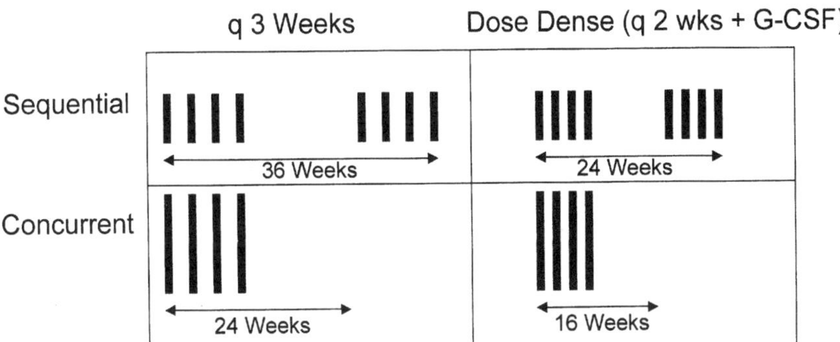

Doxorubicin 60 mg/m² i.v.

Cyclophosphamide 600 mg/m² i.v.

Paclitaxel 175 mg/m² i.v. over 3 hours

(Tamoxifen for Hormone Sensitive Disease after Chemotherapy Completed)

FIGURE 14.7 Schema of intergroup/CALGB protocol C9741 for the adjuvant chemotherapy of node-positive operated breast cancer.

same dose levels of the same drugs but in a consecutive A-T-C format (four three-week cycles of each drug); and the same A-T-C sequence but with two-week cycle lengths. The dose-dense (two-week cycle length) regimens used filgrastim after each drug administration. Just over 2000 patients joined this trial with an evaluablity rate of 98.4%.

The first results of this trial were recently published.[65] As predicted by the model, because the sequential regimens and the AC followed by paclitaxel regimens delivered identical dose levels at parallel rates of drug delivery, there was no difference in therapeutic efficacy along this axis. That is, the three drugs could be given as single agents with no loss of efficacy compared to the concurrent application of doxorubicin and cyclophosphamide. Along the other axis, in contrast, there was a major effect. The application of increased dose density resulted in a statistically significant 26% reduction in the average annual odds of recurrence and a statistically significant 31% reduction in the average annual odds of death. Benefit was seen despite the dose-dense therapies being one-third shorter in total duration of treatment.

These results seem to confirm the advantages of dose density as suggested by the simulation shown in Figure 14.6. It is important to note that all of the requisite aspects of that figure were respected in this trial: Full dose levels of active agents were used, with shortened cycle length; breast cancer grows by Gompertzian kinetics; the disease burden was small because this was a post-operative adjuvant trial.

The results of C9741 are clear and unambiguous because the study used a two-by-two factorial design with only the experimental variables distinguishing the regimens. However, it is appropriate to ask whether the benefits of dose density in C9741 will disappear with time. The answer is that they cannot. Since all patients have been followed for at least two years, the difference that is already apparent by this time cannot change. In addition, even at four years of follow-up there is a 50% diminution in the odds of recurrence, indicating that the disease-free survival curve will continue to diverge as the data mature. Finally, at the point of analysis the absolute hazard for recurrence in these patients with node-positive disease has already decreased from its highest point in the second and third years. Hence, most of the events that could be anticipated to occur over the first five years had already occurred by the time of presentation of the data.

Another concern that has been expressed is that the dose-sparse sequential regimen (A-T-C given in three-week cycle lengths) may have been so inferior that when combined with the conventional regimen of AC followed by paclitaxel in three-week cycles, it "dragged down" the three-week arms to make the dose dense two-week arms look better artificially. This, however, cannot be true since were that the case the dose-sparse sequential regimen also would have "dragged down" sequential therapy, which did not happen. In fact (as shown in the publication of these results) the two three-week regimens, sequential A-T-C and combination AC→T, are seen to be close together in terms of disease-free and overall survival, as are the two two-week regimens.

Were the dose dense regimens superior because of an immunological modulating effect of the filgrastim? This question already has been answered in the negative by the results of previous clinical trials including CALGB 9344 and NSABP B22 and 25. One-third of the patients in the CALGB trial were randomly allocated to receive doxorubicin at 90 mg/m^2 plus filgrastim in each cycle; however, these patient's results did not differ significantly from those receiving lower dose levels of doxorubicin in arms that did not employ routine filgrastim. Similarly, of the 4853 patients treated with fixed doses of doxorubicin and escalated doses of cyclophosphamide in NSABP B22 and B25, there were no differences in disease-free or overall survival despite the use of filgrastim in half of the patients (all those enrolled on B25).[23,66]

Is dose density too toxic for routine use? In actuality, the dose dense regimens were no more toxic that the three-week regimens. In contrast to many investigators' preconceived notions, less toxicity was seen in all categories except an increased use of erythrocyte transfusions in the dose-dense AC followed by paclitaxel. The increased use of transfusions in this regimen is surprising because the incidence of anemia was not increased and, therefore, currently is being investigated further by chart review. At three years of follow-up the incidence of myelodysplasia or acute myelogenous leukemia in C9741 was not increased in the two-week treatment arm compared to the three-week arm and was also the same overall as in C9344, which did not employ dose density. Hence, there is no suggestion of any increased risk of acute leukemia or myelodysplasia as a consequence of the use of filgrastim or every other week treatment.

The major beneficial effect of dose density regarding toxicity of treatment was a dramatic reduction in granulocytopenia. This led to fewer episodes of neutropenic fever with attendant expensive hospitalizations. Should dose density be adopted for wide use in the community, this would be a very desirable consequence. In addition, because the dose dense regimens were delivered over one-third less time than the three-week regimens, patients were able to complete treatment and return to their normal lives that much faster. Hence, even if dose density was not associated with major improvements in disease-free and overall survival (as it is), it would still be a preferable option by virtue of reduced toxicity.

Cautions Regarding Dose Density

As indicated above, the design of C9741 respected the requirements illustrated in Figure 14.6. Future applications of this concept cannot be expected to be successful should major deviations from these specifications be encountered. Figure 14.8, for example, illustrates that dose density, while causing greater log-kill than conventional scheduling, would not yield better clinical results if it was applied to a starting tumor size that is too large. (Mathematically, the concepts expressed in Figs. 14.3 and 14.8 are closely related.) Additionally, ineffective drugs, inadequate dose levels and lack of attention to tumor heterogeneity cannot be rescued by dose density. An unfortunate trend is to label any weekly or daily schedule "dose dense" when in fact the regimen delivers a drug amount that is intentionally reduced, because of concerns about toxicity, to a sub-optimal level. Will a dose level of z/2 mg/m^2 given weekly be more effective than z mg/m^2 given every two weeks? It will be only if the log-kill from z/2 mg/m^2 is more than 50% of the log-kill from z mg/m^2. Sadly, clinical research seldom has produced a level of detail regarding dose-response relationships useful in making such determinations.

The term *dose intensity* refers to the quantity of drug, corrected for the size of the host, delivered as a function of time, usually measured in mg/m^2/week.[67] Figure 14.9 illustrates schematically the differences between increasing dose intensity by dose escalation and by increasing dose density. As illustrated, more frequent dosing can be interpreted as a test of dose density only when the dose level and cycle number are kept constant. Failure to incorporate this concept into the design of clinical trials, as highlighted below, renders them uninterpretable for this issue.

Another potential source of confusion is the incorrect assumption that log-kill from the use of a drug will be the same if that drug in total mg/m^2 was given in one administration or in multiple fractions. If the dose intensity in mg/m^2/week related directly to efficacy in a strictly linear fashion, then twice the dose level of drug given one-half as often and one-half the number of times should be roughly

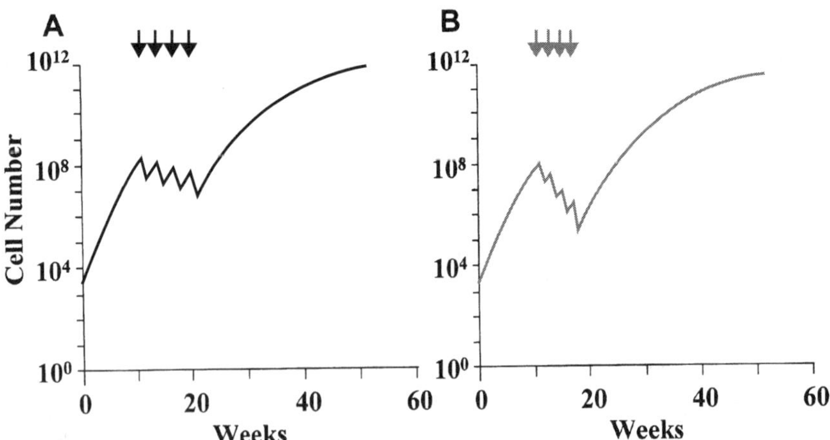

FIGURE 14.8 Dose-dense therapy of a large tumor volume. Although the increased dose rate (termed *dose density*) in panel B results in increased log-kill, rapid Gompertzian regrowth of the large residual cancer cell population produces eventual tumor growth comparable to the therapy in panel A, which has a slower dose rate (termed *dose scarcity*).

Dose intensity (mg/m^2/week) is increased when more total drug (in mg/m^2) is given over a fixed unit of time. *Dose escalation* is one way of increasing dose intensity:

or

Time

Time

Lower dose level over a certain time interval

Higher dose level over the same time interval

Dose density is another way to increase mg/m^2/week, but it does not assume a rising dose-response relationship. Density is increased when the same number of cycles at the same dose level are given over less time because of shorter inter-treatment intervals:

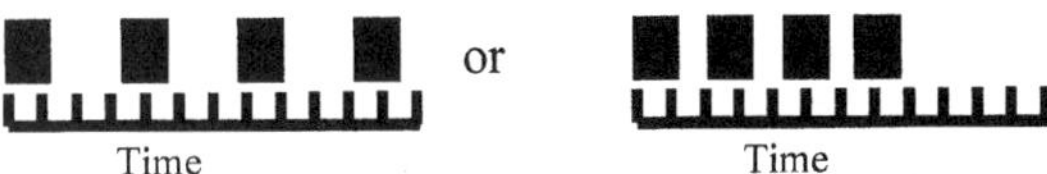

FIGURE 14.9 Relationship between dose intensity, dose escalation, and dose density.

as effective as a standard dose and schedule. That is, if the dose-response is linear, then four administrations of a drug at dose level A with an interval t between treatments should be similar in efficacy to two administrations at dose level 2A with an interval 2t between treatments. In fact, the 2A dose level plan should be a bit better because if one discounts the recovery time after the last administration, the 2A plan is actually delivered over 2t time (for a dose intensity of 4A/2t = 2A/t) while the four treatments at dose level A are given over 3t time (for a dose intensity of 4A/3t). However, this has not been demonstrated clinically for several common agents. For example, if this reasoning was valid, then four doses of cyclophosphamide 600 mg/m^2 every third week would have to be as effective as 1200 mg/m^2 every 6th week for two cycles. In fact, 1200 mg/m^2 for four cycles at three week intervals was no more effective than 600 mg/m^2, nor was 2400 mg/m^2 any more active.[23,66] This experience and a similar one with doxorubicin fail to confirm the hypothesis that dose escalation alone determines the impact of chemotherapy.[21]

An example of the subtleties one may encounter when trying to apply or evaluate dose density is illustrated by an Intergroup study (S0137) coordinated by the Southwest Oncology Group (SWOG), presented by Charles Haskell in 2002.[68] This trial was designed carefully in an era before the non-linearity of dose-response was fully appreciated. In it, patients with low-risk primary breast cancer were randomized postoperatively between two arms. The first was six three-week cycles of AC at 54 mg/m^2 of doxorubicin and 1200 mg/m^2 of cyclophosphamide. The second was four three-week cycles of 81 mg/m^2 of doxorubicin followed by three two-week cycles of 2400 mg/m^2 of cyclophosphamide. These dose levels were chosen to sum arithmetically to the same cumulative doses: 324 mg/m^2 of doxorubicin and 7200 mg/m^2 of cyclophosphamide. In this way dose intensity (mg/m^2/week) was increased in the sequential arm compared with the control arm while the total dose was held constant. The hazard for disease recurrence was 8% higher for the regimen with six cycles of AC, but this difference was not statistically significant. Can one conclude that the sequential "dose dense" regimen did not improve results? If these results are analyzed in light of data from C9344, which demonstrated that dose levels of doxorubicin greater than 60 mg/m^2 conveyed no additional log-kill, and the NSABP trials that found no advantage to doses of cyclophosphamide over 600 mg/m^2, there is no unequivocal conclusion. That is, the "conventional" arm of the SWOG trial gave six three-week cycles of doxorubicin and the "experimental" arm only four cycles at roughly equivalently effective dose levels (81 mg/m^2 being no more effective than 60 mg/m^2, which may be trivially more effective than the 51 mg/m^2 used in the conventional arm, given that C8541 found only small differences between 40 mg/m^2 and 60 mg/m^2). The conventional arm gave six three-week cycles of cyclophosphamide while the other gave only three two-week cycles, also at equivalently effective dose levels (both 2400 mg/m^2 and 1200 mg/m^2 being no more effective than 600 mg/m^2). Yet the six cycles of AC, which gave two more cycles of effective doxorubicin and three more effective cycles of cyclophosphamide, was not superior to the experimental arm. Is this because four doses of doxorubicin and three of cyclophosphamide are enough? Is it because the dose density of the cyclophosphamide in the experimental arm compensated for the fewer number of cycles? One can draw no firm conclusions from this trial, but it clearly cannot be interpreted as a negative trial regarding the concepts of sequential therapy and dose density.

Similarly, ongoing clinical trials in the adjuvant chemotherapy of breast cancer will have to be analyzed very carefully and interpreted judiciously concerning their theoretical implications. For example, an Intergroup trial (E1199), chaired by Joseph Sparano of the Eastern Cooperative Oncology Group, compares paclitaxel and docetaxel, each being administered by a three-week or a one-week schedule following four three-week cycles of AC. This study will have to be viewed with an understanding of the differences in dose level as well as schedule. That is, the dose levels for paclitaxel are 175 mg/m^2 in the three-week regimen versus 80 mg/m^2 in the weekly regimen. Is the log-kill from 80 mg/m^2 greater than one-third the log-kill from 175 mg/m^2? In the same way, how does the log-kill from 100 mg/m^2 of docetaxel each three weeks compare with 35 mg/m^2 each week? A National Cancer Institute of Canada trial (MA.21) chaired by Mark Levine contrasts epirubcicn and doxorubicin at different dose levels and schedules, with two of three arms using paclitaxel and one using 5-fluorouracil.

While this is a very important study, its asymmetry portends a fascinating but complex and possibly difficult future interpretation. An Intergroup SWOG trial (S0221) chaired by Thomas Budd compares weekly doxorubicin plus daily oral cyclophosphamide with two-weekly AC followed by weekly versus two-weekly paclitaxel, all at different dose levels (as well as different routes of administration of cyclophosphamide). This trial, also lacking the complete symmetry of C9741, will present analytic challenges. In essence, these trials were designed to compare specific regimens rather than principles that can be generalized. The results of trials comparing specific regimens can have important practical implications and are thus valuable. But because they do not control for all significant variables, they do not necessarily help us clarify principles. It is important to keep this distinction in mind even though both types of trials are needed to continue to advance the field of cancer treatment.

THE BIOLOGY OF GOMPERTZIAN GROWTH

Clearly, the above considerations call for much more clinical research evaluating new concepts of drug administration. If a two-week cycle length is preferable to a three-week cycle length, what would be the effects of a further one-third reduction to a ten-day cycle length? Is there a cycle length too short to optimize log-kill because subsequent administrations would expose cells already killed to therefore redundant treatment? Will dose density apply to other anticancer agents and other diseases that meet the criteria of being Gompertzian, at small volume, and sensitive to chemotherapy? Will these concepts prove applicable before surgery for breast cancer, where the local tumor burden is high while the systemic burden is still low? In this situation might we encounter for the first time a discrepancy between local rates of complete remission and the odds of systemic control? Is the erythrocyte transfusion requirement for 13% of patients receiving dose-dense AC followed by paclitaxel in C9741 a reproducible phenomenon, and if so, can it be prevented or ameliorated by the timely application of an erythropoietin?[69]

These are all intriguing questions, but underlying them all is the biology of Gompertzian growth and Gompertzian response to therapy. What is the molecular etiology of such patterns, and how can that be manipulated more efficiently and more safely than with toxic chemotherapy? Does chemotherapy affect all subpopulations in a heterogeneous tumor equally or—as theory suggests—are the faster-growing sub-clones more perturbed? If cancer stem cells become a proven fact, as early evidence suggests they might, what is the effect of dose dense chemotherapy and are these critical sub-populations?[70]

As we develop better methods of molecular analysis of the genes, gene products, and gene regulatory apparatus that determine the malignant phenotype, it would seem appropriate to turn our attention to the questions above, which are of theoretical as well as practical relevance.

In the history of science, phenomena that are described mathematically and then become candidates for mechanistic investigations, a style of research that has proven to bear considerable fruit over many centuries. Ideally, our clinical trial research and our laboratory studies of model systems and clinical material should converge—linked by quantitative as well as qualitative understanding—to produce more knowledge plus better ways to help our patients.

REFERENCES

1. DeVita V. Priniciples of cancer management: chemotherapy. In DeVita VT, Hellman S, Rosenberg S, eds. Cancer: Priniciples and Practice of Oncology. Philadelphia, PA: J.B. Lippincott Co., 1997:337–347.
2. Skipper HE. Laboratory models: the historical perspective. Cancer Treat Rep 1986;70:3–7.
3. Hanahan D, Weinberg R. The hallmarks of cancer [review]. Cell 2000;100:57–70.
4. Sorlie T, Tibshirani R, Parker J, et al. Repeated observation of breast tumor subtypes in independent gene expression data sets. Proc Natl Acad Sci USA 2003;100:8418–8423.
5. van de Vijver MJ, He YD, van 't Veer LJ, et al. A gene-expression signature as a predictor of survival in breast cancer. N Engl J Med 2002;347:1999–2009.
6. Sotiriou C, Neo S, McShane L, et al. Breast cancer classification and prognosis based on gene expression profiles from a population-based study. Proc Natl Acad Sci USA 2003;100: 10393–10398.
7. Skipper H, Schabel FJ, Wilcox W. Experimental evaluation of potential anticancer agents XIII: on the criteria and kinetics associated with "curability" of experimental leukemia. Cancer Chemother Rep 1964;35:1.
8. Li Y, Hively W, Varmus H. Use of MMTV-Wnt-1 transgenic mice for studying the genetic basis of breast cancer. Oncogene 2000;19:1002–1009.
9. Jackson-Grusby L. Modeling cancer in mice. Oncogene 2002;21:5504–5514.
10. Luria S, Delbruck M. Mutations of bacteria from virus sensitivity to virus resistance. Genetics 1943;28:491–511.
11. Law L. Origin of resistance of leukaemic cells to folic acid antagonists. Nature 1952;169:628.
12. Cannellos GP, DeVita VT, Gold GL, et al. Cyclical combination chemotherapy for advanced breast cancer. BMJ 1974;1:218–220.
13. DeVita VT, Young R, Canellos GP. Combination versus single agent chemotherapy: A review of the basis for selection of drug treatment of cancer. Cancer 35:98–110.
14. Hayes D, Henderson I, Shapiro C. Treatment of metastatic breast cancer: present and future prospects [review]. Semin Oncol 1995;22[suppl 5]:5–21.
15. Shapiro C, Henderson I. Adjuvant therapy of breast cancer. Hematol Oncol Clin North Am 1994;8:213–231.
16. Munster P, Hudis C. Adjuvant therapy for resectable breast cancer. Hematol Oncol Clin North Am 1999;13:391–413.
17. Sledge GW, Neuberg D, Bernardo P, et al. Phase III trial of doxorubicin, paclitaxel, and the combination of doxorubicin and paclitaxel as front-line chemotherapy for metastatic breast cancer: an Intergroup Trial (E1193). J Clin Oncol 2003;21:588–592.
18. Wood W, Budman D, Korzun A, et al. Dose and dose intensity trial of adjuvant chemotherapy for stage II, node-positive breast carcinoma. N Engl J Med 1994;330:1253–1259.
19. Budman D, Berry D, Cirrincione C, et al. Dose and dose intensity as determinants of outcome in the adjvuant treatment of breast cancer. J Natl Cancer Inst 1998;90:1205–1211.

20. Winer E, Berry D, Duggan D, et al. Failure of higher dose paclitaxel to improve outcome in patients with metastatic breast cancer—results from CALGB 9342. Proc ASCO 1998; 17:388a.

21. Henderson IC, Berry DA, Demetri GD, et al. Improved outcomes from adding sequential paclitaxel but not from escalating doxorubicin dose in an adjuvant chemotherapy regimen for patients with node-positive primary breast cancer. J Clin Oncol 2003;21:976–983.

22. Fisher B, Anderson S, DeCillis A, et al. Further evaluation of intensified and increased total dose of cyclophosphamide for the treatment of primary breast cancer: findings from National Surgical Adjuvant Breast and Bowel Project B-25. J Clin Oncol 1999;17:3374–3388.

23. Fisher B, Anderson S, Wickerham D, et al. Increased intensification and total dose of cyclophosphamide in a doxorubicin-cyclophosphamide regimen for the treatment of primary breast cancer: findings from National Surgical Adjuvant Breast and Bowel Project B-22. J Clin Oncol 1997;15:1858–1869.

24. Fisher B, Redmond C, Wickerham DL, et al. Doxorubicin-containing regimens for the treatment of stage II breast cancer: the National Surgical Adjuvant Breast and Bowel Project experience. J Clin Oncol 1989;7:572–582.

25. Fisher B, Brown AM, Dimitrov NV, et al. Two months of doxorubicin-cyclophosphamide with and without interval reinduction therapy compared with 6 months of cyclophosphamide, methotrexate, and fluorouracil in positive-node breast cancer patients with tamoxifen-nonresponsive tumors: results from the National Surgical Breast and Bowel Project B-15. J Clin Oncol 1990;8:1483–1496.

26. Breast Cancer Trialists' Collaborative Group. Polychemotherapy for early breast cancer: an overview of the randomised trials. Lancet 1998;352:930–942.

27. Adler L, Herzog T, Williams S. Analysis of exposure times and dose escalation of paclitaxel in ovarian cancer cell lines. Cancer 1994;74:1891–1898.

28. Norton L, Simon R, Brereton J, et al. Predicting the course of Gompertzian growth. Nature 1976;264:542–545.

29. Kidwell J, Howard A, Laird A. The inheritance of growth and form in the mouse. II. The Gompertz growth equation. Growth 1969;33:339–352.

30. Norton L. Mathematical Interpretation of Tumor Growth Kinetics Clinical Interpretation and Practice of Cancer Chemotherapy. In Greenspan E, ed. New York, NY: Raven Press, 1982:53–70.

31. Norton L. Biology of residual breast cancer after therapy: a kinetic interpretation. Prog Clin Biol Res 1990;354A:109–132.

32. Norton L, Simon R. Tumor size, sensitivity to therapy, and design of treatment schedules. Cancer Treat Rep 1977;61:1307–1315.

33. Stadtmauer E, O'Neill A, Goldstein L, et al. Conventional-dose chemotherapy compared with high-dose chemotherapy plus autologous hematopoietic stem-cell transplantation for metastatic breast cancer. N Engl J Med 2000;342:1069–1076.

34. Antman K, Rowlings P, Vaughan W, et al. High-dose chemotherapy with autologous hematopoietic stem-cell support for breast cancer in North America. J Clin Oncol 1997; 15:1870–1879.

35. Vahdat L, Antman K. High-dose chemotherapy with autologous stem cell support for breast cancer. Curr Opin Hematol 1997;4:381–389.

36. Berry DA, Broadwater G, Klein JP, et al. High-dose versus standard chemotherapy in metastatic breast cancer: comparison of Cancer and Leukemia Group B Trials with data from the Autologous Blood and Marrow Transplant Registry. J Clin Oncol 2002;20:743–750.

37. Norton L. Implications of kinetic heterogeneity in clinical oncology. Semin Oncol 1985;12: 231–249.

38. Nabholtz J, Pienkowski T, Mackey J, et al. Phase III trial comparing TAC (docetaxel, doxorubicin, cyclophosphamide) with FAC (5-fluorouracil, doxorubicin, cyclophosphamide) in the adjuvant treatment of node positive breast cancer (BC) patients: interim analysis of the BCIRG 001 study. Proc Am Soc Clin Oncol 2002;21:141a.

39. Buzdar A, Singletary S, Valero V, et al. Evaluation of paclitaxel in adjuvant chemotherapy for patients with operable breast cancer: preliminary data of a prospective randomized trial. Clin Cancer Res 2002;8:1073–1079.

40. Goldie JH, Coldman AJ. A mathematical model for relating drug sensitivity of tumors to their spontaneous mutation rate. Cancer Treat Rep 1979;63:1727–1733.

41. Goldie JH, Coldman AJ, Gudauskas GA. Rationale for the use of alternating non-cross-resistant chemotherapy. Cancer Treat Rep 1982;66:439–449.

42. Dang C, Gilewski T, Surbone A, et al. Cytokinetics. In Kufe DW, Weichselbaum RR, Bast RC Jr, et al., eds. London, UK: BC Decker, 2003:645–668.

43. Norton L, Simon R. The Norton-Simon hypothesis revisited. Cancer Treat Rep 1986: 70:163–169.

44. Norton L, Day R. Potential innovations in scheduling of cancer chemotherapy. In Vincent J, DeVita T, Hellman S, Rosenberg SA, eds. Important Advances in Oncology 1991. Pennsylvania, PA: JB Lippincott Company, 1991:57–72.

45. Buzzoni R, Bonadonna G, Valagussa P, et al. Adjuvant chemotherapy with doxorubicin plus cyclophosphamide, methotrexate, and fluorouracil in the treatment of resectable breast cancer with more than three axillary lymph nodes. J Clin Oncol 1991;9:2134–2140.

46. Bonadonna G, Zambette M, Valagussa P. Sequential or alternating doxorubicin and CMF regimens in breast cancer with more than three positive nodes. JAMA 1995;273:542–547.

47. Poole C, Earl H, Dunn J, et al. NEAT (National Epirubicin Adjuvant Trial) and SCTBG BR9601 (Scottish Cancer Trials Breast Group) phase III adjuvant breast trials show a significant relapse-free and overall survival advantage for sequential ECMF. Proc Am Soc Clin Oncol 2003;22:4 (abstr #13).

48. Muss H, Woolf S, Berry D, et al. Older women with node positive (N+) breast cancer (BC) get similar benefits from adjuvant chemotherapy (Adj) as younger patients (pts): The Cancer and Leukemia Group B (CALGB) experience. Proc Am Soc Clin Oncol 2003;22:4 (abstr #11).

49. Mamounas E, Bryant J, Lembersky B, et al. Paclitaxel (T) following doxorubicin/cyclophosphamide (AC) as adjuvant chemotherapy for node-positive breast cancer: Results from NSABP B-28. Proc Am Soc Clin Oncol 2003;22:4 (abstr #12).

50. NIH Consensus Development Panel. National Institutes of Health Consensus Development Conference statement: adjuvant therapy for breast cancer, November 1-3, 2000. J Natl Cancer Inst Monogr 2001;30:5–15.

51. Perloff M, Norton L, Korzun A, et al. Postsurgical adjuvant chemotherapy of stage II breast carcinoma with or without crossover to a noncross-resistant: A CALGB study. J Clin Oncol 1996;14:1589–1598.

52. Hutcheon A, Heys S, Sarkar TK, and the Aberdeen Breast Group. Neoadjuvant docetaxel in locally advanced breast cancer. Breast Cancer Treat Rep 2003;79(Suppl 1):519–524.

53. Crown J, Raptis G, Hamilton N, et al. High-dose chemotherapy of breast cancer: current status and developmental strategies. Eur J Cancer 1995;31A:809–811.

54. Rodenhuis S, Bontenbal M, Beex LV et al. High dose chemotherapy with hematopoietic stem-cell rescue for high-risk breast cancer. N Engl J Med 2003;349:7–16.

55. Peters W, Rosner G, Vredenburgh J, et al. A prospective, randomized comparison of two doses of combination alkyating agents (AA) as consolidation after CAF in high-risk primary breast cancer involving ten or more axillary lymph nodes (LN): preliminary results of CALGB 9082/SWOG 9114/NCIC MA-13 [abstr.] Proc Am Soc Clin Oncol 1999;18:2a.

56. Bergh J, Wiklund T, Erikstein B, et al. Tailored fluorouracil, epirubicin, and cyclophosphamide compared with marrow-supported high-dose chemotherapy as adjuvant treatment for high-risk breast cancer: a randomised trial. Scandinavian Breast Group 9401 study. Lancet 2000;356:1384–1391.

57. Tallman MS, Gray R, Robert NJ, et al. Conventional adjuvant chemotherapy with or without high-dose chemotherapy and autologous stem-cell transplantation in high-risk breast cancer. N Engl J Med 2003;349:17–26.

58. Crown J, Norton L. Potential strategies for improving the results of high-dose chemotherapy in patients with metastatic breast cancer. Ann Oncol 1995;6[suppl 4]:21–26.

59. Crown J, Perey L, Lind M, et al. Superiority of tandem high-dose chemotherapy (HDC) versus optimized conventionally-dosed chemotherapy (CDC) in patients (pts) with metastatic breast cancer (MBC): The International Randomized Breast Cancer Dose Intensity Study (IBDIS 1). Proc Am Soc Clin Oncol 2003;22:23 (abstr #88).

60. Tallman MS, Gray R, Robert NJ, et al. Conventional adjuvant chemotherapy with or without high-dose chemotherapy and autologous stem-cell transplantation in high-risk breast cancer. N Engl J Med 2003;349:17–26.

61. Hudis C, Seidman A, Baselga J, et al. Sequential dose-dense doxorubicin, paclitaxel, and cyclophosphamide for resectable high-risk breast cancer: feasibility and efficacy. J Clin Oncol 1999;17:93–100.

62. Hudis C, Fornier M, Riccio L, et al. 5-year results of dose-intensive sequential adjuvant chemotherapy for women with high-risk node-positive breast cancer: a phase II study. J Clin Oncol 1999;17:1118.

63. Fornier MN, Seidman AD, Theodoulou M, et al. Doxorubicin followed by sequential paclitaxel and cyclophosphamide versus concurrent paclitaxel and cyclophosphamide: 5-year results of a phase II randomized trial of adjuvant dose-dense chemotherapy for women with node-positive breast carcinoma. Clin Cancer Res 2001;7:3934–3941.

64. Gabrilove J, Jakubowski A, Scher H, et al. Effect of granulocyte colony-stimulating factor on neutropenia associated morbidity due to chemotherapy for transitional-cell carcinoma of the urothelium. N Engl J Med 1988;318:1414–1422, 1988.

65. Citron ML, Berry DA, Cirrincione C, et al. Randomized trial of dose-dense versus conventionally scheduled and sequential versus concurrent combination chemotherapy as postoperative adjuvant treatment of node-positive primary breast cancer: first report of Intergroup Trial C9741/Cancer and Leukemia Group B Trial 9741. J Clin Oncol 2003;9:81.

66. Fisher B, Anderson S, DeCillis A, et al. Further evaluation of intensified and increased total dose of cyclophosphamide for the treatment of primary breast cancer: findings from National Surgical Adjuvant Breast and Bowel Project B-25. J Clin Oncol 1999;17: 3374–3388.

67. Hryniuk W, Figueredo A, Goodyear M. Applications of dose intensity to problems in chemotherapy of breast and colorectal cancer. Semin Oncol 1987;14[suppl 4]:3–11.

68. Haskell C, Green S, Sledge G, et al. Phase III comparison of adjuvant high-dose doxorubicin plus cyclophosphamide (AC) versus sequential doxorubicin followed by cyclophosphamide (A→C) in breast cancer patients with 0-3 positive nodes (intergroup 0137) [abstr.]. Proc Am Soc Clin Oncol 2002;21:142a.

69. Case D, Bukowski R, Carey R, et al. Recombinant human erythropoietin therapy for anemic cancer patients on combination chemotherapy. J Natl Cancer Inst 1993;85:801–806.

70. Dontu G, Al-Hajj M, Abdallah A, et al. Stem cells in normal breast development and breast cancer. Cell Prolif 2003;36[suppl 1]:59–72.

Chapter 15

Current Status of Total Mesorectal Excision for Rectal Cancer

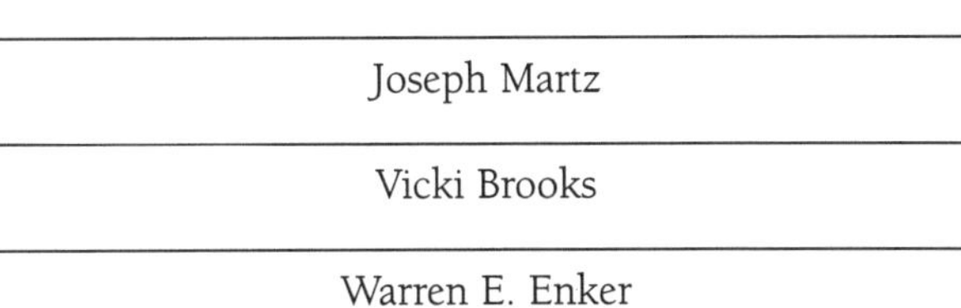
Joseph Martz

Vicki Brooks

Warren E. Enker

Rectal cancers are resected with the goals of cure, that is, the resection of all regional disease and the prevention of spread, and the prevention of local or pelvic recurrence. The rectum is contained within the posterior visceral compartment of the pelvis. Together, the rectum and the mesorectum are an integral unit that is contained within a defining sheath or circumferential boundary known as the visceral layer of the pelvic fascia (VLPF).[1,2] Within the mesorectal fat are located the superior rectal vessels, and the majority of the lymph nodes that, if involved by cancer, would constitute regional disease.

The majority of patients with rectal carcinoma are symptomatic. Most patients (65%–85%) present with either full thickness penetration of the rectal wall (T3 or T4) or with mesorectal lymph node involvement (T any N1-2 M0).[3] This represents either stage II or stage III disease, and is defined as regional disease. In 1963, Morson et al identified that 60% of patients with transmural penetration of the bowel wall (T3) had mesorectal lymph node involvement.[4] In addition to lymph nodes, Reynolds et al identified non-nodal foci or "mesorectal deposits" in association with 5 of 21 (24%) Dukes B tumors and mesorectal deposits and/or lymph node metastases in 12 of 23 (52%) Dukes C patients.[5] In some cases these were situated within millimeters of the circumferential or "lateral" edges of the regional "container" that is defined by the VLPF. These findings strongly suggested that the mesorectum is the repository for regional lymph node spread or of any type of resectable curable spread outside of the rectal wall, and strongly influenced both the rationale and the outcomes of total mesorectal excision (TME) for rectal cancer.

While the treatment of rectal cancer is based upon the principle of eradicating regional disease, not all pelvic disease is restricted to the mesorectum. In some cases, lateral spread also constitutes a part of the natural history. As early as 1940, Coller and McIntyre studied the pattern of lymph node involvement in rectal cancer using fat-clearing methods.[6] As expected, 63% of the patients had lymph node metastases within the mesorectum (stage III). Of the specimens obtained from the 19 patients with distal rectal cancers, 11 (58%) harbored lymph node metastases; 5 within the mesorectum only, and 6 (32%) within the mesorectum and to the lateral internal iliac nodes along the pelvic side wall. In the modern era, Morikawa et al evaluated specimens from the resection of 171 cancers (38 rectosigmoid, 68 upper rectal, and 65 lower rectal) also studied by lymph node clearing.[7] The overall rate of lymph node metastases was 57.3%, in the same range as prior studies, with 33.3% of T1 rectal cancers having involved lymph nodes. Hida et al reported similar findings.[8]

CLINICAL PRESENTATION AND REGIONAL DISEASE

Most mesorectal lymph node involvement is situated either directly adjacent or proximal to the primary tumor. Occasionally, skip disease, that is, proximal or apical nodes positive with adjacent nodes negative, is observed. In order to include all potentially curable lymph node involvement in a resection and for purposes of sphincter-preserving reconstruction, proximal ligation of the inferior mesenteric artery and vein is commonly practiced.[3] It is critical that the surgeon also focus on the extent of the lymph node spread that may involve the mesorectum distal to or below the primary cancer. It is the potential for mesorectal spreads that should determine the extent of *en bloc* distal mesorectum to be resected as the "distal margin," and not the extent of distal intramural spread. While the extent of distal intramural spread seems to get more publicity or attention, it is of considerably less importance in the pathophysiology of recurrent disease than is distal mesorectal disease. Scott et al evaluated specimens from 20 curative resections of tumors within 18 cm of the anal verge.[9] Distal mesorectal spread of cancer was seen in 5 of 18 (28%) specimens. One of the five specimens exhibited distal intramural spread of malignant cells to 2 cm beyond the macroscopic edge. However, four (20%) of the specimens exhibited tumor cell spread in the mesorectum as far as 3 cm from the distal edge of the tumor, with or without associated mural extension. In general the degree of extramural or mesorectal spread will exceed the degree of distal intramural spread. Hida et al performed an analysis of 198 specimens using lymph node enhancing, fat-clearing methods to evaluate distal spread.[8] Distal intramural spread was only observed in 10.6% of patients, extending up to 2 cm in the case of proximal rectal cancers and 1 cm in the case of distal rectal tumors. Distal intramural spread was not observed in T1 or T2 tumors. However, distal mesorectal nodal metastases were identified in 20% of T3 patients with distal lymph node metastases being present as far as 4 cm below the distal edge of the primary tumor. Overall, 24% of patients had involvement of the mesorectum distal to the tumor. The maximum distance from the primary carcinoma to a metastatic lesion was >2 cm in five of these 12 individuals and was 5 cm. in one patient. According to these data, patients with T3 lesions undergoing curative resections (the majority of patients with symptomatic disease) should have a distal margin of 5 cm of *mesorectum* resected, in order to provide a curative resection.

Within the mesorectum, nodal metastases or focal deposits may be situated centrally or immediately adjacent to the primary tumor, or they may be found peripherally, that is, close, within millimeters of the lateral circumferential margins of the mesorectum. Clearly, the surgeon is faced with eradicating regional, as opposed to local or mural disease in the overwhelming majority of patients. Strict adherence to these principles constitutes the pathologic foundation for the resection of rectal cancers according to the principles of TME.

Position Statement

The observations by Coller et al,[6] Scott et al,[9] Hida et al,[8] Reynolds et al,[5] and others[10] confirmed the risks that distal mesorectal metastases may exist, in addition to radial and proximal metastases. They confirm the importance of respect for the circumferential margins, as defined by the VLPF,[11] and of resecting the rectum and the mesorectum as an integral unit for a distance of *not less* than 5 centimeters distal to the lowest palpable edge when dealing with primary tumors, which are situated in the mid-rectum or above. TME can only be accomplished in conjunction with a complete rectal mobilization[3,12,13] from the sacral promontory down to the anal canal, that is, the anal hiatus within the levator ani muscles.

DEFINITIONS OF THE RECTUM

In clinical practice, the rectum is defined both by anatomic guidelines and by accepted, practical conventions; these definitions and issues have been reviewed elsewhere.[11] Anatomically, the rectum is the distal portion of the large bowel that is extra-peritoneal. From a rectal cancer standpoint, a marked difference in the incidence of local recurrence has been noted for cancers below versus above 11 to 12 cm.[14] In the pre-TME era, these data were corroborated by others, leading the GI Tumor Study Group[15] and other Cooperative groups to adopt the 12-centimeter margin as the defining criterion for rectal cancers in assigning patients to adjuvant therapy trials.[15–17]

TRADITIONAL SURGICAL MANAGEMENT

Hstorically, rectal cancer has been treated by some form of local, that is, transanal or perineal resection. Until the early part of the 20th century, few cases were reported to involve both resection of the primary tumor and its predictable pathways of lymph node spread. Since 1908, the guiding principles have been based upon the resection of the primary tumor and of its lymphatic distribution, principles that were first elucidated by the autopsy dissections and by the surgical experience of Sir Ernest Miles.[18] Sphincter-preserving operations (SPOs) were introduced by Dixon in the late 1930s.[19]

From the late 1940s to the 1970s, low anterior resection, defined as a resection of the rectum with an extra-peritoneal anastomosis, was perfected by the efforts of many.[20] Division of the so-called "lateral ligaments" assured complete mobilization of the rectum, making SPOs possible for mid-rectal cancers, for the first time. Prior to that time, most SPOs were really performed for cancers of the recto-sigmoid or distal sigmoid colon. At the same time, surgeons devoted to the treatment of rectal cancer began adopting the use of sharp, anatomically-driven pelvic dissections, performed under direct vision. Many of these advances were accomplished by specialty Services at major, high-volume institutions. In the U.S., despite progress generated by specialty Services, the overwhelming majority of patients with rectal cancer continued to undergo traditional operations, performed using blunt dissection without regard for anatomic pathways, These operations are associated with a high incidence of pelvic recurrence, poor survival, a high incidence of permanent colostomy, impotence and bowel or bladder dysfunction.[3] As a result of conventional surgery, even up to the present time, worldwide local recurrence rates have consistently averaged 30% to 40%[21] and, in some locally advanced cases, either overall or stage-related local failure rates were reported to be much higher.[22,23] Traditional five-year survival rates have ranged from 27% to 42%.[15,24–26]

PATHOPHYSIOLOGY OF PELVIC RECURRENCE

Many theories have been advanced to explain the causes of pelvic recurrence of rectal cancer, including, the implantation of shed tumor cells at the anastomosis[27] and the up-regulation of tumor growth at the anastomosis.[28] In keeping with the rare incidence of true "anastomotic" recurrences, Morson et al showed that so-called "local recurrences" after rectal excision were, in fact, pelvic recurrences located outside of the bowel lumen.[4] It is important to realize that early in the development of TME, this point was well emphasized by Heald et al, as they developed their philosophy or approach to rectal cancer and the importance of the mesorectum.[13] Most recurrences are stage-related, with known risk factors of mural penetration or nodal involvement. Minor risk factors for local pelvic recurrence include extramural vascular, lymphatic or perineural invasion.[15] These pathologic risk factors suggested decades ago,[4] or even earlier, that the major cause of pelvic recurrence affecting the majority of such patients is the inadequate resection of regional mesorectal disease.

Inadequate resection occurs because of the prevalence of blunt or conventional resection. Despite the introduction of sharp pelvic dissection for rectal cancer along anatomically defined planes, even today, most "conventional" resections of rectal cancers that are performed still utilize "blunt" surgical techniques that fail to mobilize the rectum along definable tissue planes. Anatomic pelvic dissections have demonstrated that the bluntly dissecting hand behind the rectum, in the retro-rectal space, encounters the dense, two-layered recto-sacral fascia at about the level of S3-S4.[2,29] Continued attempts to get past this impediment frequently shear into or violate the mesorectum, creating a grossly visible tear or an obvious defect in the surgical margin. This tear shears lymph nodes or metastatic deposit-containing fat away from the bulk of the mesorectum, leaving cancer-bearing mesorectal fat attached to the pelvic sidewall, the sacrum, etc. This persistent residual disease, referred to as a positive lateral or circumferential margin, serves as the nidus for "local recurrence" that usually becomes clinically evident within eighteen months.[30]

Since 1979, a series of clinical studies have been undertaken to determine the role of two factors in the prevention of local pelvic recurrence: the importance of achieving uninvolved lateral or circumferential surgical margins, and the pathophysiologic basis for the extent of proximal, lateral and distal mesorectal excision.[31,32] These studies demonstrated the importance of the circumferential margins of resection and a reduced rate of local, pelvic recurrence in patients undergoing a wide, sharp pelvic dissection.[32]

Heald and coworkers attributed some element of pelvic recurrence to microscopic foci of disease left behind in the distal mesorectum several centimeters distal to the apparent lower edge of a rectal cancer.[13] As previously indicated, Morson et al[4] related the incidence of pelvic recurrence to the extent of mural penetration or nodal involvement. Despite the attempts of both Heald et al[13] and of Enker et al[3] to prove that pelvic recurrences results from surgical failure, these attempts lacked a pathologic correlation until the mid-1980s. In 1986 Quirke et al reported on the analysis of the resected specimens from 52 patients, with a minimum follow-up of two years using whole mount cross sections.[33] All patients had undergone what were deemed by their surgeons to be "curative" resections using conventional modes of blunt pelvic dissection. Significant missing portions of the mesorectum, gouged out of what should be the intact or unviolated contour of the mesorectal fat were observed, and involved lateral resection margins were identified in 14 (27%) of the specimens. The operating surgeons did not suspect such pathology findings. Not surprisingly, 85% of the patients with positive margins (12 of 14) developed a pelvic recurrence. Quirke et al attributed their documentation of this relationship to their change in the method of handling the surgical specimen, which allowed the pathologist to evaluate the relationship between the extent of disease and the surgical margins of resection.[33]

Subsequently, Ng et al reported on 80 patients undergoing proctectomy for cancer with a median follow-up of 26.6 months.[34] The lateral resection margins were positive in 20% of cases. Among those undergoing "curative resections" the pelvic recurrence rate was 17% in patients with uninvolved margins and 60% in those with involved margins ($P < .001$). These data correlated well with the work of Quirke et al.[33]

Adam et al extended Quirke's series and reported a prospective study of 190 patients undergoing conventional operations (that is, blunt dissection) with a median follow-up of five years.[35] These pathologists introduced a protocol for the processing of rectal cancer specimens, involving serial transverse and coronal sections, measuring the closest point where any tumor (such as, nodal disease, non-nodal implants or venous invasion) approached the lateral margin, and defining a margin of <1 mm as a positive margin. Local recurrence and survival rates were correlated with margin status. Positive lateral margins were identified in 36% of cases and in 25% of those undergoing curative resections. The local recurrence rates were 64% in patients with involved circumferential margins versus 9% in those with uninvolved margins, overall, and 66% versus 8%, respectively, in those undergoing curative resection. The hazard ratio for recurrence based upon a positive circumferential margin was 12.23. Similarly, the overall five-year life-table survival was 15% in those with involved margins and 66% in those with uninvolved margins (24% vs. 74% in curative resections). Pelvic recurrence was directly related to inadequate surgical resection with involved circumferential margins.

Position Statement

The implications of Quirke's findings together with the findings of the preceding clinical and pathological studies are that rectal cancers must be resected as a regional unit of the affected rectum and mesorectum, with uninvolved and unviolated circumferential margins of resection if one is to reduce the incidence of pelvic recurrence. This is one of the foundations of "mesorectal excision."

TOTAL MESORECTAL EXCISION

With the advent of mesorectal excision using sharp technique, improvements in local recurrence rates and in the survival rates of patients with rectal cancer have been observed over the past two decades. These improvements are the primarily the result of advances in surgical technique. Currently referred to as TME, this technique of resection for rectal cancer has resulted in a new platform of improved surgical results with dramatically improved cancer-related and functional outcomes.[3,36–38]

In our experience the technique of TME utilizes precise, sharp dissection in the anatomically defined areolar tissue between the visceral and parietal layers of the pelvic fascia[35] performed under direct vision.

Several studies have described total mesorectal excision, including: TME,[13,37,38,39] TME with autonomic nerve preservation,[3,21,40] mesorectal excision or sharp perimesorectal dissection[41] or extra-fascial excision.[12] Each title describes a specific author's version of the operation or some area of specific emphasis. The precise method of sharp dissection, under direct vision, leaves the gonadal vessels, ureters, iliac vessels, sacral veins, pelvic autonomic nerves, and pelvic wall musculature peripheral to the parietal fascia, minimizing the risk of damage to these structures[36] and preserving their functions.

The planes of dissection that define a curative resection also define preservation of the autonomic nervous system. Particularly in the male, blunt or random dissections may lead to Inferior hypogastric plexus (also known as the pelvic autonomic nerve plexus) or nerve injury and sexual or urinary dysfunction.[40] The autonomic nerves of the pelvis are intimately associated with the lateral edges of the mesorectum and the pelvic fascial layers, and because of the narrow pelvis they are particularly vulnerable in male patients. The act of rectal excision also requires a constant focus on the anatomy of the autonomic nerves in order to preserve both urinary and sexual functions, hence the focus in our Service on TME with autonomic nerve preservation (ANP).[39]

Position Statement

Heald et al define TME as an excision of the entire rectum and the mesorectal package down to the ano-rectal junction, resecting an intact mesorectum with unviolated boundaries. Based on the works of Havenga et al,[2] Quirke et al,[33] Hida et al,[8] Reynolds et al,[5] Enker et al define TME as a resection of the rectum utilizing sharp dissection between the visceral and the parietal layers of the pelvic fascia, to a minimum resection of 5 cm of the *mesorectum* that is situated distal to the lowest edge of the primary tumor, whether or not that ends up at the ano-rectal junction.[31] The *sine qua non* of any form of TME is the complete mobilization of the rectum from the sacral promontory to the anal hiatus that is located within the levator ani muscles of the pelvic floor. All techniques utilize sharp dissection and, to a greater or lesser extent, all reported methods follow the defined areolar plane between the visceral and parietal layers of the pelvic fasciae.

HISTORICAL DEVELOPMENT AND OUTCOMES OF TME

In the United Kingdom

In 1982, Heald and associates described patients in whom the risk of local recurrence of cancer was attributed to minute foci of adenocarcinoma located in the mesorectum distal to the lower edge of a rectal cancer. Initially, they advocated a specific dissection of the distal mesorectum off the back of the muscular tube of rectal wall, including the distal mesorectum in the resected specimen. Access to the distal mesorectum was obtained by dissection along the anatomic, areolar plane of the pelvis described above, and a consecutive series of patients undergoing excision of the entire mesorectum was reported with a very low incidence of pelvic recurrence.[13] Much of what today is understood about the natural history of rectal cancer and of the surgical approach that can address this problem effectively, is foretold by the authors in this article.

In 1992, Heald and Karanjia reported a five-year actuarial local recurrence rate of 3.5% in 152 patients undergoing curative anterior resections.[37] In 1998, the Basingstoke experience was updated with a report concerning 519 patients with rectal cancer resections.[38] Patients were included with lesions situated within 15 cm of the anal verge, and mean follow-up was 8.3 years. Adjuvant or neoadjuvant treatment was rarely utilized. The overall pelvic recurrence rates at five and ten years were 6% and 8%, respectively, primarily in patients undergoing anterior resection. Pelvic recurrence rates of 17% and 36% at five and ten years, respectively, were observed in patients undergoing APR. MacFarlane et al reported on the subset of "high risk" patients with preoperative stages that would prompt others to use neoadjuvant therapy, that is, T3 or T4, N0, or N1 disease.[39] As opposed to their 1998 report, all of the cancers represented in this report were located within 12 cm of the anal verge. These two factors—preoperative stage and definition of the rectum—allowed the authors to compare their results to the "high risk" patients undergoing conventional surgery with either postoperative radiation or radiation and chemotherapy through the North Central Cancer Treatment Group (NCCTG), based out of the Mayo Clinic.[42] The median follow-up was 7.7 years. The life table analysis calculated five-year survival was 5% and the overall recurrence rate was 22%. In contrast, the local recurrence rate in the NCCTG study was 25%, and was reduced to 13% by radiation and chemotherapy. The overall recurrence rate for Dukes C patients exceeded 60% in the conventional surgery plus RTCRx study. In this study, MacFarlane et al emphasized that adjuvant therapy could not make up for the deficiencies of conventional surgery, when compared to the results obtained by TME alone.

In 1998, Heald and colleagues summarized their pioneering work on TME, reviewing the Basingstoke experience from 1978 to 1997.[38] During that period, 519 patients were entered into a prospective consecutive case series involving 465 anterior resections, 37 APRs, and 10 Hartmann's resections. Of the 465 LARs, 407 had low stapled anastomoses, thus qualifying as TMEs (in accordance with the authors' use of the term). Dukes stage distributions were: 102 Dukes A (19.6%), 167 Dukes B (32.2%), 142 Dukes C (27.4%), and 108 Dukes D (20.8%; residual disease or metastases). Cancer-specific survival for all 519 patients undergoing surgery was 68% at five years. Local recurrence or persistent disease was evident in 6% at five years and 8% at ten years. In the patients who were treated for cure, the cancer-specific survival at five years was 80%, and for non-curative procedures, 31%. (It must be noted that the latter number is curiously somewhat higher than other experiences worldwide with a 5-year survival of 7%–10% in stage IV disease.[38])

Stage-specific rates of local recurrence or of cancer-specific survival were not provided in this publication, nor, for that matter, in the seminal 1993 publication from the same authors.[39] The absence of these data reduced the usefulness of their otherwise excellent results, as subsequent discussions of the effectiveness of TME in the control of regional disease were compromised, particularly in discussions that related to the use of adjuvant therapy. In the absence of stage-related subset analysis, the overall results may be criticized as being dependent upon the fraction of patient in the series with Dukes A or stage D disease. In their 1998 report,[38] 40% of their patients had either localized, that is, highly curable disease (Dukes A) or metastatic (Dukes D or stage IV) disease with a shorter median life span.[38] In the long run, both stages I and IV are far less likely to result in local recurrences than are stages II or III.

In the United States

The historical development of TME in the United States begins with the work of Coller et al in 1940.[6] They reported on the pattern of lymph node metastases associated with primary rectal cancers using a fat-clearing method reported by Gilchrist and David in 1938.[43] Of the specimens obtained from the 19 patients with distal rectal cancers, 11 (58%) harbored lymph node metastases; 5 within the mesorectum only, and 6 (32%) within the mesorectum and to the lateral internal iliac nodes along the pelvic side wall. These findings prompted Coller et al to recommend that the traditional Miles resection[18] be widened in scope to include ligation of the inferior mesenteric artery at its origin, resection of the sigmoid mesentery and the entire mesorectum, along with an *en bloc* internal iliac lymphadenectomy. Coller et al are credited with having introduced sharp dissection, under direct vision, along the medial adventitial plane of the internal iliac veins as the lateral circumferential planes of dissection for primary rectal cancers.

His student, Dr. George E. Block, whose career at the University of Chicago spanned the period of 1960 to 1993, faithfully practiced Coller et al's preachings. Indeed, the results of abdomino-perineal resection (APR) or low anterior resections (LARs) with lateral pelvic lymphadenectomy and without adjuvant radiation therapy were reported in 1979[31] and again in 1990.[30] Enker and coworkers reported that sharp pelvic dissection and wide anatomic resection of rectal cancers was associated with dramatically lower rates of pelvic recurrence than were the prevailing conventional, bluntly performed operations characterized by non-anatomical margins.[31] In 1990, Michelassi et al summarized this experience, reviewing the outcomes of surgery in 853 patients undergoing surgery for colorectal cancers from 1965 to 1981 at the University of Chicago. Local recurrences were related to depth of mural invasion, location in the rectum less than 12 cm from the anal verge (12%) and lymphatic or capillary micro invasion.[30]

Despite these results, lateral pelvic dissection remained a technically challenging operation that was associated with an increased incidence of bleeding due to iliac vein injury, and with a prominent incidence of impotence and of neurogenic bladder due to autonomic nerve injury. In 1973, Lee, Maurer and Block indicated that these consequences were a logical outcome of rectal cancer surgery and that, based upon cadaver dissections, any dissection lateral to the pelvic peritoneum made the autonomic nerves vulnerable to injury.[44]

In the mid-1970s, stimulated by the works of Lee et al,[44] and of Tsuchiya and Ohki[45] and of Walsh[46] outlining the possibilities of autonomic nerve preservation, Enker undertook the modification of Block's operation in several respects, using the following postulates and principles:

1. The primary goals of resection would be cure of rectal cancer and the prevention of local recurrence. To achieve cure and local control would require proximal, circumferential, and distal margins free of tumor, in keeping with the natural history and the pathophysiology of the disease, that is, resectable and curable regional spread by either direct extension or lymph node metastases.
2. Skeptical of the conclusions of the 1973 paper on pelvic dissection, that impotence and neurogenic bladder were inevitable outcomes of rectal cancer surgery,[44] Enker sought to develop a plane of pelvic dissection medial to the autonomic nerves. The pelvic fascial dissections of Waldeyer,[29] together with the modern practices of Tsuchiya and Ohke[45] and of Walsh,[46] suggested that a plane of dissection should be possible that would resect the rectum and its mesorectum as an intact, unviolated specimen while sparing the pelvic autonomic nerves, along with bladder and sexual functions. Dissection along these planes and the preservation of intact nerves and of an intact mesorectum could only be fulfilled by a sharp dissection, in keeping with the original recommendation of Coller et al.[6]
3. The incidence of spread to the lateral pelvic lymph nodes, although a reality, was historically quite rare. Universally applied, lateral pelvic lymphadenectomy would subject 100% of patients to the risk of high morbidity while fewer that 10% would benefit from the added dissection by the removal of positive lateral nodes. Proving this point, the most recent data from Japan indicates a 9.4% incidence of lateral nodal involvement in over 10,000 patients undergoing lateral pelvic lymphadenectomy. Only 33% of the patients with lateral nodal involvement survived the cancer, making the overall benefit of the added dissection (1/3 of the 9.4%) only 3%.[47]
4. Since the overwhelming majority of spread within the boundaries of the mesorectum was either lateral or cephalad, a generous margin of the distal mesorectum, divided at right angles to the rectal wall and to the plane of dis-

section, should allow for a safe use of sphincter-preservation in the majority of patients with cancers of the mid-rectum. Subsequently, this postulate is supported by the work of Hida et al,[8] demonstrating that 20% of patients with T3 lesions harbor lymph node metastases in the distal mesorectum, as far as four cm distal to the palpable lowest edge of the primary tumor. A margin of 5 cm of distal mesorectum should be adequate in the overwhelming majority of resections that are dealing with regional (as opposed to mural or localized) disease that is present in 85% of curable patients.

5. The visceral layer of the pelvic fascia (VLPF) surrounds the rectum and the mesorectum, while, for the most part, the iliac vessels and the autonomic nerves lie outside the parietal layer of the pelvic fascia (PLPF). Sharp dissection between these two fascial layers should allow one to accomplish the goals outlined above.

Beginning in 1978, Enker and co-workers used the clinical material then available in an effort to shed light on the concept of achieving uninvolved circumferential margins of resection as a logical basis for the surgery of rectal cancer. Papers published in 1979[31] and in 1984[32] were intended to demonstrate that the circumferential margins of resection were the most important element defining an adequate resection for rectal cancer. In both papers we used a documented lateral pelvic lymphadenectomy as the only available, objective definition of a "radical" or so-called "wide" lateral dissection. Neither study was intended to evaluate the potential benefits of lateral internal iliac node dissection, nor where they in any way intended as support for the concept. Instead, both articles reflected the use of sharp dissection under direct vision along definable planes of the pelvis with supposedly negative lateral margins of resection. Together, both studies served as a logical foundation for the next clinical step: the systematic sharp dissection between the visceral and the parietal planes of the pelvic fascia. Both papers lacked today's standards of the pathologic correlation that were ultimately published by Quirke et al in 1986.[33]

In 1995, Enker and colleagues reported stage-related survival and local recurrence rates, in a consecutive series of Dukes B and C patients undergoing TME that was in progress since 1979. These data were prospectively gathered in a longitudinal database, and compared 246 "high risk" patients to the 171 patients reported by MacFarlane et al[39] in 1993. All of the patients had cancers situated within 12 cm of the anal verge, and conformed to TNM stages T3N0M0 or TanyN1or N2M0, or Dukes B and C lesions, that is, regional disease that would be considered eligible for adjuvant therapy trials in the same manner as was evaluated by MacFarlane et al in 1993.[39] Patients were not excluded for "locally advanced" disease and curative resections were defined as the removal of all gross disease.

Overall, the five-year Kaplan-Meier estimate of pelvic recurrences was 7.3%, and it was 5.7% in the absence of subsequent metastatic disease. Risk factors included nodal status and perineural invasion, but there was no correlation between local recurrence and tumor height (distance from the anal verge) or with LAR versus APR. The rate of distant failure was 23.6% and the five-year survival rate for this "high risk" group was 74.2%. Comparable figures from the NCCTG included LR rates of 13% to 25% and a rate of distant metastases of 64% in node positive patients.

This article provided our first report of survival and local recurrence rates by stage of disease in statistically reasonable cohorts. At a median follow-up of six years, the survival and local recurrence rates for Dukes B cancers (T3N0M0, 99 patients) were 86.7% and 3%, and for node positive patients (Tany N1or N2 M0, 147 patients) were 64% and 10%, respectively. The total operative mortality was 0.8%. Patients undergoing abdominoperineal resection were analyzed separately.[47] Their operative mortality was 2%, the five-year survival was 60% ($P < .001$ compared to 81% for patients who underwent LAR), and was attributable to the presence of positive nodes. Local recurrences were observed in 8 of 148 patients (an actuarial rate of 8%, P = NS) without metastases, and ranged from 5% in T3N0M0 to 21% in patients with stages TanyN1orN2M0.

Michelassi and co-workers[48] have reported on their experience with 73 patients undergoing TME for lesions located within 10 cm of the anal verge. Five-year actuarial survival was 65% for node positive patients, and local recurrences were observed in 3.1% of curable patients. Tumor stage and vascular/lymphatic invasion were significantly associated with recurrence. Circumferential lesions, adjacent organ invasion and location within 5 cm of the anal verge were significantly associated with AP resection.

CURRENT PERSONAL EXPERIENCE WITH TME

A total of 744 consecutive patients have undergone TME for primary rectal cancers situated within 12 cm of the anal verge, through October of 2003. Between October 1979 and December 31, 1998, 544 of these patients had a median follow up of 5.2 years, and no patients were excluded for locally advanced disease. Three hundred and seventy-eight have undergone a low anterior resection (69.5 %), including colo-anal anastomoses, while 166 patients have undergone AP resection (30.5%). Three hundred and nineteen patients (58.6%) were male and the median age was 61. The cancer-related five-year survival is 73.5% for 537 of 544 patients with known follow-up. The five-year local recurrence free survival is 94.8%, for a five-year local recurrence rate of 5.2% (23 of 537 patients). Both survival and local recurrence free survival are stage-related. The cancer-free survival following low anterior resection is 76.1% while the cancer-free survival following AP resection is 60.1% ($P = .001$). Local recurrence-free survival after LAR for stages T3N1orN2M0 is 93.6%, and after AP resection is 92.4% (P = NS). After APR, there is a slightly higher incidence of local failure (e.g., Tany N1-2M0 after LAR = 8.3% vs. TanyN1-2M0 after APR = 15%); however, it does not reach statistical significance. These numbers remain consistent with our initial reports of the results of TME in a high-risk population of Dukes B and C patients.[3] These data suggest that the continued excellent results of TME represent a stable platform for the testing of adjuvant therapy in Cooperative group trials.

MULTI-SURGEON TRIALS

After the reports of Heald et al and of Enker et al, the question was raised as to whether the technology of TME was transferable or if these results would prove to be strictly operator dependent. While the surgeon was ultimately proven to be a critical variable in patient outcome, clearly, the operation could be taught to others either inside or outside of the context of a clinical trial setting.

Arbman et al[49] reported on a multi-surgeon trial in Sweden, comparing 230 patients undergoing curative resections for rectal cancer between 1990 and 1992, with 211 patients who underwent conventional operations between 1984 and 1986. The series was largely devoid of adjuvant therapy. The local recurrence rate for the TME group was 6% versus 14% in the conventional group. These data are entirely comparable to the results of TME or to comparisons between TME and conventional surgery as performed in single-surgeon trials.

Havenga et al[21] reported on a prospective but not randomized data, in which the volume of patients was accrued by examining the results of four surgeons practicing TME (691 patients) versus the results of the West Netherlands Cancer Center (720 patients) where conventional surgery was practiced up to the point of the study. All patients had stage II or III rectal cancers situated within 12 cm of the anal verge, and were resected for cure.

The local recurrence rates for the TME groups were from 4% to 9% versus the conventional surgery group of 32% to 35%. The five-year cancer-specific survival was 75% to 80% versus 52%. These differences persisted for each stage and through multivariate analyses.

In 2001, Kapiteijn et al reported on over 1800 patients undergoing TME who were randomized to either receive or not receive short course radiation therapy during the week prior to surgery.[50] In order to assure surgical quality control, TME-certified proctors scrubbed with experienced surgeons at the participating Dutch hospitals under the clinical trials auspices of the Dutch Colorectal Study Group, and the Department of Surgery at the University of Leiden. At two years, the overall local recurrence rate was 5%, 8% for patients not undergoing pre-operative radiation therapy, and 2% for those who did undergo preoperative treatment ($P \leq .01$). For the purpose of this publication, the local recurrence rate of 5% is identical with those reported by single surgeon studies and by other multi-surgeon trials.

In a multi-center trial from Germany, Kockerling et al evaluated 1581 curative resections performed from 1985 to 1991 as TME was being introduced regionally.[51] Patients were compared to a historical conventional surgery control group from 5 to 10 years earlier. Over the periods of the trial, the local recurrence rates declined form 39.4% to 9.8% (P = .0001) and the five-year survival increased from 50% to 71% (P < .0001).

In a study of 681 patients undergoing sphincter-preserving operations on a multi-surgeon specialty service, Enker and co-workers reported a five-year actuarial local recurrence rate of 4% along with a cancer-related five-year survival rate of 81% (N = 34).[41] In this study, no significant differences were noted between tumor variables and recurrence including T stage, location of tumor, and pathologic features.

Hermanek and Hermanek addressed the issue of inter-surgeon variability as a prognostic factor in rectal cancer, and concluded that higher rates of local control and of survival can be expected of surgeons performing TME.[52] There was no clear correlation between surgical volume and outcome, and inter-institutional variation simply reflected the inter-surgeon variability. Of greatest importance in the factors determining outcome is the adequacy of the mesorectal excision, the absence of intra-operative complications, such as tumor perforation. Quality assurance of both surgery and pathology are required in order to assess the outcomes.

Bulow and co-workers recently reported on 311 patients with mobile cancers situated within 15 cm form the anal verge undergoing TME with curative intent, using a subsequent series of patients who underwent conventional operations as part of a separate trial (Danish RANX05) as a historical control group.[53] The authors accepted the limitations of randomization based upon ethical considerations at the time of the study. The study included patients undergoing both low anterior resection (LAR) and abdomino-perineal resection (APR). The cumulative three-year local recurrence rate was 11% after TME, compared with 30% in the historical control group. The crude three-year survival was 77% in the TME group and 62% in the conventional group. Local recurrence was found in 5 of 14 patients with a circumferential margin of 1 mm compared with 21 of 259 patients with a circumferential margin of 2 mm or more (P = .03).

All in all, whether in single surgeon experiences that introduced the concept of TME or in the multi-surgeon studies that have followed, the data support the premise that TME is the correct operation for treating rectal cancer, as supported by both the local recurrence rates, and the survival rates. The same can be said for the reduction of long-term morbidity, in association with TME.

Position Statement

1. Single surgeon, multi-surgeon and multi-institutional trials of TME whether or not they have been controlled for adjuvant therapy, or stratified by height and or stage, all have demonstrated local recurrence rates of only 2% to 10% compared with the 30% to 40% rates of local recurrence that are associated with traditional surgery.

2. Mature studies, that is, studies with five years or more of median follow-up, also have reported dramatically lower rates of metastatic disease associated with the surgical elimination of all regional disease, suggesting that the benefit of TME is not limited to the elimination of LR alone.
3. All surgical series should report their results by stage of disease, that the utility of TME may be analyzed in the setting of regional disease and that the data may be utilized in defining the role of adjuvant or neoadjuvant therapy.

PATHOLOGY IN SUPPORT OF TME

Institutions supporting the standardized use of TME are generally evolving to the use of the Quirke methodology for the handling and sectioning of rectal cancer specimens.[33,54] Transverse serial sectioning of the partially fixed specimen allows the pathologist to report the presence of uninvolved, microscopically involved or grossly involved circumferential margins. Each of these is designated as R0, R1 or R2 resections, respectively, and carries a significant prognostic value, as outlined above.

In general, these criteria are consistent with the approved guidelines for pathological evaluations that are set out by the College of American Pathology (CAP) in accordance with the *AJCC/UICC TNM Classification*, published in 2002.[55] In addition, accurate lymph node counts are critical to colorectal cancer staging. Joseph et al[56] studied 1585 patients undergoing either left or right hemicolectomy. The evaluation of fewer than ten nodes was required to achieve a <25% probability of true nodal negativity in T3 and T4 patients. When examining the specimens of T1 and T2 patients, however, to achieve the same degree of probability required the examination of 25 to 30 nodes per specimen. Based upon the work of Herrera-Ornelas,[57] the average total number of nodes potentially available for examination was deemed to be 44 to 46 per resected right or left colon specimen. Survival was statistically related to the number of lymph nodes resected or examined. While patient factors and surgeon factors are thought to influence the lymph node count from case to case, meticulous pathologic evaluation should set standards that yield a respectable median count when audited longitudinally. Herrera and Villareal[58] have further determined that 50% of the lymph nodes that are affected by rectal cancer are <5 mm in size, setting minimum size criteria of 2 to 3 mm for documenting accurate examination of the resected specimen.

Imaging Studies

Standard imaging techniques, that is, ultrasound, computerized axial tomography (CAT) scanning, CAT-positron emission tomography (CAT-PET) scanning, and standard magnetic resonance imaging (MRI), all have advocates in the staging of rectal cancer. The identification of transmural invasion is generally accurate, with the exception of distinguishing T2 versus microscopic T3 lesions. The identification of involved lymph nodes in the mesorectum continues to elude any satisfactory degree of accuracy, because of the diminutive size of involved nodes.[58] More recently, Brown and colleagues[59] reported a significant advance using high-resolution MRI for preoperative staging. Ninety-eight patients undergoing TME were assessed prospectively for the T and N stage, and other associated adverse pathologic risk factors. Correlation was made with histopathology on matched whole-mount sections of the resected specimen. There was 94% agreement between MRI and pathological T stage, and 84% agreement between MRI and pathological N stage. Circumferential, that is, surgical margin involvement was accurately predicted by MRI in 92% of cases. Extramural venous invasion in vessels >3 mm was correctly identified in 15 of 18 specimens, and stage T4 (peritoneal perforation) was correctly noted in seven of nine cases preoperatively.[59] High-resolution MRI shows promise as a more accurate tool for preoperative staging than current modalities. From a surgeon's standpoint, viewing high-resolution MR images that, unlike ultrasound, are not operator-dependent, which are anatomically-oriented and in which planes of pelvic anatomy are eminently discernible (i.e., the visceral layer surrounding the mesorectum) can only speak to a promising future for this modality in association with TME and the use of neoadjuvant therapy. All of these studies must be viewed as extensions of the examining finger, and the surgeon must place the imaging findings in the context of the natural history of rectal cancer, and not rely on imaging studies alone for preoperative staging.

ADJUVANT THERAPY IN THE CONTEXT OF TME

Postoperative Adjuvant Therapy

The role of adjuvant therapy in the context of TME remains controversial, and studies are in progress to outline the roles of radiation and chemotherapy, where TME provides such good local control.[50,60] Treatment benefit will have to be weighed against short-term and long-term morbidities before we know where this issues stands.

Selecting patients for postoperative RTCRx or for chemotherapy alone is a dilemma. In both Dukes B and C cases, the incidence of distant metastases outweighs the incidence of local recurrence after TME.[3,11,39] While radiation therapy traditionally has earned a role in the prevention of local recurrence, its role in TME versus conventional surgery needs to be worked out on the stable, new surgical platform provided by the growing use of TME.

It is customary to treat node-positive rectal cancer patients with adjuvant RTCRx. In 1995, Enker et al raised several questions regarding the use of adjuvant therapy, based upon the clinical results obtained with TME.[3] In 99 patients with T3N0M0 or Dukes B carcinomas, the local recurrence rate was only 3%, with only one patient undergoing radiation therapy. According to these data, the traditional view that radiation therapy is warranted in T3 lesions[15,42] is open to challenge when the patient has undergone TME, and when thorough pathological evaluation has confirmed T3N0M0, stage II, or Dukes B disease. Merchant et al have reported similarly low rates of local pelvic recurrence in T3N0M0 patients, such as, 2% to 3%, without the addition of adjuvant therapy.[61] Instead, selecting the appropriate patients for systemic chemotherapy, such as patients with extramural venous invasion, lymphatic vascular or peri-neural invasion, etc., would seem to be more profitable, that compromising the opportunity for full dose chemotherapy with whole pelvic irradiation.

When it comes to node-positive rectal cancer, current standards call for radiation and chemotherapy, if the patient has undergone an R_0 TME and if all of the pathological assessment is up to the CAP standards. However, randomized and properly stratified adjuvant therapy trials have never been conducted in which the outcome of patients with T3N1M0 disease are compared between two groups; one receiving chemotherapy and radiation, the other chemotherapy alone. In the views of this author (WEE) given the results achieved by TME alone without adjuvant therapy, such a study would be both warranted and ethical.

Neoadjuvant Therapy

Preoperative radiation and chemotherapy (RTCRx) has been studied in multiple centers in the interest of down staging that is dependent upon blood supply to the primary tumor. Other goals include the reduction of primary tumor volume, facilitating resectability with negative margins, enhancing the likelihood of sphincter-preservation, and the reduction of radiation therapy-related short- and long-term morbidities. Pathologic complete responses to treatment have been the important end point of these trials, and have proven to be durable responses, long-term cure.[67]

Selecting patients for preoperative treatment remains a dilemma. On the one hand, patients with N1 or N2 disease continue to defy preoperative staging. Both statistically and pathologically, it is well established that 60% of patients with T3 lesions harbor lymph node metastases.[4,8,58] By imaging criteria, however, the detection of lymph node involvement in the individual patient remains anything but a certainty. Ultrasound studies may detect enlarged (>1 cm) lymph nodes in up to 60% of patients undergoing preoperative study. Nevertheless, Herrera and Villareal have reported that 50% of cancer-involved lymph nodes are histologically proven to be smaller than 5 mm, a size that is not generally visible to ultrasound detection.[58]

On the other hand, Enker et al[3] and Merchant et al[61] have both reported that after TME resection of stage T3N0 rectal cancers, patients have extremely low rates of local pelvic recurrence, for example, 2% to 3%, without the addition of adjuvant therapy. Treating all patients with T3 rectal cancers with preoperative radiation therapy would seem to be excessive, and the successful treatment of patients who really stand to benefit from neoadjuvant therapy is strongly dependent on clinical selection as well as imaging results.

We select potentially curable patients for neoadjuvant therapy using the following criteria:

1. Marginally resectable lesions. Knowing the natural history of rectal cancer, there is a concern that despite a TME resection, proceeding directly to surgery in locally advanced cases, could result in a microscopically positive or close margin, an R1 resection. Many of these lesions are ideally suited to a combined modality, or a multidisciplinary program of neoadjuvant therapy, R0 resection, and intraoperative radiation therapy.[62] In such cases, high-resolution MRI, or CAT scan combined with PET scan imaging may be extremely useful in evaluating the extent of pretreatment disease, and in evaluating the response to neoadjuvant therapy.[59]
2. Distal rectal cancer, defined as all ≥T3 cancers situated within 5 cm of the anal verge. The natural history of these lesions tends to be more aggressive than the natural history of more proximal lesions. This includes a higher likelihood of mesorectal as well as lateral, that is, internal iliac and obturator lymph node spread.[8,47] This includes anorectal adenocarcinomas.
3. Circumferential, obstructing, or perforated lesion.
4. Poorly differentiated or undifferentiated carcinoma on preoperative biopsy. This includes evidence of signet-ring features, small cell lesions, or other adverse pathological features.

Generally, neoadjuvant therapy applied to patients with locally advanced lesions has been considered successful in reducing tumor volume and in down staging. Delaney and co-workers reported on a series of patients treated with preoperative RTCRx, undergoing TME for T3 rectal cancers at the Cleveland Clinic.[63] Survival was increased from 58% to 82% in node-negative patients with lesions less than 8 cm from the anal verge. Complete responders to RTCRx were not documented.

Garcia-Aguilar and co-workers reported on a series of locally advanced lesions treated pre-operatively by RTCRx, including 168 patients who underwent radical resection by TME; 161 of the patients underwent curative resection.[64] The mean follow-up was 37 months. Ninety-seven patients (58%) achieved ultrasound measurable preoperative down staging. None of the pathologic complete responders (CRs) has recurred local or distantly. A pathologic CR was associated with improved local control and survival in patients undergoing mesorectal excision.

Brown et al studied 89 patients undergoing preoperative RTCRx and radical resection in a retrospective trial that included TME for lower third lesions and tumor-specific TME for middle or upper third lesions.[65] All rectal lesions were situated below the peritoneal reflection. Twenty-one patients (24%) achieved a complete pathologic response. By ultrasound criteria, stage III patients were less likely to achieve complete pathologic responses to preoperative treatment than Stage II. CRs demonstrated only a trend toward improved survival and decreased recurrence compared with non-CRs (95% vs. 74%) due to the small number of patients reaching five-year follow-up at the time of their analysis. The median f ollow-up time for CR was 23.5 months and 31 months for the non-CRs.

Horgan and Finlay felt that preoperative RTCRx should be reserved for patients with locally advanced lesions to enhance the likelihood of margin-free resection.[66] Ruo et al, however, recently reported that the complete responses observed after RTCRx are durable, with no evidence of long-term recurrence.[67] Enker et al had the same experience, making preoperative RTCRx extremely valuable to some patients. The issue is appropriate patient selection, and the decision will rest upon good imaging or on the development of selective markers that have evaded definition to this point. Janjan et al reviewed the current literature on neoadjuvant therapy.[68] Dramatic issues of changing to TME from conventional surgery, along with the integration of neoadjuvant therapy are insightfully reviewed by Soreide et al.[69]

Laparoscopic TME

Several authors have embarked upon selected series of patients in whom they have performed TME laparoscopically. While this is an operation that reflects the skills of these authors, laparoscopic TME is generally applicable to only a small proportion of the patients with rectal cancers. Certainly, cancers of the distal sigmoid, >12 to 18 cm form the anal verge, are approachable laparoscopically. In cancers of the true rectum, ≥10 to 12 cm from the anal verge, other issues arise, including sphincter-preservation. This is particularly the case in situations where this decision can only be made after complete rectal mobilization. Laparoscopic APR is an ideal operation under most circumstances, where loss of the sphincter is a certainty. Nevertheless, accurate preoperative staging, the presence of regional or locally advanced disease that defies detection by current imaging techniques, matching the extent of resection to the disease, adjacent organ invasion and resection, are all issues surrounding laparoscopic TME, even in the best of hands. Currently, the best series recently on this subject indicate that when TME is performed laparoscopically, in a manner that is identical to the open operation, there are no differences in the rates of survival or local recurrence. These issues have been recently reviewed[70] and are currently under study in various centers.[71–76]

REFERENCES

1. Godlewski G, Prudhomme M. Embryology and anatomy of the anorectum. Surg Oncol Clin North Am 2000;80:319–343.

2. Havenga K, DeRuiter MC, Enker WE, Welvaart K. Anatomical basis of autonomic nerve-preserving total mesorectal excision for rectal cancer. Br J Surg 1996;83:384–388.
3. Enker WE, Thaler HT, Cranor ML, Polyak T. Total mesorectal excision in the operative treatment of carcinoma of the rectum. J Am Coll Surg 1995;181:335–346.
4. Morson BC, Vaughn EG, Bussey HJR. Pelvic recurrences after excision of the rectum for carcinoma. BMJ 1963;2:13–18.
5. Reynolds JV, Joyce WP, Dolan J, et al. Pathological evidence in support of total mesorectal excision in the management of rectal cancer. Br J Surg 1996;83:1112–1115.
6. Coller FA, Kay EB, MacIntyre RS. Regional lymphatic metastases of carcinoma of the rectum. Surgery 1940;8:294–311.
7. Morikawa E, Yasutomi M, Shindou K. Distribution of metastatic lymph nodes in colorectal cancer by the modified clearing method. Dis Colon Rectum 1994;37:219–223.
8. Hida J, Yasutomi M, Maruyama T, et al. Lymph node metastases detected in the mesorectum distal to carcinoma of the rectum by the clearing method: justification of total mesorectal excision. J Am Coll Surg 1997;184:584–588.
9. Scott N, Jackson P, Al-Jaberi T, et al. Total mesorectal excision and local recurrence: a study of tumour spread in the mesorectum distal to the rectal cancer. Br J Surg 1995;82:1031–1033.
10. Gilchrist RK, David VC. A consideration of the pathological factors influencing five year survival in radical resection of the large bowel and rectum for carcinoma. Ann Surg 1947;126:421–438.
11. Murty M, Enker WE, Martz J, et al. Current status of total mesorectal excision and autonomic nerve preservation in rectal cancer. Semin Surg Oncol 2000;19:321–328.
12. Bissett IP, Hill GL. Extrafascial excision of the rectum for cancer: A technique for the avoidance of complications of rectal mobilization. Semin Surg Oncol 2000;18:207–215.
13. Heald RJ, Husband EM, Ryall RDH. The mesorectum in rectal cancer surgery: the clue to pelvic recurrence. Br J Surg 1982;69:613–616.
14. Pilipshen SJ, Heilweil M, Quan SHQ. Patterns of pelvic recurrence following definitive resections of rectal cancer. Cancer 1984;53:1354–1362.
15. Gastrointestinal Tumor Study Group. Prolongation of the disease-free interval in surgically treated rectal carcinoma. N Engl J Med 1985;312:1465–1472.
16. Enker WE. Cancer of the rectum. Operative management and adjuvant therapy. In: Fazio VW, ed. Current Therapy in Colon and Rectal Surgery. Toronto, Canada: B.C. Decker, 1990:120–129.
17. Enker WE. Sphincter-preserving operations for rectal cancer. Oncology 1996;10:1673–1689.
18. Miles EW. A method of performing abdomino-perineal excision for carcinoma of the rectum and of the terminal portion of the pelvic colon. Lancet 1908;2:1812.
19. Dixon CF. Anterior resection for malignant lesions of upper part of rectum and lower part of sigmoid. Ann Surg 1948;128:425–442.
20. Deddish MR, Stearns MW. Anterior resection for carcinoma of the rectum and rectosigmoid area. Ann Surg 1961;154:961–966.
21. Havenga K, Enker WE, Norstein J, Moriya Y, et al. Improved survival and local control after total mesorectal excision or D3 lymphadenectomy in the treatment of primary rectal cancer: an international analysis of 1411 patients. Eur J Surg Oncol 1999;25:368–374.
22. Tepper JE, Cohen AM, Wood WC, et al: Postoperative radiation therapy for rectal cancer. Int J Radiat Oncol Biol Phys 1987;3:5–10.
23. Glimelius B, Isacsson U, Jung B, Pahlman L. Radiotherapy in addition to radical surgery in rectal cancer. Acta Oncol 1995;34:565–570.

24. Fisher B, Wolmark N, Rockette H, et al. Postoperative adjuvant chemotherapy or radiation therapy for rectal cancer: results from NSABP protocol R-01. J Natl Cancer Inst 1988;80: 21–29.

25. Gastrointestinal Study Group. Adjuvant therapy of colon cancer: results of a prospectively randomized trial. N Engl J Med 1984;310:737–743.

26. Minsky BD. The role of adjuvant radiation therapy in the treatment of colorectal cancer. Hem Oncol Clin North Am 1997;11:679-697.

27. Gordon-Watson C. Origin and spread of cancer of the rectum in surgical treatment. Lancet 1983;i:239–245.

28. Williamson RCN, Davis PW, Bristol JB, Wells M. Intestinal adaptation and experimental carcinogenesis after partial colectomy: increased tumour yields are confined to the anastomosis. Gut 1982;23:316–325.

29. Church JM, Raudkivi PJ, Hill GL. The surgical anatomy of the rectum—a review with particular relevance to the hazards of rectal mobilization. Int J Colorect Dis 1987;2:158–166.

30. Michelassi F, Vannucci L, Ayal JJ, et al. Local recurrence after curative resection of colorectal adenocarcinoma. Surgery 1990;108:787–792.

31. Enker WE, Laffer UT, Block GE. Enhanced survival of patients with colon and rectal cancer is based upon wide anatomic resection. Ann Surg 1979;190:350–360.

32. Enker WE, Philipsen SJ, Heilweil ML, et al. En bloc pelvic lymphadenectomy and sphincter preservation in the surgical management of rectal cancer. Ann Surg 1986;203:426–433.

33. Quirke P, Durdey P, Dixon MF. Local recurrence of rectal adenocarcinoma due to inadequate surgical resection. Lancet 1986;i:996–999.

34. Ng IOL, Luk ISC, Yuen ST, et al. Surgical lateral clearance in resected rectal carcinomas: a multivariate analysis of clinicopathological features. Cancer 1993;71:1972–1976.

35. Adam IJ, Mohamdee MO, Martin IG, et al. Role of circumferential margin involvement in the local recurrence of rectal cancer. Lancet 1994;344:707–711.

36. Enker WE. Total mesorectal excision with sphincter and autonomic nerve preservation in the treatment of rectal cancer. Curr Tech Gen Surg 1996;5:1–8.

37. Heald RJ, Karanjia ND. Results of radical surgery for rectal cancer. World J Surg 1992; 16:848–857.

38. Heald RJ, Moran BJ, Ryall RD, et al. Rectal cancer—the Basingstoke experience of total mesorectal excision, 1978-1997. Arch Surg 1998;133:894–899.

39. McFarlane JK, Ryall RDH, Heald RJ. Mesorectal excision for rectal cancer. Lancet 1993; 341:457–460.

40. Enker WE. Potency, cure, and local control in the operative treatment of rectal cancer. Arch Surg 1992;127:1396–1402.

41. Enker WE, Merchant N, Cohen AM, et al. Safety and efficacy of low anterior resection for rectal cancer—681 consecutive cases from a special service. Ann Surg 1999;230:544–554.

42. Krook JE, Moertel CG, Gunderson L, et al. Effective surgical adjuvant therapy for high-risk rectal carcinoma. N Engl J Med 1991;324:709–715.

43. Gilchrist, RK, David VC. Lymphatic spread of carcinoma of the rectum. Ann Surg 1938;108:621.

44. Lee JF, Maurer VM, Block GE. Anatomic relations of pelvic autonomic nerves to pelvic operations. Arch Surg 1973;107:324–328.

45. Tsuchiya S, Ohki,S. Radical surgery for rectal cancer with preservation of the pelvic autonomic nerves: symposium on colon and rectal cancer. Presented at the East-Asia Collegium Internationale Chirurgica Digestivae, Feb 26, 1992; Taipei, Taiwan.

46. Walsh PC. Radical prostectomy, preservation of sexual function, cancer control. The controversy. Urol Clin N Am 1987;14:663–673.
47. Enker WE, Havenga K, Polyak T, et al. Abdominoperineal resection via total mesorectal excision and autonomic nerve preservation for low rectal cancer. World J Surg 1997;21:715–720.
48. Arenas RB, Fichera A, Mhoon D, Michelassi F. Total mesorectal excision in the surgical treatment of rectal cancer. Arch Surgery 1998;133:608–611.
49. Arbman G, Nilsson E, Hallböök O, Sjödahl R. Local recurrence following total mesorectal excision for rectal cancer. Br J Surg 1996;83:375–379.
50. Kapiteijn E, Marijnen CAM, Nagtegaal I, et al. Preoperative radiotherapy combined with total mesorectal excision for resectable rectal cancer. N Engl J Med 2001;345:638–646.
51. Kockerling F, Reymond M, Altendor-Hofmann A, et al. Influence of surgery on metachronous distant metastases and survival in rectal cancer. J Clin Oncol 1998;16:324–329.
52. Hermanek P, Hermanek PJ. Role of the surgeon as a variable in the treatment of rectal cancer. Semin Surg Oncol 2000;19:329–335.
53. Bulow S, Christensen IJ, Harling H, et al. Recurrence and survival after mesorectal excision for rectal cancer. Danish TME Study Group and RANX05 Colorectal Cancer Study Group. Br J Surgery 2003;90:974–980.
54. Birbeck KF, Macklin CP, Tiffin NJ, et al. Rates of circumferential resection margin involvement vary between surgeons and predict outcomes in rectal cancer surgery. Ann Surg 2002;235:449–457.
55. AJCC Cancer Staging Manual, 6th ed. New York, NY: Springer-Verlag, 2002:113–131.
56. Joseph NE, Sigurdson ER, Hanlon AL, et al. Accuracy of determining nodal negativity in colorectal cancer on the basis of the number of nodes retrieved on resection. Ann Surg Oncol 2003;10:213–218.
57. Herrera-Ornelas L. Metastases in small lymph nodes from colon cancer. Arch Surg 1987; 122:1253–1256.
58. Herrera L, Villareal JR. Incidence of metastases from rectal cancer in small lymph nodes detected by a clearing method. Dis Colon Rectum 1992;35:783–788.
59. Brown G, Radcliffe AG, Newcombe RG, et al. Preoperative assessment of prognostic factors in rectal cancer using high-resolution magnetic resonance imaging. B J Surg 2003;90:355–364.
60. Sauer R, German Rectal Cancer Group. Adjuvant versus neoadjuvant combined modality treatment for locally advanced rectal cancer: first results of the German Rectal Cancer Study (CAO/ARO/AIO-94). Int J Rad Biol Phys 2003;57[suppl 2]:124.
61. Merchant WB, Guillem JG, Paty PB, et al. T3N0 rectal cancer: results following sharp mesorectal excision and no adjuvant therapy. J. Gastrointest Surg 1999;3:642–647.
62. Hu KS, Harrison LB. Results and complications of surgery combined with intra-operative radiation therapy for the treatment of locally advanced or recurrent cancers in the pelvis. Semin Surg Oncol 2000;18:269–278.
63. Delaney CP, Lavery IC, Brenner A, et al. Preoperative radiotherapy improves survival in patients undergoing total mesorectal excision for stage T3 low rectal cancers. Ann Surg 2002; 236:203–207.
64. Garcia-Aguilar J, Hernandez de Anda E, Sirivongs P, et al. A pathologic complete response to preoperative chemoradiation is associated with lower local recurrence and improved survival in rectal cancer patients treated by mesorectal excision. Dis Colon Rectum 2003;46:298–304.
65. Brown CL, Ternent CA, Thorson AG, et al. Response to preoperative chemoradiation in stage II and III rectal cancer. Dis Colon Rectum 2003;46:1189–1193.
66. Horgan AF, Finlay IG. Preoperative staging of rectal cancer allows selection of patients for preoperative radiotherapy. Br J Surg 2000;87:575–579.

67. Ruo L, Tickoo S, Klimstra DS, et al. Long-term prognostic significance of rectal cancer response to preoperative radiation and chemotherapy. Ann Surg 2002;236:75–81.

68. Janjan NA, Khoo VS, Abbruzzese J, et al. Tumor downstaging and sphincter preservation with preoperative chemoradiation in locally advanced rectal cancer: the MD Anderson experience. Int J Rad Oncol Biol Phys 1999;44:1027–1038.

69. Soreide O, Norstein J. Local recurrence after operative treatment of rectal carcinoma: a strategy for change. J Am Coll Surg 1997;184:84–92.

70. Enker WE, Rosser JC, Noyan E. Laparoscopic colectomy: an evolving art. In DeVita VT, Hellman S, Rosenberg SA, ed. Progress in Oncology, 2003. Boston, MA: Jones and Bartlett, Publishers, 2003:314–341.

71. Morino M, Parini U, Giraudo G, et al. Laparoscopic total mesorectal excision: a consecutive series of 100 patients. Ann Surg 2003;237:335–342.

72. Bretagnol F, Rullier E, Couderc P, et al. Technical and oncological feasibility of laparoscopic total mesorectal excision with pouch coloanal anastomosis for rectal cancer. Colorect Dis 2003;5:451–453.

73. Koda K, Saito N, Oda K, et al. Evaluation of lateral lymph node dissection with preoperative chemo-radiotherapy for the treatment of advanced middle to lower rectal cancers. Int J Colorectal Dis 2003, In Press.

74. Poulin EC, Schachta CM, Gregoire R, et al. Local recurrence and survival after laparoscopic mesorectal resection for rectal adenocarcinoma. Surg Endosc 2002;16:989–995.

75. Weiser MR, Milsom JW. Laparoscopic total mesorectal excision with autonomic nerve preservation. Semin Surg Oncol 2000;18:265–268.

76. Mehigan BJ, Monson JRT. Laparoscopic rectal-abdominoperineal resection. Surg Oncol Clin North Am 2001;10:611–623.

Index

A

B

C

D

E

F

G

H

I

K

L

M

N

O

P

R

S

T

U

V

W

X

INDEX OF TABLES